Shoulder Fractures in Context

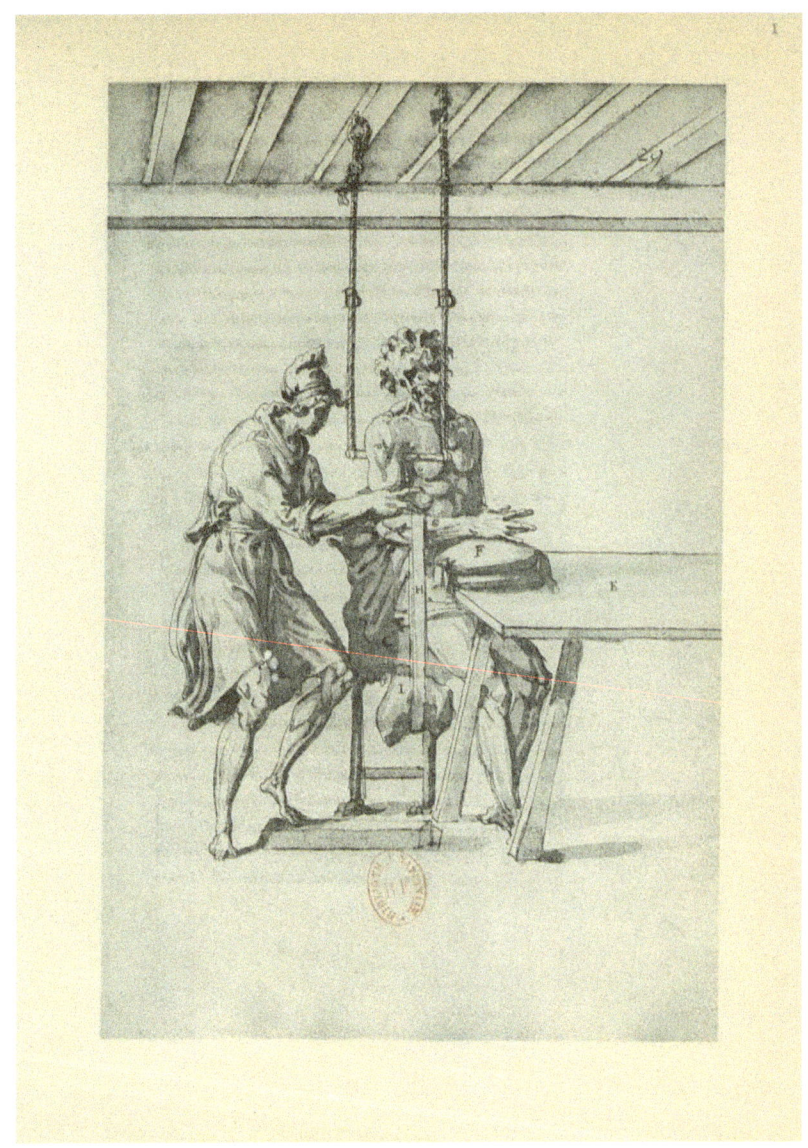

Renaissance interpretation of the Hippocratic method for reducing fractures of the proximal humerus. Illustration attributed to Francesco Primaticcio (1504–1580). (Reproduced with permission of the Bibliothèque nationale de France. Any commercial reuse requires authorization from the Bibliothèque nationale de France)

Stig Brorson

Shoulder Fractures in Context

Controversies in Orthopaedic Surgery

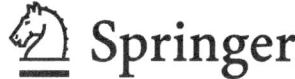

Stig Brorson
Centre for Evidence-Based Orthopaedics
Zealand University Hospital and Department
of Clinical Medicine, University of Copenhagen
Koege, Denmark

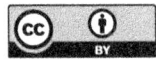

ISBN 978-3-031-93603-6   ISBN 978-3-031-93604-3   (eBook)
https://doi.org/10.1007/978-3-031-93604-3

This work was supported by Zealand University Hospital, Department of Orthopaedic Surgery, Køge, Denmark.

© The Editor(s) (if applicable) and The Author(s). 2025. This book is an open access publication

Open Access This book is licensed under the terms of the Creative Commons Attribution 4.0 International License (http://creativecommons.org/licenses/by/4.0/), which permits use, sharing, adaptation, distribution and reproduction in any medium or format, as long as you give appropriate credit to the original author(s) and the source, provide a link to the Creative Commons license and indicate if changes were made.
The images or other third party material in this book are included in the book's Creative Commons license, unless indicated otherwise in a credit line to the material. If material is not included in the book's Creative Commons license and your intended use is not permitted by statutory regulation or exceeds the permitted use, you will need to obtain permission directly from the copyright holder.
The use of general descriptive names, registered names, trademarks, service marks, etc. in this publication does not imply, even in the absence of a specific statement, that such names are exempt from the relevant protective laws and regulations and therefore free for general use.
The publisher, the authors and the editors are safe to assume that the advice and information in this book are believed to be true and accurate at the date of publication. Neither the publisher nor the authors or the editors give a warranty, expressed or implied, with respect to the material contained herein or for any errors or omissions that may have been made. The publisher remains neutral with regard to jurisdictional claims in published maps and institutional affiliations.

This Springer imprint is published by the registered company Springer Nature Switzerland AG
The registered company address is: Gewerbestrasse 11, 6330 Cham, Switzerland

If disposing of this product, please recycle the paper.

This book is dedicated to my patients.

Foreword

Stig Brorson considers me as an expert (i.e., someone with a lot of experience) in shoulder fractures and he gave me the honor of forewording his book. I hope he will forgive me to be biased, as a designer of techniques and implants for the treatment of proximal humerus fractures (PHFs).

Proximal humerus fractures (PHFs) are the third most common fractures, following hip and wrist fractures. With the aging of the world's population, we are going to face a "tsunami" of shoulder fractures … and we are not ready because we still have more questions than answers. The book of Stig Brorson is arriving just in time to help us seeing clearer and further.

As all orthopedic/trauma surgeons, I have encountered and dealt with many shoulder fractures from the very beginning of my career. And, like many surgeons, I have often been dissatisfied with the results of the different treatment options, especially when seeing how crippling a badly treated shoulder fracture can be. This led naturally to questioning all the aspects of shoulder fractures, from biomechanics to classification and, of course, care and treatment. Then finding answers through clinical studies and putting the insight gained into the development of implants and care options to improve the outcomes. While thoroughly examining and taking into consideration the existing knowledge base, I cannot deny a tiny part of intuition, the condensation of knowledge and experience.

Stig has looked at the question from a different standpoint, he encompasses the past, the present, and asks for the evidence of what works to help the future. With this book, Stig has done a huge favor to everyone who is interested in shoulder fractures, giving us an all-embracing, documented, and thought-provoking compass to shoulder fractures.

Stig has made a tremendous work to show that there is no (or little) *clinical evidence* in the diagnosis and treatment of shoulder fractures. However, the "lack of evidence," often provided by the literature, should be interpreted with caution. For instance, there is no evidence that surgical treatment of PHFs could be better than conservative treatment. However, in most series, the diagnosis of the type of fractures is incorrect, and this is even obvious when looking at the figures provided by the authors in their articles. In other words, many studies are comparing "apples with bananas." In my (expert) opinion, the mistake is to use the AO classification for the diagnosis of PHFs instead of the "4-part" classification, described by Codman and popularized by Neer. While the first one is a *descriptive* classification, the other is a "*concept*" rather than a classification, but this concept is helpful for the diagnosis and the indication. A PHF should *not* be seen as a *puzzle* to reconstruct, but rather as a *rotator cuff tear* to repair. This means that the fracture anatomy and the displacement of the bony parts should be viewed from a *soft tissue perspective*. How can we prove this?... Unfortunately, neither I nor Stig can do it. We see here both the limits of evidence-based medicine and expertise.

Another merit of Stig is to scientifically demonstrate that, despite 30 years of use, there is high-quality clinical evidence that locking plates did not improve the results of treatment of PHFs and led to high rates of complications and reoperations, even in the hands of proponents and "experts." This is a very kind conclusion. In my experience, locking plates not only do not improve the outcomes of treatment of PHFs, but "*it burns the bridge*" because of what I have termed "*the terrible triad*" after plating of PHFs: posterior GT migration, humeral head necrosis, and glenoid destruction. In other words, and in agreement with Stig's work, I strongly believe that the locking plate is a "*false good idea*" for the treatment of PHFs.

Stig also demonstrates that there is no evidence of superiority between internal fixation with a locking plate versus a locking IM nail. In other words, IM nails are no better than locking plates, and this is not surprising for me: most series compare the results of locking plates with those of first or second generation IM nails, which are both based on *humeral head fixation* instead of *tuberosity fixation*. The biggest conceptual mistake is to operate a PHF with the primary goal of fixing the humeral head. The shoulder is not the hip! The primary goal should not be to fix the humeral head but rather to fix the greater tuberosity (GT). Why? For at least two reasons: firstly, because the humeral head does not need to be fixed once the tuberosities are reconstructed, and secondly, because we know how to replace the humeral head (in case of necrosis) with a prosthesis, while we don't know how to deal with a massive, irreparable, and retracted posterosuperior rotator cuff tear (after posterior migration of the GT). IM nails that have a screw directed toward the head with locking technology "burn the bridge" in the same way that plates do. In my experience, the use of third generation IM nail (tuberosity-based fixation) is a real game changer.

Stig also questions the value of hemiarthroplasty (HA) and reverse shoulder arthroplasty (RSA) for the treatment of PHFs and, once again, he is right. We still have to demonstrate that any of these implants is better than no implant. Well-designed prospective randomized studies are lacking. But again, the studies available should be interpreted with caution. In many series, the tuberosities are poorly or not correctly fixed to the implants, and not surprisingly, the results are poor, and the rates of complications/reoperations are high. Furthermore, most series report the results of classical implants (used for osteoarthritis) with bulky metaphysis that prevents tuberosity healing. Again, in my experience, the use of "low profile" implants, specifically designed for the treatment of PHFs (i.e., reverse fracture prosthesis), with a standardized technique of tuberosity fixation, is also a game changer.

Finally, Stig points out that in very few clinical series, the type of trauma, the type of patients, and the degree of osteopenia are considered. It is not the same to deal with a 3- or 4-part fracture in a 30-year-old patient with good bone quality who had a ski accident (i.e., a high-energy trauma) and a

70-year-old woman with severe osteoporosis who fell down from her height in her apartment (i.e., a low-energy trauma). Furthermore, besides the functional results, clinical studies should report on the quality of life, the rate of complications, and reoperations to allow unbiased comparisons. As we can see, the number of parameters that should be considered in the decision-making process for a PHF is high. Despite this, I am optimistic: the future is bright. Artificial intelligence (AI) will help us soon to improve our diagnosis and our decision-making process to choose the best technique and implants. The combination of human intuition, clinical experience, and the power of calculation of AI will provide the most efficient results.

This book is about much more than shoulder fractures. It describes a new philosophy about how we should look at PHFs in terms of diagnosis and treatment. This book is a "must read" in a time where teaching and training of young surgeons is often provided by the industry, whose interest is to push them to operate on all cases and use as many implants (plates, IM nails, prostheses) as possible. On the one hand, this book shows us that a nonsurgical approach can be recommended for many shoulder fractures with good functional results and almost no risk of complications and reoperations. It is always important to remember what has been forgotten. On the other hand, this book emphasizes that well-performed surgery (ORIF or prosthesis) in carefully selected patients and fractures can provide excellent results with low risks of complications and reoperations.

This book already has its prominent place on my bookshelf, and I will put it in the hands of all those who deal with this controversial question. Orthopedic surgeons, including those in training (residents and fellows), as well as medical doctors and physiotherapists should read this wonderful work of art, science, and philosophy.

Hopefully, this book will help surgeons to think differently of shoulder fractures and prevent them from performing useless or even detrimental surgical procedures. In a certain way, this book is reminding us of the most important rule in Medicine, that we should never forget: "First, do no harm!".

Thank you, Stig for giving us such a wonderful present.

Professor of Orthopaedic Surgery
and Traumatology, Past-President
of SECEC (European Society
for Shoulder & Elbow Surgery)
ICR-Institut de Chirurgie Réparatrice
Nice, France

Pascal Boileau

Foreword

Stig Brorson is to be congratulated for writing an excellent book on proximal humeral fractures, referred to in the book as shoulder fractures. It is important to study proximal humeral fractures as analysis has shown that they are common fractures particularly in females where they are the third most common fracture. In a rapidly aging population, they are becoming more common, and they are in fact the second most common fracture in males and the third most common fracture in females aged 65 years or more. As the aging population becomes healthier the incidence of these fractures is going to increase and surgeons are going to be faced with an increasing number of proximal humeral fractures. It is therefore important to analyze how these fractures are treated and to determine how improvements in treatment can be made.

The book is divided into six basic sections dealing with important aspects of proximal humeral fractures. These are morphology and epidemiology, history, fracture patterns and classification, management, the benefits and problems associated with treatment, and the success of modern treatment methods.

The epidemiology of proximal humeral fractures is carefully outlined. It is pointed out that shoulder fractures are common injuries, especially in older people and are associated with increased mortality. They are also associated with other secondary osteoporotic fractures. The morphology and classifications of proximal humeral fractures are described from Ancient Egypt to modern times. There are excellent accounts of the old pre-radiological classifications and careful analyses of modern classifications such as the Neer and AO classifications. The advantages and disadvantages of both these classifications, and more modern classifications, are described in detail. Surgeons will find the descriptions of ancient Egyptian, Greek, and Roman, and more modern medieval, classifications and treatment methods to be of considerable interest as many surgeons in these times had an excellent understanding of fracture morphology and complications. Advances in classification and surgical treatment after the invention of anesthesia and aseptic wound treatment are also described.

The main message that many surgeons should take from this book is that Stig Brorson is quite clear that there is little justification for the increased use of locking plates and reverse shoulder arthroplasties particularly in older patients. He points out that there is little evidence that locking plates or reverse shoulder arthroplasties confer benefit over nonoperative treatment in older patients and they are associated with a higher complication rate. He states that it is increasingly clear that in two-, three-, and four-part fractures in older people surgery is not indicated. He also reports that social and psychological factors are more important than fracture-related factors in recovery in older people. He believes that a recent increase in surgical treatment has been driven by a belief in the benefits of surgery, a lack of awareness of the evidence, and effective marketing. He describes many modern surgeons as academic bonesetters who may not feel the need to follow evidence regarding surgical treatment. We need to develop better measures of outcome and undertake better studies of the treatment of these fractures.

I recommend that surgeons treating fractures read this book as it contains excellent information about the history and current management of proximal humeral fractures, but it also outlines areas where the next generation of surgeons can improve their treatment.

Honorary Professor, University of Edinburgh
Edinburgh, Scotland, Great Britain

Charles Court-Brown

Preface

The treatment of shoulder fractures has provoked discussion for over 3000 years—and the debate continues. Although recent decades have certainly seen substantial advancements in orthopedic implants and procedures, and made surgical options available for many patients and injuries, the enthusiasm for new surgical treatments has not been accompanied by thorough testing of their benefits and harms. Randomized clinical trials have been conducted within the last 15 years, but they have not demonstrated the expected superiority of surgery over nonsurgical treatment. This disparity has led to a growing tension between evidence and practice and presents a challenge to the exercise of evidence-based practice.

In this book, I will discuss how orthopedic surgeons think and act when practice does not align with the best evidence. The primary focus will be on the treatment of shoulder fractures, but I will also touch on aspects of the evolution of orthopedic knowledge and practice.

Some orthopedic interventions *remain controversial* despite a growing number of high-quality trials reporting no difference in effect when compared to nonsurgical treatment. The treatment of displaced shoulder fractures is a conspicuous example. In the orthopedic literature, it has become a cliché that the treatment of shoulder fractures remains controversial. A PubMed search conducted in July 2024 using the search terms ("Shoulder Fractures"[Mesh]) AND (controvers*[Text Word]) revealed 139 articles describing the treatment of shoulder fractures as controversial. A search in Google Books using the words "proximal humerus controversial" revealed 34 textbooks referring to this controversy.

This repeatedly mentioned controversy can no longer be ascribed to any lack of evidence of treatment outcomes. In the latest Cochrane review, my colleagues and I identified 47 randomized trials, 10 of which compared surgical and nonsurgical treatments [1]. The studies unanimously found surgical interventions to be no superior to nonsurgical treatments. We have, that is to say, moved from *no evidence of a difference* to *evidence of no difference*. Current evidence is quite clear that surgery should no longer be routine for shoulder fractures in older people—but, surprisingly, in most countries, the number of surgeries has only increased. It is not clear quite how much documentation might be required to de-implement a surgical intervention introduced without high-quality evidence.

Disagreement between advocates of surgical and nonsurgical treatment is not new. In his presidential address to the British Orthopaedic Society of

1912, Sir Robert Jones summarized the evidence of his time: "Statistics do not seem to throw much light on the vexed question whether or not it is better to operate on fractures of the surgical neck of the humerus, for the percentages of good results are nearly equal by each method" [2].

Since Sir Robert Jones's time, it has become generally established that displaced long bone fractures require anatomical reduction and stable fixation, as stated in the AO principles from the late 1950s [3]. The persistent adherence to surgical solutions for any trauma case calls for reflection. In this book, I will explore the history of the debate on the treatment of shoulder fractures and question whether adherence to the principles of long bone fracture management adds value to older people with osteoporotic shoulder fractures.

The book is divided into six parts, comprising 17 chapters. Each chapter begins with an abstract and can be read independently or as part of the book. Part I introduces the fracture, its morphology, and epidemiology. The first chapter 1 discusses inconsistencies in basic descriptive terms and proposes a common terminology. The second chapter 2 provides an overview of epidemiological knowledge, including incidences, prevalences, and trends in surgical activity. Chapter 3 contains an illustrated introduction to the most common fracture patterns.

The second part includes a history of shoulder fractures from the earliest known surgical texts (Chap. 4) through Medieval and Renaissance sources (Chap. 5) to the early twentieth century. The current understanding of pathoanatomy was laid down in the first half of the nineteenth century (Chap. 6). Anesthesia and aseptics were introduced in the mid-nineteenth century, followed by radiology at the end of that century. Osteosynthesis became an option in the early twentieth century (Chap. 7).

The historical chapters are based on my reading and interpretation of primary sources. In guiding my search for these, I am indebted to encyclopedias on surgical history, in particular *Histoire de la chirurgie en occident depuis le VIe jusqu'au XVIe siècle* by Jean Joseph-Francois Malgaigne (1870) [4], *Geschichte der Chirurgie und ihrer Ausübung* by Ernst Julius Gurlt (1898) [5], and *Fractures: A History and Iconography of Their Treatment* by Leonard Peltier (1990) [6]. Whenever possible, I have referred to English translations of the texts. Covering more than three millennia of surgical history in four chapters may appear somewhat hazardous. I have focused on authors addressing shoulder fracture diagnosis, classification, or treatment, and I encourage readers to use the historical review as a sourcebook for further reading.

In Part III, I discuss the challenges faced by medical practitioners in understanding and interpreting imaging-based fracture patterns and developing hierarchies and classification systems. I also question the current use of radiographic classifications as the sole basis for making surgical treatment decisions: the shadow of a bone on a screen, I believe, is an insufficient guide for patient-centered and evidence-based decision-making. Chapter 8 covers cognitive processes and fundamental principles in classifying shoulder fractures; Chapter 9 examines the underlying assumptions behind the Neer and AO classifications; Chapter 10 offers a critical review of the current literature on observer agreement and discusses its clinical implications.

Part IV addresses the growing tension between evidence and practice. The development of orthopedics has been driven by the persistent efforts of orthopedic surgeons to develop implants and procedures. Most clinical studies on shoulder fractures published today are either non-comparative case series of surgical interventions or series with historical controls. Unable to provide unbiased estimates of treatment effects, these designs are inadequate for the justification of surgical practice: specifically, they cannot tell us whether the surgery under study is better than no surgery. Industrial sponsors are reluctant to support clinical trials with nonsurgical comparators, which may bias the choice of clinical research questions. In Chap. 11, I discuss the abundance of meta-analyses; these frequently arrive at different conclusions, even when based on the same primary data. While the number of network meta-analyses is increasing, they cannot bridge the knowledge gap due to unmet essential methodological preconditions.

Although they are rare, there have been game-changing events in the treatment of shoulder fractures. Recent examples include the introduction of locking plate technology and the extended use of reverse arthroplasty in fracture treatment. Both technologies were widely used for over a decade before they were tested in randomized trials. Chapter 12 considers why orthopedic surgeons persist with the use of locking plates in older people despite reports of high failure rates and an absence of benefits compared to nonsurgical treatment. In Chap. 13, I critically analyze the clinical evidence supporting the increasing use of reverse shoulder arthroplasty in shoulder fractures.

In Part V, I focus on measuring the benefits and harms after shoulder fracture treatment. Chapter 14 reviews commonly used assessment tools and their properties in a clinical setting, challenging the traditional preference for objective assessments. Validated complication terms are essential for weighing benefits and harms. Chapter 15 provides an overview of the scientific literature's multiple overlapping, and sometimes conflicting, complication terms and suggests a consensus-based approach to facilitate comparative studies. Chapter 16 discusses the lack of follow-up data, especially for non-surgically treated patients, and recommends systematically collecting outcome data for all patients, regardless of their treatment. In the closing chapter, I discuss the tension between learned medicine and surgical practice within the broader context of intellectual history, proposing future evidence-based treatment paths for patients with shoulder fractures. I also introduce the concept of the *academic bonesetter*—a practitioner who integrates surgical skills with academic proficiency.

This book recommends a nonsurgical approach for most shoulder fractures. Implementing evidence-based practice will likely decrease the number of surgical procedures for proximal humerus fractures in older people. Still, we have no reason to believe that the sum of orthopedic procedures will decrease. While I have no intention to discredit orthopedic surgery or my fellow surgeons, I believe it is essential to acknowledge that the best evidence does not always guide clinical decision-making. Poorly performed surgery on the right indications does not add value to patients, nor does well-performed surgery on the wrong indications.

The book is a compilation and a rethinking of my clinical and academic work. Many patients have generously provided valuable insights and the motivation to write it. Conversations with fellow surgeons and academic peers have shaped my approach to this common injury. I want to express my gratitude to Asbjørn Hróbjartsson, Hanne Andersen, Thomas Juul Sørensen, Kenneth Holtz, Zaid Issa, Hans Gottlieb, and Line Houkjær for discussions on earlier versions of the book. I am grateful to the late Charles Neer (1917–2011) for his encouragement during my early years in shoulder research. I want to express my gratitude to 62 co-authors from 10 countries who contributed to 42 of my papers published between 2000 and 2024, revisited during the writing of this book. I, however, take full responsibility for the errors or uncertainties it contains.

Finally, I am a great fan of orthopedic surgery. Well-performed surgery for the right patients, on the right indications, at the right time, can provide excellent value to patients and society. This book is not about the neglect of surgery; this book is about the neglect of evidence.

Copenhagen, Denmark
August 2024

Stig Brorson

References

1. Handoll HH, Elliott J, Thillemann TM, Aluko P, Brorson S. Interventions for treating proximal humeral fractures in adults. Cochrane Database Syst Rev. 2022;6(6):CD000434. Available from: https://www.cochranelibrary.com/cdsr/doi/10.1002/14651858.CD000434.pub5/abstract.
2. Jones R. Presidential address on the present position of treatment of fractures. Br Med J. 1912;2:1589–94.
3. Müller ME, Allgöwer M, Willenegger H. Technik der Operativen Frakturenbehandlung. Berlin: Springer; 1963.
4. Malgaigne J-F. Histoire de la chirurgie en Occident depuis le VIe jusqu'au XVIe siècle et histoire de la vie et des travaux d'Ambroise Paré. Paris: Baillière; 1870. Available from: https://archive.org/details/histoiredelachir00malg/.
5. Gurlt E. Geschichte der Chirurgie und ihrer Ausubung: Volkschirurgie – Alterthum – Mittelalter – Renaissance (Vol. 1–3). Berlin: Hirschwald; 1898. Available from: https://archive.org/details/geschichtederchi01gurl/.
6. Peltier LF. Fractures: a history and iconography of their treatment. San Francisco: Norman Publishing; 1990.

Ethics Approval Primary data has been included in Chap. 16 as part of a prospective cohort study approved by The Scientific Ethics Committee, Region Zealand, Denmark (jr. no. EMN-2021-07413).

Competing Interests The author has no competing financial or nonfinancial interests in relation to the content of the book.

Contents

Part I What Is a Shoulder Fracture?

1 Shoulder Fractures: A Brief Guide to Terminology 3
   1.1 Introduction 3
   1.2 Shoulder Fracture.................................... 4
   1.3 Dislocated or Displaced?............................. 4
   1.4 Subluxation of the Humeral Head 5
   1.5 Complexity... 5
   1.6 Comminution 6
   1.7 Part, Group, or Class? 6
   1.8 Instability 6
   1.9 Conservative... 6
   1.10 Pseudoarthrosis, Delayed Union, or Nonunion? 7
   1.11 Complication 7
   1.12 Elderly or Old?...................................... 7
   1.13 Frailty, Sarcopenia, and History of Falls 8
   1.14 Perspectives 8
   References... 9

2 The Epidemiology of Shoulder Fractures.................... 11
   2.1 Introduction 11
   2.2 Incidence 11
   2.3 Prevalence Matters................................... 12
   2.4 National Trends in Surgical Treatment 13
   2.5 Registry-Based Data 14
   2.6 Osteoporosis... 14
   2.7 Perspectives 16
   References... 16

3 The Morphology of Shoulder Fractures: An Iconography 19
   3.1 Introduction 19
   3.2 Patterns of Displacement............................. 19
   3.3 Anatomical Neck Fractures 20
   3.4 Translated Surgical Neck Fractures.................... 21
   3.5 Impacted Surgical Neck Fractures..................... 25
   3.6 Tuberosity Fractures................................. 27

	3.7	Fractures of the Humeral Neck and the Greater Tuberosity........	27
	3.8	Fractures of the Humeral Neck and Both Tuberosities	29
	3.9	Fracture-Dislocations................................	30
	3.10	Articular Surface Fractures	31
	3.11	Perspectives	32
		References..	32

Part II History: Shoulder Fractures from Ancient Egypt to the Early Twentieth Century

4 Pre-radiological Diagnostics and Classification of Shoulder Fractures 37
  4.1 Introduction 37
  4.2 Ancient Egypt 37
  4.3 Ancient Greece..................................... 40
  4.4 Ancient Rome 41
  4.5 Medieval Sources................................... 42
  4.6 Renaissance Sources 43
  4.7 French Hospital Surgery in the Eighteenth Century 44
  4.8 Perspectives 45
  References... 46

5 Interventions for Shoulder Fractures from Ancient Egypt to the Eighteenth Century......................... 49
  5.1 Introduction 49
  5.2 The Edwin Smith Papyrus 49
  5.3 Human Remains................................... 50
  5.4 The Hippocratic Corpus............................. 51
  5.5 Galen's Commentaries to Hippocrates.................. 54
  5.6 Medieval Treatments 54
  5.7 Renaissance Surgery 55
  5.8 The End of the Hippocratic Legacy 56
  5.9 Perspectives 57
  References... 58

6 Pathoanatomical Conceptions of Shoulder Fractures in the Nineteenth Century 61
  6.1 Introduction 61
  6.2 The French Pathoanatomical School 61
  6.3 Sir Astley Cooper................................... 62
  6.4 Robert William Smith 63
  6.5 Joseph-Francois Malgaigne 65
  6.6 Ludwig Thudichum's Pathoanatomical Classification....... 66
  6.7 Theodor Kocher.................................... 66
  6.8 Perspectives 69
  References... 69

	7	**Radiology and the Advent of Surgical Interventions for Shoulder Fractures**	71
		7.1 Introduction	71
		7.2 Skeletal Radiology	71
		7.3 The Short Rotators and the Subacromial Bursa	72
		7.4 Codman on Fractures	72
		7.5 The Four-Part Classification	73
		7.6 Early Surgical Interventions	75
		7.7 Perspectives	77
		References	77

Part III Classification: Knowing and Telling a Fracture

	8	**Why Do We Classify Shoulder Fractures?**	81
		8.1 Introduction	81
		8.2 Morphological Fracture Classification	82
		8.3 Clinical Properties of a Fracture Classification System	83
		8.4 Implications of Radiology-Based Classifications	83
		8.5 Telling a Fracture	85
		8.6 Philosophical Considerations	86
		8.7 Perspectives	87
		References	87
	9	**Imaging-Based Shoulder Fracture Classification Systems**	89
		9.1 Introduction	89
		9.2 Historical Context	89
		9.3 The First Neer Classification (1970)	91
		9.4 Early Criticism of the Neer Classification (1993)	93
		9.5 Neer's Second Response to His Critics (2002)	94
		9.6 The AO Classification System (1990, 2007, and 2018)	95
		9.7 Criticism of the AO Classification System	97
		9.8 Perspectives	98
		References	98
	10	**Why Do We Disagree When Classifying Shoulder Fractures?**	101
		10.1 Introduction	101
		10.2 Classification in Everyday Clinic	101
		10.3 Measures of Agreement	102
		10.4 An Introduction to Observer Studies	103
		10.5 The Landscape of Observer Studies	104
		10.6 Limitations of Observer Studies	105
		10.7 What Are the Clinical Implications of Disagreement on Classification?	105
		10.8 Translation of Categories Between Classification Systems	106
		10.9 Perspectives	107
		References	108

Part IV Management: Eminence Meets Evidence

**11 Interventions for Shoulder Fractures:
The Evidence Base** 113
    11.1   Introduction 113
    11.2   Randomized Trials................................ 113
    11.3   A Failed Trial..................................... 116
    11.4   The Evidence Base for Rehabilitation Interventions 116
    11.5   Systematic Reviews and Meta-analyses.................. 116
    11.6   Multiple Overlapping Meta-analyses................... 118
    11.7   Methodological Flexibility............................ 119
    11.8   Network Meta-analyses 120
    11.9   Perspectives 121
    References....................................... 123

**12 The Rise and Fall of an Implant: Locking Plates
in Shoulder Fractures** 127
    12.1   Introduction 127
    12.2   The Biomechanical Properties of Locking Plates 128
    12.3   How Does a Rigid Implant Work in an Osteoporotic
           Humeral Head? 129
    12.4   Indications for Locking Plate Osteosynthesis 131
    12.5   The Evidence Base for Locking Plates in Shoulder
           Fractures in Elderly 132
    12.6   Failure of Locking Plate Osteosynthesis 133
    12.7   The Locking Plate Epidemic 134
    12.8   Perspectives 135
    References....................................... 136

**13 The Use of Reverse Shoulder Arthroplasty
in Shoulder Fractures** 139
    13.1   Reverse Shoulder Arthroplasty in Fracture
           Management...................................... 139
    13.2   The Evidence Base for Reverse Shoulder
           Arthroplasty in Fracture Management................... 141
    13.3   The Limited Impact of a Negative Finding 142
    13.4   The "Red Wine Effect" of Fracture Prostheses 143
    13.5   "The Surgeon's Fallacy" 143
    13.6   Perspectives 144
    References....................................... 145

Part V Benefits and Harms

14 Outcome After Shoulder Fractures........................ 151
    14.1   Introduction 151
    14.2   The Landscape of Outcome Assessment Instruments 151
    14.3   Properties of Outcome Assessment Instruments 152
    14.4   The Constant-Murley Score and Its Limitations 152

14.5	Patient-Reported Outcomes	154
14.6	Perspectives	154
	References	155

15 Complications After Shoulder Fractures ... 157
- 15.1 Introduction ... 157
- 15.2 Complications After Non-surgical Treatment of Shoulder Fractures ... 157
- 15.3 Complications After Surgical Treatment of Shoulder Fractures ... 158
- 15.4 Toward a Core Event Set for Complication Reporting ... 158
- 15.5 Radiographic Monitoring ... 159
- 15.6 What Is a Radiological Complication? ... 160
- 15.7 Malunion: Friend or Foe? ... 163
- 15.8 Impairment of Rotational Mobility and Proprioception ... 165
- 15.9 Perspectives ... 165
- References ... 165

16 Bridging the Evidence-Practice Gap in Shoulder Fracture Management ... 167
- 16.1 Introduction ... 167
- 16.2 Barriers to Accommodate Evidence ... 167
- 16.3 Can Orthopedic Surgeons Change Behavior? ... 168
- 16.4 What Happens If We Do Not Operate? ... 169
- 16.5 Previous Prospective Cohort Studies ... 169
- 16.6 The Danish Cohort ... 171
- 16.7 Preliminary Outcome Data from the Danish Cohort ... 172
- 16.8 Perspectives ... 174
- References ... 174

Part VI Conclusions

17 Shoulder Fractures in Context: The Academic Bonesetter ... 179
- 17.1 Introduction ... 179
- 17.2 The Historic Bonesetter ... 179
- 17.3 Poor Practice and Iatrogenic Injury ... 180
- 17.4 Professional Ethics ... 181
- 17.5 The Academic Bonesetter ... 182
- 17.6 Future Directions ... 183
- 17.7 Perspectives ... 183
- References ... 184

About the Author

Stig Brorson is a clinical professor of orthopedic surgery at the University of Copenhagen and serves as a consultant shoulder surgeon at Zealand University Hospital in Denmark. He has a PhD in medical philosophy and a doctoral degree focusing on fractures of the proximal humerus. His research encompasses various aspects of proximal humerus fractures, including their cultural history, epidemiology, classification, diagnosis, decision-making, evidence-based treatment, outcome assessment, prognosis, and complications. He has supervised national and international multi-center studies and has compiled the current evidence in clinical guidelines, systematic reviews, and meta-analyses. Brorson advocates for evidence-based clinical practice and supports patient involvement in clinical decision-making. He has questioned the benefits of surgical interventions for shoulder fractures in older adults and argued for the de-implementation of low-value orthopedic procedures. In his clinical practice, he treats around 250 older individuals with shoulder fractures each year, with about 5% undergoing surgery.

Part I

What Is a Shoulder Fracture?

Shoulder Fractures: A Brief Guide to Terminology

1.1 Introduction

Shoulder fractures comprise a heterogeneous group of injuries that affect the upper end of the humerus. The head of the humerus articulates with the glenoid, a part of the scapular bone; jointly, they form the bony structure of the shoulder joint, also known as the glenohumeral joint. The shoulder joint is a ball-and-socket joint that offers a wide range of motion. The articular capsule, the fibrocartilage rim, the biceps tendon, the negative pressure within the joint, and the ligaments contribute to the stability of the joint. Superficial and deep muscles play a crucial role in the morphology of shoulder fractures.

A shoulder fracture is most frequently defined by its appearance on an anterior-posterior radiograph. The fracture determines the pathology, while the shoulder or the proximal humerus is the topological determinant. While no anatomical landmarks distinguish the proximal humerus from the humerus shaft, the two may be distinguished by a method known as *Heim's square* (Fig. 1.1).

In an elderly person, the trauma mechanism is typically a low-energy trauma following a standing fall. Swelling, severe pain, and lack of shoulder mobility are key symptoms. Although the fracture is at the shoulder level, discoloration and swelling are often seen at the arm and chest due to migration of the fracture hematoma (Fig. 1.2).

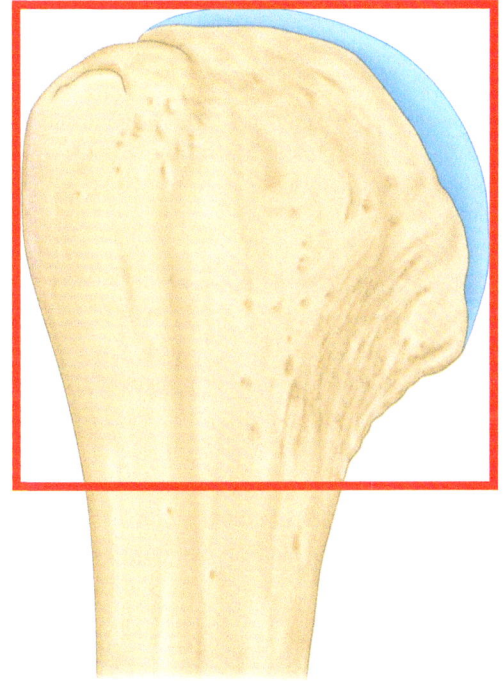

Fig. 1.1 The square definition of the proximal humerus. The widest part of the humeral head is measured to obtain the square. The lower endpoint of the square demarcates the proximal humerus from the shaft

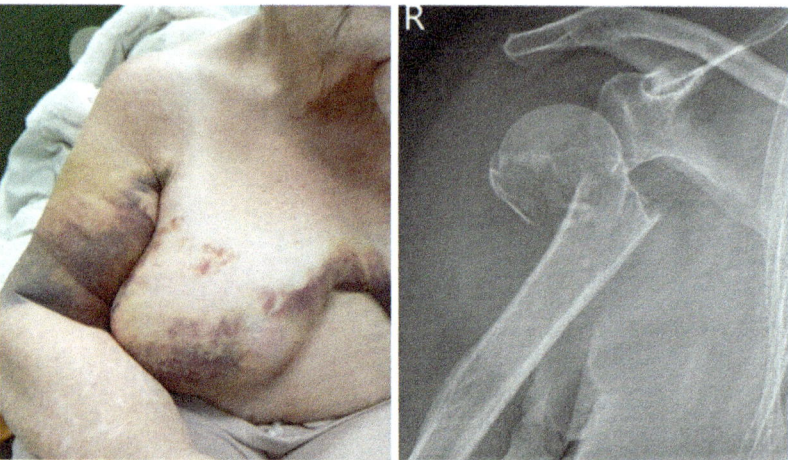

Fig. 1.2 A typical clinical appearance and the corresponding anterior-posterior radiograph in an elderly female with a medially translated surgical neck fracture

Below, I will briefly discuss some standard terms used for pathoanatomical descriptions, treatment decisions, and outcome analysis. Finally, I will discuss some important terms used to define the fracture population.

1.2 Shoulder Fracture

The term *shoulder fracture* has been used interchangeably with *proximal humerus fracture* or *proximal humeral fractures* since the early twentieth century. Before the mid-nineteenth century, it was challenging to distinguish proximal humerus fractures from other traumatic shoulder conditions due to the lack of pathoanatomical studies and radiology. Given the substantial evolution of medical knowledge and technology over the centuries, it is difficult to compare injuries from different periods; compound fractures of the humerus were discussed in medical texts in ancient Egypt, Greece, and Rome, for instance—but these injuries and the mechanisms causing them may differ from those we see today. Even today, there is uncertainty on the definition of proximal humerus fractures, especially if fracture lines cross the surgical neck. It can even be challenging to determine whether the head of the humerus is inside or outside the glenoid. This book deals with fractures on the humeral side of the shoulder. For brevity, *shoulder fracture* will be used synonymously with *proximal humerus fracture*.

1.3 Dislocated or Displaced?

In orthopedic terminology, the term *dislocated* refers to any fractured bone that is out of place. This can create issues when describing the morphology of shoulder fractures. Displacement, as defined by Charles Neer (1917–2011), is present when at least two of the four anatomical parts of the proximal humerus (Fig. 7.1) are displaced by at least 1 cm or angled by at least 45° [1]. Although this definition has limitations in clinical practice, it offers a common language for communication regarding fractures. Shoulder fracture morphology is simplified into a binary distinction: *minimally displaced* or *displaced*. The term *dislocated* violates this distinction and confuses fractures with fracture-dislocations. Fracture-dislocations are severe but rare injuries calling for orthopedic action. Neurovascular structures in the axilla and upper limb function are in danger when the broken humeral head is outside the capsule. In this book, the term *displaced* is preferred. *Dislocated* is restricted to cases explicitly dealing with fracture-dislocations.

1.4 Subluxation of the Humeral Head

Subluxation is a poorly defined radiological term that describes a humeral head positioned lower than expected in the glenoid cavity on plain radiographs, CT, or MRI scans. Luxation is misleading because the humeral head is still inside the capsule. On the lateral view, the humeral head is found low but not anteriorly or posteriorly to the glenoid. The phenomenon is common in acute fracture cases and is often reversed after mobilization of the rotator cuff (Fig. 1.3). In impacted fractures, the humeral head is depressed, frequently resulting in an inferior appearance of the humeral head.

1.5 Complexity

Complexity can refer to the morphology of a shoulder fracture: a four-part fracture is more complex than a two-part fracture, for example, and an intraarticular fracture is more complex than an extraarticular fracture. Some associate complexity with dislocation or comminution, while others link it to neurovascular involvement. In surgical communities where the treatment of choice is open reduction and internal fixation, *complexity* can refer to the expected difficulty in reconstruction surgery. In the latest Arbeitsgemeinschaft für Osteosynthesefragen/Orthopaedic Trauma Association (AO/OTA) classification revision, the term *complex* has been

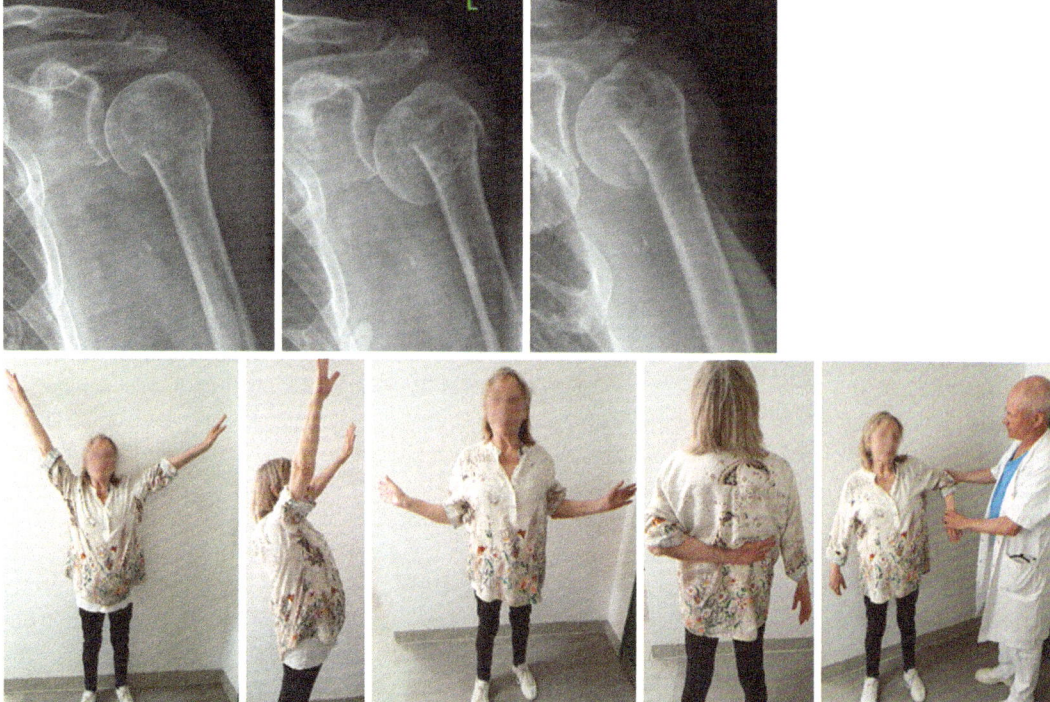

Fig. 1.3 Subluxation of the humeral head in a 71-year-old female with a surgical neck fracture. During the first week, the fracture collapsed into varus, and the head was found low in the glenoid cavity. After rehabilitation, the rotator cuff was reactivated, and the humeral head became better centered. The impaction of the humeral head remained. Radiographs at admission, 1 and 12 weeks. Clinical photos at 12 weeks

replaced by *multifragmentary*—a change that does little to aid clarity [2].

1.6 Comminution

Comminution is a commonly used but poorly defined descriptive term. Radiologists use the term to report that the fracture has more than two bony fragments. It has limited value for clinicians unless the description is within the frame of Codman's four anatomical parts. Some use the term for three- and four-part fractures, while others for metaphyseal comminution. This ambiguity is further confused by other terms such as *multipart*, *multifragment*, or *multi-segment*. These terms play a role in clinical decision-making, and explicitly defining them in clinical and scientific contexts is essential.

1.7 Part, Group, or Class?

Descriptive terms referring to pathoanatomical classification systems (Chap. 9) are often used interchangeably in the scientific literature and may cause confusion and the imperfect transmission of information. Commonly used terms include *part*, *segment*, *fragment*, *type*, *group*, *subgroup*, *class*, or *category*. *Type*, *group*, and *subgroup* are associated with the AO/OTA classification [3]. *Part* and *segment* are related to the Neer classification [1] based on Codman's four anatomical parts of the proximal humerus [4]. *Category* and *class* are neutral to the classification system and can be used in fracture communication if accompanied by a specification. As discussed in Chap. 10, substantial inconsistencies between classification systems can make translation between systems impossible and diminish the external validity of clinical research.

1.8 Instability

Instability is a term used to describe the expected course of a fracture. In a clinical context, it refers to the surgeon's interpretation of a radiograph, evaluation of the stability of the fracture, selection of an implant for the specific fracture pattern, and prediction of the patient's prognosis. Ultimately, the stability of a shoulder fracture can be assessed under fluoroscopy by manipulating the fracture while the patient is anesthetized. While this procedure was the standard in the 1960s and 1970s, it has been replaced by advanced imaging modalities or simply by operating on all radiographically displaced fractures.

A fracture is often considered unstable if the fracture morphology changes between two radiographic assessments. With the tendency of displaced shoulder fractures to settle and consolidate, however, especially within the first few weeks, changes in the radiographic appearance do not automatically indicate the need for surgical intervention. The concept of stability is based on a specific surgical tradition; it is not a natural property of the fracture. If a fracture is deemed unstable, it requires surgery. Conversely, if you believe a fracture requires surgery, you will likely classify it as unstable. A two-part surgical fracture with medial translation (Fig. 1.2) may be considered unstable by a surgeon who is familiar with locking plates, for example, even if that fracture might offer good potential for natural healing and function. Figure 1.3 shows a fracture proven unstable due to secondary varus collapse within the first week after injury. Despite this, the patient can still have a good clinical outcome. High-quality clinical data to challenge our assumptions about fracture stability is needed. Without modifying our clinical perspective based on the best evidence, we risk continuing to perform unnecessary or even harmful surgery.

1.9 Conservative

In orthopedic terminology, *conservative* treatment commonly refers to any treatment not involving open surgery. This includes closed reduction, bandaging, supervised or non-supervised training, watchful neglect, or neglect. Since the term can lead to the imperfect transmission of information if different stakeholders interpret it differently, this book uses *non-surgical* or *nonoperative* rather than conservative, accompanied by a treatment specification. It should be noted that before the advent of anesthetics and antiseptics in the mid-nineteenth century (Chap. 6), any procedure involving a medical practitioner or described by a medical writer was termed *surgical* or *operative*, even if it was not invasive in a modern sense. For many modern surgeons, the term conservative is used to demarcate the group of patient cases outside the surgeon's interest. However, even if only some 10% of cases require surgery, the remaining patients still need medical attention. The challenge lies in identifying the few cases that do require surgery—which needs a thorough evaluation of the entire population of patients with shoulder fractures.

1.10 Pseudoarthrosis, Delayed Union, or Nonunion?

Pseudoarthrosis is commonly used to describe a condition lacking radiological bony healing after a fracture. This may result in the formation of a *false joint* with the creation of a synovial membrane and joint fluid. This is typically identified through radiographs and defined by the duration of failed healing. In clinical use, the term *pseudoarthrosis* overlaps with the conditions of delayed union or nonunion. Radiographs cannot reveal the pathoanatomical changes or the clinical symptoms, and biomechanical factors such as weight-bearing need to be considered, calling for different treatment strategies for upper and lower extremity fractures. While some disturbances in the healing process may not show any symptoms, severe pain can still occur even if a fracture seems to have healed perfectly on radiographs. Therefore, the terms pseudoarthrosis, *delayed union*, and *nonunion*, as diagnosed on radiographs, are not very useful as indications for surgery or in clinical research (Fig. 15.1). The strength of fibrous healing is often underestimated, as is the strength and pain relief after lateral and posterior callus bridging and endosteal callus formation (Figs. 3.9 and 3.10).

CT scans are sometimes used to confirm the progress of healing after a shoulder fracture. However, in older people with osteoporosis and non-surgically treated displaced fractures, complete and rapid healing cannot be expected. It is more relevant to monitor the appearance of lateral and endosteal callus bridging and decreasing symptoms rather than relying on advanced imaging. MRI scans will show bone edema and incomplete healing. Lack of radiological healing is commonly found for an extended period.

Some commonly agreed definitions for the reading and interpretation of images may be helpful for more standardized reporting and study comparison. In an international consensus protocol for radiological monitoring of proximal humerus fractures, my colleagues and I asked 129 shoulder surgeons to define fracture healing. Eighty-nine percent agreed on the definition of mineralized callus circumferentially around the fracture on at least two orthogonal radiographs or CT scans. Delayed union was defined as occurring at 3 months in the absence of bridging callus on at least one of four cortices on two orthogonal radiographs or CT scans. Nonunion was defined as an absence of callus on more than two cortices after 6 months [5]. The definitions must be validated for clinical and scientific purposes.

1.11 Complication

Validated complication terms are necessary if we are to improve patient safety and to balance benefits and harms in clinical decision-making—but the literature on shoulder fractures offers us a poor definition of a term as common as *complication* itself. Complication, *event*, *adverse event*, *unfavorable event*, *harm*, and *failure* are used interchangeably, usually without further specification. Chap. 15 discusses the implications of poorly defined complication terms in the scientific literature and proposes a standardized reporting guideline. A consensus-based list of standardized event terms is available [6].

1.12 Elderly or Old?

Most studies on shoulder fractures define and report the study population according to chronological age. Substantial differences in age limits can be found in the orthopedic literature, with

95% of orthopedic studies using chronological age as the only definition of the population [7]. The age limit for classification as *elderly* varies between 50 and 80 years in orthopedic studies, with 65 being the most common cutoff value. Age contributes to fracture risk independent of osteoporosis [8]. In low-energy shoulder fractures, age and sex serve as proxies for osteoporosis. But it is challenging to compare results between clinical studies if age limits differ. In randomized trials on shoulder fractures, the lower age limit varies from 18 [9] to 80 years [10]. Most studies include only patients aged 60 or above, while evidence-based recommendations in younger populations are lacking. The United Nations defines individuals as elderly if they are 65 or older. The limit reflects life expectancy and socioeconomic factors [11]. In Africa, a person is defined as elderly if they are 50 years or older. In this book, a person is considered elderly at 60 years.

Some people find the term elderly disrespectful, while others consider it more polite than *old*. The sources cited in this book inconsistently use both terms. As a result, both terms will be found in text, citations, and references. I hope not to offend any readers using either term.

1.13 Frailty, Sarcopenia, and History of Falls

It is essential to consider factors other than age and osteoporosis in relation to the healing of injury and patient recovery. There is an overlap in the biology of *osteoporosis*, *frailty*, *sarcopenia*, and the geriatric *syndrome of falls*. A frail *phenotype* has been described, consisting of (1) weight loss, (2) exhaustion, (3) low energy expenditure, (4) slow gait speed, and (5) weak grip strength [12]. Several frailty scoring systems and interpretations are in clinical and scientific use. While these may be important determinants for patient outcome after shoulder fractures, validation in this specific fracture population is required. Systemic sarcopenia and a history of falls are other important prognostic factors. Muscular functionality is age-dependent. The condition of the deep and superficial muscles acting on the shoulder joint is an important determinant of rehabilitation potential. *Geriatric* designates medical care for older people, aged 65 years and over. Among individuals of this age living in the community, about a third suffer a fall within a year. The rate increases to half of individuals aged 80 and above [13]. Fall risk is a better predictor of fragility fractures than osteoporosis, and fall assessment is indicated after shoulder fractures in older people [14]. A prospective cohort study found that *kinesiophobia*—the fear of movement—after a week post-injury was the strongest predictor of limitations after 6 months [15].

1.14 Perspectives

The use of vague or poorly defined terms poses a challenge for clinical practice and research. In this chapter, I have briefly discussed some of the terms commonly causing confusion. I recommend the use of the following descriptive terms for fracture morphology: the four anatomical *parts* or *segments* defined according to Codman; *displacement* defined according to Neer; and *dislocation* reserved for injuries including joint dislocation. *Complexity* should be restricted to the description of Codman's four parts, and the notion of *subluxation* can be omitted. The terms *type*, *group*, and *subgroup* should be used within the AO classification, while *parts*, *segments*, and *categories* should be used in the Neer classification. Radiology-based assessment of fracture healing in older people with shoulder fractures is secondary to patient history, clinical examination, and the patient's treatment preferences. Radiology should not be used as the sole indication for surgery as *malunion* and *nonunion* seem to be surprisingly well tolerated. When defining the aging fracture population, age and sex can serve as proxies for osteoporosis. Other important predictive factors include a history of falls, kinesiophobia, sarcopenia, and frailty. The fracture population will be more thoroughly characterized in the next chapter.

References

1. Neer CS. Displaced proximal humeral fractures. I. Classification and evaluation. J Bone Joint Surg Am. 1970;52(6):1077–89.
2. Meinberg EG, Agel J, Roberts CS, Karam MD, Kellam JF. Fracture and dislocation classification compendium – 2018. J Orthop Trauma. 2018;32(Suppl 1):S1–170. Available from: https://journals.lww.com/jorthotrauma/fulltext/2018/01001/fracture_and_dislocation_classification.1.aspx
3. Marsh JL, Slongo TF, Agel J, Broderick JS, Creevey W, DeCoster TA, et al. Fracture and dislocation classification compendium – 2007: Orthopaedic trauma association classification, database and outcomes committee. J Orthop Trauma. 2007;21(10 Suppl):S1–133. Available from: https://journals.lww.com/jorthotrauma/abstract/2007/11101/fracture_and_dislocation_classification_compendium.1.aspx
4. Codman EA. The shoulder: rupture of the supraspinatus tendon and other lesions in or about the subacromial bursa. Malabar: T. Todd; 1934. Available from: https://wellcomecollection.org/works/k83a3rba
5. Lambert S, Brorson S, Joeris A, Durchholz H, Moro F, Audigé L. International consensus for a core radiological monitoring protocol of proximal humerus fractures. Injury. 2022;53(10):3326–31. Available from: https://www.sciencedirect.com/science/article/pii/S0020138322005010
6. Audigé L, Brorson S, Durchholz H, Lambert S, Moro F, Joeris A. Core set of unfavorable events of proximal humerus fracture treatment defined by an international Delphi consensus process. BMC Musculoskelet Disord. 2021;22(1):1002. Available from: https://bmcmusculoskeletdisord.biomedcentral.com/articles/10.1186/s12891-021-04887-1
7. Sabharwal S, Wilson H, Reilly P, Gupte CM. Heterogeneity of the definition of elderly age in current orthopaedic research. Springerplus. 2015;4:516. Available from: https://www.ncbi.nlm.nih.gov/pmc/articles/PMC4573966/
8. Falaschi P, Marsh D. Orthogeriatrics: the management of older patients with fragility fractures. Springer Nature Switzerland AG; 2021. Available from: https://link.springer.com/book/10.1007/978-3-030-48126-1
9. Rangan A, Handoll H, Brealey S, Jefferson L, Keding A, Martin BC, et al. Surgical vs nonsurgical treatment of adults with displaced fractures of the proximal humerus: the PROFHER randomized clinical trial. JAMA. 2015;313(10):1037–47. Available from: https://jamanetwork.com/journals/jama/fullarticle/2190987
10. Lopiz Y, Alcobía-Díaz B, Galán-Olleros M, García-Fernández C, Picado AL, Marco F. Reverse shoulder arthroplasty versus nonoperative treatment for 3- or 4-part proximal humeral fractures in elderly patients: a prospective randomized controlled trial. J Shoulder Elb Surg. 2019;28(12):2259–71.
11. United Nations. Leaving no one behind in an ageing world. World Social Report 2023. Available from: https://www.un.org/development/desa/dspd/wp-content/uploads/sites/22/2023/01/2023wsr-chapter1-.pdf
12. Martin FC, Ranhoff AH. Frailty and sarcopenia. In: Falaschi P, Marsh D, editors. Orthogeriatrics. Springer; 2021. p. 53–65. Available from: https://www.ncbi.nlm.nih.gov/books/NBK565582/.
13. Eurosafe. Active ageing through preventing falls. 2015. Available from: https://www.eurosafe.eu.com/uploads/inline-files/JointDeclaration_Sept2015.pdf
14. Adachi JD, Berger C, Barron R, Weycker D, Anastassiades TP, Davison KS, et al. Predictors of imminent non-vertebral fracture in elderly women with osteoporosis, low bone mass, or a history of fracture, based on data from the population-based Canadian Multicentre Osteoporosis Study (CaMos). Arch Osteoporos. 2019;14(1):53. Available from: https://scite.ai/reports/predictors-of-imminent-non-vertebral-fracture-vJKEXzW
15. Jayakumar P, Teunis T, Williams M, Lamb SE, Ring D, Gwilym S. Factors associated with the magnitude of limitations during recovery from a fracture of the proximal humerus: predictors of limitations after proximal humerus fracture. Bone Joint J. 2019;101-B(6):715–23.

Open Access This chapter is licensed under the terms of the Creative Commons Attribution 4.0 International License (http://creativecommons.org/licenses/by/4.0/), which permits use, sharing, adaptation, distribution and reproduction in any medium or format, as long as you give appropriate credit to the original author(s) and the source, provide a link to the Creative Commons license and indicate if changes were made.

The images or other third party material in this chapter are included in the chapter's Creative Commons license, unless indicated otherwise in a credit line to the material. If material is not included in the chapter's Creative Commons license and your intended use is not permitted by statutory regulation or exceeds the permitted use, you will need to obtain permission directly from the copyright holder.

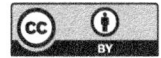

The Epidemiology of Shoulder Fractures

2.1 Introduction

Within the European Union (EU-27), the population of people aged 65 years or more is expected to increase from 90.5 million at the start of 2019 to 129.8 million by 2050. During this period, the number of people aged 75–84 is projected to expand by 56.1%, while those aged 65–74 are projected to increase by 16.6% [1]. National differences in demography exist even within the EU. It has further been estimated that 9 million osteoporotic fractures were sustained globally in the year 2000 (in men and women aged 50 or above), with more than 700,000 involving the humerus; of these, 250,000 were in Europe [2].

Shoulder fractures are common injuries, especially in elderly people. In the most cited epidemiological studies from the last century, shoulder fractures account for 4–6% of all fractures [3, 4]. More than 70% are seen in women, and the fracture is closely related to osteoporosis [5].

Increased mortality after shoulder fractures was found in a Swedish population, with a median survival of 9 years reported compared to 12 years in a matched population without a shoulder fracture. The lifetime risk of suffering a proximal humerus fracture in a female aged 50 years was 13% [5]. In the group aged 65 or above, 94% of the fractures were related to falls from standing height [6].

2.2 Incidence

Valid estimates of epidemiological measures are contingent on valid registration. Data should be reported from all treating institutions (coverage), and all data should be reported (completeness). Further, it is important to validate that fracture coding accurately represents the relevant fracture (positive predictive value) [7]. Unique identification of patients is a prerequisite for linking databases. Incidence rates, defined as the number of shoulder fractures per 100,000 persons per year, can be calculated based on discharge diagnosis and population statistics. The reported incidences may differ according to the definition of the fracture population, the background population, and the period under study.

A Finnish study of 79,676 shoulder fractures reported an incidence of 105 per 100,000 person-years in a population aged 16 or above in the years 1997–2019 [8]. Among those aged 80 and over, the incidence was 405 per 100,000 person-years. An increase in incidence throughout the study period was reported. In Finland, a threefold increase in incidence between 1970 and 2002 has been reported [9], but the incidence seems to have stabilized [10]. Following the increasing aging population, the absolute number of fractures may still increase despite a stable incidence. A study of a fracture population from Scotland

(n = 4786) collected over 2 years reported an incidence of 392 per 100,000 person-years in females aged 65 or above. In females aged 80 and above, the incidence was 520 per 100,000 person-years [11]. In a Danish study of 137,436 cases from the national patient registry between 1996 and 2018, my colleagues and I found an overall incidence rate of 138 per 100,000 person-years in persons aged 18 or above [12]. In females aged 60 years or above, the incidence was 500 per 100,000 person-years. The incidence remained stable throughout the period.

National differences in reported incidences can partly be attributed to variations in definitions of the fracture population and the quality of discharge data. The Danish study used discharge data for reimbursement, with high completeness and nationwide coverage [13]. To confirm the accuracy of the diagnosis, my colleagues and I reviewed medical charts. We found the positive predictive value for the diagnosis of proximal humerus fractures to be 91% [7].

2.3 Prevalence Matters

What is the prevalence of shoulder fractures? How many people are affected by them at a given time point? Prevalence may refer to the number of new cases within a defined period, but the number of symptomatic cases in the population is unknown. While some patients may recover fully and regain shoulder function within 6 weeks, others may experience complications from their fracture or treatment that can last for years. Patient-reported outcome data are needed to characterize the affected fracture population—but such data are generally available only through a few arthroplasty registries. I have argued that the accuracy of our assumptions about prevalence directly impacts the quality of our clinical decisions [14]. When we hear hoofbeats, it is knowledge of prevalence that allows us to assess whether we can expect to meet a horse or a zebra. We adapt our choices to the evidence we have, and if the available epidemiological data are misleading, cognitive bias may arise.

When treating shoulder fractures, one of the critical factors to consider is whether the fracture is displaced. This binary distinction guides our treatment choices and helps us make prognostic assessments. Orthopedic surgeons generally agree that minimally displaced fractures should not be operated on. In his iconic 1970 paper, Charles Neer (1917–2011) defined a fracture as displaced if two or more of the four anatomical parts of the proximal humerus are displaced at least 1 cm or angled at least 45° [15]. Applying this simple binary distinction has implications for the validity of the classification items. In an observer study, my colleagues and I reported a mean kappa value for interobserver agreement of 0.41 in identifying displacement [16]. This indicates that the level of agreement between observers is closer to chance than to complete agreement. Observer variation remains challenging for imaging-based classification systems and will be discussed in Part III.

Any statement concerning the prevalence of displaced fractures is specific to a population. The underlying population characteristics should be known. In the half-century since Charles Neer stated that "this group [minimally displaced fractures] constitutes over 85 percent of proximal humeral fractures" [15], the consensus in the orthopedic literature followed that 85% of all proximal humerus fractures were minimally displaced and could be treated without surgery. Neer's statement has two implications. First, we would expect displaced fractures to be rare occurrences; second, if a displaced fracture is identified, we will tend to approach it surgically. In this section, I will explore the origins of Neer's assertion to explain why it is misleading and how it can affect the quality of clinical decision-making.

Charles Neer wrote his seminal works while affiliated with Columbia-Presbyterian Medical Center, New York. Between 1953 and 1967, he followed up 300 patients with displaced shoulder fractures. The mean age of his cohort was 10 years lower than that in later studies (Table 2.1) [17]. All patients were treated under anesthesia. Despite this, the claim that 85% of fractures have

Table 2.1 The prevalence of minimally displaced fractures in five fracture populations

Study	Fractures (n)	Minimally displaced fractures (%)	Age (mean and range)
Neer (1970) [15]	300	85	56 (22–89)
Court-Brown (2001) [18]	1027	49	66 (13–98)
Tamai (2009) [19]	509	36	65 (18–95)
Roux (2012) [20]	329	43	70 (16–97)
Bahrs (2014) [21]	815	14	66 (19–99)

been minimally displaced has remained unquestioned for the last 50 years. The only reference used in support of Neer's statement was a single study that included pediatric fractures but did not provide any details about the fracture morphology. Since then, other epidemiological studies have been unable to confirm Neer's findings.

Since 1970, Neer's authoritative statement has been repeated in numerous scholarly papers and orthopedic textbooks. This may have led to clinicians underestimating the number of displaced fractures they encounter in their clinics when expecting to find only 15%. Furthermore, if displacement is used as the sole indication for surgery, many patients may undergo unnecessary surgical procedures.

2.4 National Trends in Surgical Treatment

The optimal surgery rate in patients with shoulder fractures is not known. It cannot be determined without including the patient's values and preferences. Radiographically based treatment plans assigning an implant to a fracture pattern may appeal to surgeons. However, fixing the fracture or replacing the joint cannot be expected to add value unless aligned with the best available evidence and patient preferences. Surgeons' preferences for surgery and surgical implants change over time. A diverse body of papers has reported the proportion of surgical treatment performed on patients with shoulder fractures and temporal changes. They are briefly reviewed below.

A national study from Germany reported a 39% increase in surgery between 2007 and 2016 [22]. Osteosynthesis was preferred in 72% of the surgeries. In 2016, 35,000 surgeries were performed in Germany, with a locking plate being the preferred implant. A more recent study from Germany analyzed billing data from a health insurance company between 2005 and 2021 and found 81,909 cases of shoulder fractures in individuals aged 65 and older. Of these cases, 46% were treated surgically. The study also noted a steep increase in the utilization of reverse shoulder arthroplasties over the years, with fewer complications reported, prompting a recommendation for broader implementation of reverse shoulder arthroplasties [23].

In the Swedish population, the proportion of surgically treated females increased from 12% in 2001 to 17% in 2012 [24]. In South Korea, the surgery rate increased from 25% to 37% between 2008 and 2016 [25]. The preference for locking plates rose from 72% to 82% in the same period. The percentage of those surgically treated in the United States has been reported to increase from 35% in 2004 to 41% in 2012 [26]. Substantial differences in surgery rates between states and centers can be found.

In the Danish population, my colleagues and I found that 87% of all shoulder fractures were treated non-surgically between 1996 and 2018. The surgery rate increased to 17% in 2013 and gradually declined to 11% in 2018. In patients aged 60 or above, the surgery rate declined from 17% in 2013 to 10% in 2018 [12]. Among the surgically treated cases, 42% received a locking plate; 34% received a hemiarthroplasty or a reverse arthroplasty, and 25% were treated with other surgical methods. In patients aged 60 or above, locking plates were used in half of the cases. The use of hemiarthroplasty declined while reverse arthroplasty increased. A similar trend can be found in the Finnish population [27]. The incidence of surgery rose from 5.1 to 19.6/100,000 person-years between 1987 and 2016. From 2002, osteosynthesis became increasingly popular, with a more than threefold increase in the incidence. In 2019, the overall incidence of surgery had fallen to 13/100,000 person-years, primarily driven by a decrease in locking plate osteosynthesis [8]. Trends of decreasing surgical activity have been reported in Australia. Operative treatment decreased from 33% in 2008 to 23% in 2017 [28]. Among the operatively treated, the locking plate rate slightly decreased, while reverse arthroplasty steeply increased at the cost of hemiarthroplasty.

The reasons behind the increasing use of locking plates and reverse arthroplasties are unclear and cannot be derived from epidemiological studies. However, some factors can be suggested as possible contributors. Local or national reimbursement practices may encourage surgical treatment strategies, for instance. Some surgeons may be worried about budgeting for their clinics and securing their income, while the influence of implant industry promotions on surgeon behavior cannot be overlooked. National traditions—the widespread use of osteosynthesis in German-speaking countries, for example—are also reflected in the surgery rates. Other factors may include a strong belief in biomechanical reasoning, passed-down practice, or limited access to high-quality evidence. A different case mix may also explain differences in surgery rates. Despite a lack of supporting clinical evidence, surgical activity continues to increase in many countries.

2.5 Registry-Based Data

National and international healthcare databases and registries provide valuable data on patients treated with joint replacement. Unfortunately, patients treated with head-preserving techniques or without surgery are usually not followed up systematically. National fracture registries are rare; only a few collect patient-reported outcome data [29]. The number of shoulder arthroplasty registries is increasing, but patient-reported outcomes are rarely recorded. Instead, implant survival rates are used as an indicator of treatment success. In a Nordic dataset covering 6756 fracture prostheses, my colleagues and I found a satisfactory low revision rate of 4% [30]. However, this is not very informative for the outcome in the remaining 96% of the patients.

The absence of revision is a poor proxy for treatment success. Revision surgery can be a relief for a patient with a painful prosthesis. Conversely, if revision surgery is not performed, it can have unbearable consequences for the patient. Revision rates reflect surgeons' willingness to perform revisions. Surgeons may avoid revising clinical failures or cases that require demanding surgery. To better understand patient outcome, it is necessary to obtain patient-reported data. It has proven difficult to obtain satisfactory completeness for patient questionnaires. In a study based on the Danish Shoulder Arthroplasty Registry, my colleagues and I obtained a completeness of about 60% [31]. The rate of revision was 4%. However, when using a patient-reported questionnaire (WOOS) to study patient-reported shoulder function, we found that 25% of patients had less than half of their shoulder function remaining. In 11% of patients, the Western Ontario Osteoarthritis of the Shoulder Index (WOOS) score was below 30% of a full shoulder function.

2.6 Osteoporosis

Bone quality is a crucial factor in shoulder fractures. Independent risk factors for shoulder fractures include bone mineral density and previous fractures [6]. In preliminary data from my clinic, in a series of 300 patients aged 50 or older who experienced a low-energy shoulder fracture, we found that 40% had manifest osteoporosis, defined as a T-score below −2.5 according to dual-energy X-ray absorptiometry (DEXA). An additional 39% had varying degrees of osteopenia, defined as a T-value between −2.5 and −1. The remaining 21% had a normal bone mineral density.

Although these numbers may be comparable with a matched background population, they have important clinical implications for patients, healthcare providers, and society. The risk of a subsequent fragility fracture is considerably higher after a shoulder fracture, particularly

Fig. 2.1 The risk of a second major osteoporotic fracture (95% CI) after the index fracture in women aged 75. The risk is very high immediately after the index fracture and remains higher than in the background population. The dashed line represents the risk of suffering the first major osteoporotic fracture in the background population [36]. (With permission from Springer Nature)

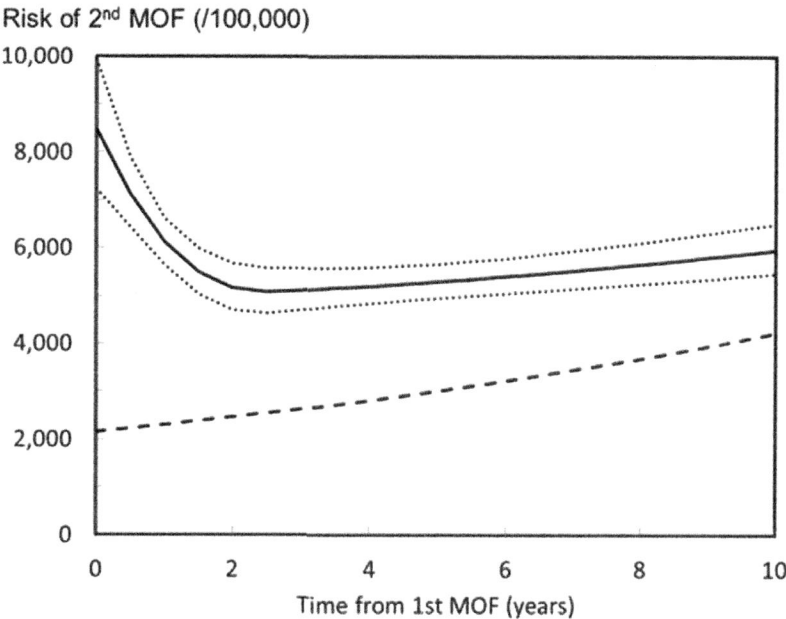

within the first 2 years. This *imminent fracture risk* highlights the importance of identifying osteoporosis in older people with low-energy shoulder fractures (Fig. 2.1) [32]. The imminent fracture risk estimates the increased risk of a second major osteoporotic fracture after the index fracture. This is the rationale behind Fracture Liaison Service [33], which seeks to assess fracture risk in patients who have suffered a fragility fracture and to provide medical treatment if needed. I have argued that a treatment gap currently exists in secondary fracture prevention after shoulder fractures [34, 35]. If fracture care providers had a stronger interest in secondary prevention, many fragility fractures, including hip fractures, could be prevented. This would benefit patients and society.

A typical *fracture career* in an osteoporotic female may include a wrist fracture at the age of 61, a shoulder fracture at the age of 69, and a hip fracture at the age of 81 [37]. Fragility fractures of the lumbar spine are underdiagnosed, and their onset and prevalence are not fully known. When an elderly patient experiences a shoulder fracture, the prevention of further fractures becomes crucial. Even though the patient may recover from the shoulder fracture, there remains a risk of a devastating hip fracture. In a female population aged 65 or above, the risk of a subsequent hip fracture was increased more than five times in the first year after a shoulder fracture [38]. A Medicare-based study of a female population aged 65 or above reported a 15.7% (95% CI 15.2–16.2) refracture rate within 2 years after a proximal humerus fracture. After 5 years, the cumulated refracture rate rose to 31.8% (95% CI 28.8–34.8) [39].

Most orthopedic surgeons agree that preventing secondary fractures after a hip fracture is important. This involves managing osteoporosis and preventing falls. However, not all elderly individuals who suffer from shoulder fractures receive the same level of attention. They are often treated with varying protocols by different doctors in outpatient clinics. It is unknown how many older people with shoulder fractures do not receive osteoporosis checkups. In a Danish hip fracture population, 28% of patients reported having at least one fragility fracture in the previous decade. Wrist and shoulder fractures accounted for 70% of these fractures [40].

Extensive literature exists on assessing local bone quality at the proximal humerus. Surprisingly, these studies aim to predict screw purchases for operative fixation of the fractures, not the prevention of hip fractures. This situation is unfortunate for two reasons. First, it shifts the focus away from secondary fracture prevention. Second, it promotes unnecessary surgical practices. As a result, patients may undergo unnecessary osteosynthesis while remaining at a substantial risk of a potentially preventable hip fracture. Surrogate measures for assessing the local bone quality of the proximal humerus have become popular to aid in preoperative planning. The *Tingart measure* [41] and the *deltoid tuberosity index* [42] can be determined from cortical thickness and calculated from plain radiographs. Local assessment may even be preferred to the evaluation of the axial skeleton as DEXA examination of the central skeleton may poorly reflect the bone quality of the proximal humerus [43].

2.7 Perspectives

The review reveals substantial national and regional differences in surgery rates. While the ideal surgery rate for shoulder fractures in older people cannot be derived from epidemiological data, a rough estimate can be made based on results from randomized trials. Randomized trials have been unable to demonstrate the superiority of surgery in two-, three-, and four-part fractures in older people. A comprehensive epidemiological study that categorized fractures using the Neer and AO classification systems found that 49% of fractures were displaced [18]. Most surgeons agree that minimally displaced fractures should be treated non-surgically. If we follow the evidence and treat two-part surgical neck fractures (28%), three-part greater tuberosity fractures (9%), and four-part fractures (2%) without surgery, about 12% is left for surgical consideration. This may represent an upper limit for surgery. Among the remaining displaced fracture patterns not covered by randomized trials, some older people with isolated tuberosity fractures may be treated non-surgically, while some younger patients may be treated surgically.

The high refracture rates after shoulder fractures in older people are a major concern for patients, the healthcare system, and society. Orthopedic surgeons have historically prioritized surgical interventions at the proximal humerus rather than secondary fracture prevention. The number of preventable hip fractures suffered remains unknown. In this chapter, I have argued that evaluating the bone mineral density of the axial skeleton is essential after shoulder fractures in older people, regardless of the type of fracture or the treatment provided [35].

References

1. European Commission. Aging Europe – statistics on population developments. Available from: https://ec.europa.eu/eurostat/statistics-explained/index.php?title=Ageing_Europe_-_statistics_on_population_developments
2. Johnell O, Kanis JA. An estimate of the worldwide prevalence and disability associated with osteoporotic fractures. Osteoporos Int. 2006;17(12):1726–33.
3. Buhr AJ, Cooke AM. Fracture Patterns. Lancet. 1959;273(7072):531–6.
4. Knowelden J, Buhr A, Dunbar O. Incidence of Fractures in persons over 35 years of age. A report to the M.R.C. Working Party on Fractures in the elderly. Br J Prev Soc Med. 1964;18(3):130–41.
5. Kanis JA, Johnell O, Oden A, Sembo I, Redlund-Johnell I, Dawson A, et al. Long-term risk of osteoporotic fracture in Malmö. Osteoporos Int. 2000;11(8):669–74.
6. Olsson C, Nordqvist A, Petersson CJ. Increased fragility in patients with fracture of the proximal humerus: a case control study. Bone. 2004;34(6):1072–7.
7. Karimi D, Houkjær L, Gundtoft P, Brorson S, Viberg B. Positive predictive value of humeral fractures in the Danish National Patient Registry. Dan Med J. 2023;70(4) Available from: https://ugeskriftet.dk/dmj/positive-predictive-value-humeral-fractures-danish-national-patient-registry
8. Leino OK, Lehtimäki KK, Mäkelä K, Äärimaa V, Ekman E. Proximal humeral fractures in Finland: trends in the incidence and methods of treatment between 1997 and 2019. Bone Joint J. 2022;104-B(1):150–6.
9. Palvanen M, Kannus P, Niemi S, Parkkari J. Update in the epidemiology of proximal humeral fractures. Clin Orthop Relat Res. 2006;442:87–92.
10. Kannus P, Niemi S, Sievänen H, Parkkari J. Stabilized incidence in Proximal humeral fractures of elderly women: Nationwide statistics from Finland in 1970–2015. J Gerontol A Biol Sci Med Sci. 2017;72(10):1390–3.
11. Court-Brown CM, Clement ND, Duckworth AD, Aitken S, Biant LC, McQueen MM. The spectrum of fractures in the elderly. Bone Joint J. 2014;96-B(3):366–72.

References

12. Brorson S, Viberg B, Gundtoft P, Jalal B, Ohrt-Nissen S. Epidemiology and trends in management of acute proximal humeral fractures in adults: an observational study of 137,436 cases from the Danish National Patient Register, 1996–2018. Acta Orthop. 2022;93:750–5. Available from: https://actaorthop.org/actao/article/view/4578
13. Schmidt M, Schmidt SAJ, Sandegaard JL, Ehrenstein V, Pedersen L, Sørensen HT. The Danish National Patient Registry: a review of content, data quality, and research potential. Clin Epidemiol. 2015;7:449–490. Available from: https://www.dovepress.com/the-danish-national-patient-registry-a-review-of-content-data-quality%2D%2Dpeer-reviewed-article-CLEP
14. Brorson S. How many shoulder fractures are displaced? How a misleading statement became orthopedic knowledge. Acta Orthop. 2023;94:328–9. Available from: https://actaorthop.org/actao/article/view/13651
15. Neer CS. Displaced proximal humeral fractures. I. Classification and evaluation. J Bone Joint Surg Am. 1970;52(6):1077–89.
16. Brorson S, Bagger J, Sylvest A, Hrobjartsson A. Low agreement among 24 doctors using the Neer-classification; only moderate agreement on displacement, even between specialists. Int Orthop. 2002;26(5):271–3. Available from: https://www.ncbi.nlm.nih.gov/pmc/articles/PMC3620992/
17. Brorson S. Proximal humeral fractures. In: Court-Brown C, McQueen MM, Swiontkowski MF, Ring D, Friedman SM, Duckworth A, editors. Musculoskeletal trauma in the elderly. Taylor & Francis Group; 2017. p. 257–71.
18. Court-Brown CM, Garg A, McQueen MM. The epidemiology of proximal humeral fractures. Acta Orthop Scand. 2001;72(4):365–71. Available from: https://actaorthop.org/actao/article/view/20079
19. Tamai K, Ishige N, Kuroda S, Ohno W, Itoh H, Hashiguchi H, et al. Four-segment classification of proximal humeral fractures revisited: a multicenter study on 509 cases. J Shoulder Elb Surg. 2009;18(6):845–50. Available from: https://www.sciencedirect.com/science/article/pii/S1058274609000834
20. Roux A, Decroocq L, El Batti S, Bonnevialle N, Moineau G, Trojani C, et al. Epidemiology of proximal humerus fractures managed in a trauma center. Orthop Traumatol Surg Res. 2012;98(6):715–9. Available from: https://www.sciencedirect.com/science/article/pii/S1877056812001570?via%3Dihub
21. Bahrs C, Stojicevic T, Blumenstock G, Brorson S, Badke A, Stockle U, et al. Trends in epidemiology and patho-anatomical pattern of proximal humeral fractures. Int Orthop. 2014;38(8):1697–704. Available from: https://www.ncbi.nlm.nih.gov/pmc/articles/PMC4115093/
22. Klug A, Gramlich Y, Wincheringer D, Schmidt-Horlohé K, Hoffmann R. Trends in surgical management of proximal humeral fractures in adults: a nationwide study of records in Germany from 2007 to 2016. Arch Orthop Trauma Surg. 2019;139(12):1713–21.
23. Katthagen JC, Raschke MJ, Fischhuber K, Iking J, Marschall U, Sußiek J, et al. Conservative versus operative treatment of Proximal Humerus Fractures in older individuals. Dtsch Arztebl Int. 2024;121(14):454–60. Available from: https://www.aerzteblatt.de/int/archive/article/240186
24. Sumrein BO, Huttunen TT, Launonen AP, Berg HE, Felländer-Tsai L, Mattila VM. Proximal humeral fractures in Sweden—a registry-based study. Osteoporos Int. 2017;28(3):901–7.
25. Jo Y-H, Lee K-H, Lee B-G. Surgical trends in elderly patients with proximal humeral fractures in South Korea: a population-based study. BMC Musculoskelet Disord. 2019;20(1):136. Available from: https://bmcmusculoskeletdisord.biomedcentral.com/articles/10.1186/s12891-019-2515-2
26. Sabesan VJ, Lombardo D, Petersen-Fitts G, Weisman M, Ramthun K, Whaley J. National trends in proximal humerus fracture treatment patterns. Aging Clin Exp Res. 2017;29(6):1277–83. Available from: https://link.springer.com/article/10.1007/s40520-016-0695-2
27. Huttunen TT, Launonen AP, Pihlajamäki H, Kannus P, Mattila VM. Trends in the surgical treatment of proximal humeral fractures – a nationwide 23-year study in Finland. BMC Musculoskelet Disord. 2012;13(1):261. Available from: https://bmcmusculoskeletdisord.biomedcentral.com/articles/10.1186/1471-2474-13-261
28. McLean AS, Price N, Graves S, Hatton A, Taylor FJ. Nationwide trends in management of proximal humeral fractures: an analysis of 77,966 cases from 2008 to 2017. J Shoulder Elb Surg. 2019;28(11):2072–8.
29. Bergdahl C, Wennergren D, Swensson-Backelin E, Ekelund J, Möller M. No change in reoperation rates despite shifting treatment trends: a population-based study of 4,070 proximal humeral fractures. Acta Orthop. 2021;92(6):651–7. Available from: https://actaorthop.org/actao/article/view/1445
30. Brorson S, Salomonsson B, Jensen SL, Fenstad AM, Demir Y, Rasmussen JV. Revision after shoulder replacement for acute fracture of the proximal humerus. Acta Orthop. 2017;88(4):446–50. Available from: https://actaorthop.org/actao/article/view/9694
31. Amundsen A, Rasmussen JV, Olsen BS, Brorson S. Low revision rate despite poor functional outcome after stemmed hemiarthroplasty for acute proximal humeral fractures: 2,750 cases reported to the Danish Shoulder Arthroplasty Registry. Acta Orthop. 2019;90(3) Available from: https://actaorthop.org/actao/article/view/529
32. Pinedo-Villanueva R, Charokopou M, Toth E, Donnelly K, Cooper C, Prieto-Alhambra D, et al. Imminent fracture risk assessments in the UK FLS setting: implications and challenges. Arch Osteoporos. 2019;14(1):12. Available from: https://www.ncbi.nlm.nih.gov/pmc/articles/PMC6398567/

33. Fuggle NR, Kassim Javaid M, Fujita M, Halbout P, Dawson-Hughes B, Rizzoli R, et al. In: Falaschi P, Marsh D, editors. Fracture risk assessment and how to implement a fracture liaison service. Cham (CH); 2021. p. 241–56. Available from: https://www.ncbi.nlm.nih.gov/books/NBK565570/.
34. Skjødt MK, Ernst MT, Khalid S, Libanati C, Cooper C, Delmestri A, et al. The treatment gap after major osteoporotic fractures in Denmark 2005-2014: a combined analysis including both prescription-based and hospital-administered anti-osteoporosis medications. Osteoporos Int. 2021;32(10):1961–71.
35. Brorson S. Who should care about the patient's next fracture? A treatment gap after shoulder fractures in the elderly. Acta Orthop. 2023;94:514–5. Available from: https://actaorthop.org/actao/article/view/21273
36. Johansson H, Siggeirsdóttir K, Harvey NC, Odén A, Gudnason V, McCloskey E, et al. Imminent risk of fracture after fracture. Osteoporos Int. 2017;28(3):775–80.
37. Bergh C, Möller M, Ekelund J, Brisby H. 30-day and 1-year mortality after skeletal fractures: a register study of 295,713 fractures at different locations. Acta Orthop. 2021;92(6):739–45. Available from: https://actaorthop.org/actao/article/view/1451
38. Clinton J, Franta A, Polissar NL, Neradilek B, Mounce D, Fink HA, et al. Proximal humeral fracture as a risk factor for subsequent hip fractures. J Bone Joint Surg Am. 2009;91(3):503–11.
39. Balasubramanian A, Zhang J, Chen L, Wenkert D, Daigle SG, Grauer A, et al. Risk of subsequent fracture after prior fracture among older women. Osteoporos Int. 2019;30(1):79–92.
40. Frederiksen A, Abrahamsen B, Johansen PB, Sørensen HA. Danish, national cross-sectional observational study on the prevalence of prior major osteoporotic fractures in adults presenting with hip fracture-limitations and scope for fracture liaison services in prevention of hip fracture. Osteoporos Int. 2018;29(1):109–14.
41. Tingart MJ, Apreleva M, von Stechow D, Zurakowski D, Warner JJ. The cortical thickness of the proximal humeral diaphysis predicts bone mineral density of the proximal humerus. J Bone Joint Surg Br. 2003;85(4):611–7.
42. Spross C, Kaestle N, Benninger E, Fornaro J, Erhardt J, Zdravkovic V, et al. Deltoid tuberosity index: a simple radiographic tool to assess local bone quality in Proximal Humerus Fractures. Clin Orthop Relat Res. 2015;473(9):3038–45. Available from: https://www.ncbi.nlm.nih.gov/pmc/articles/PMC4523505/
43. Lee SY, Kwon S-S, Kim TH, Shin S-J. Is central skeleton bone quality a predictor of the severity of proximal humeral fractures? Injury. 2016;47(12):2777–82.

Open Access This chapter is licensed under the terms of the Creative Commons Attribution 4.0 International License (http://creativecommons.org/licenses/by/4.0/), which permits use, sharing, adaptation, distribution and reproduction in any medium or format, as long as you give appropriate credit to the original author(s) and the source, provide a link to the Creative Commons license and indicate if changes were made.

The images or other third party material in this chapter are included in the chapter's Creative Commons license, unless indicated otherwise in a credit line to the material. If material is not included in the chapter's Creative Commons license and your intended use is not permitted by statutory regulation or exceeds the permitted use, you will need to obtain permission directly from the copyright holder.

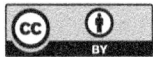

The Morphology of Shoulder Fractures: An Iconography

3.1 Introduction

The morphology of a displaced proximal humerus fracture reflects the deforming forces acting on the fracture parts. The forces acting on a surgical neck fracture differ from those affecting tuberosity fractures. A radiograph or CT scan of the fracture anatomy shows the state of the soft tissue but is often interpreted as a bone problem only. The key to understanding displaced shoulder fractures lies in the delicate balance between the superficial and deep muscles surrounding the shoulder. Rational treatment strategies require an understanding of soft tissue pathology, whether approached surgically or non-surgically. In older people, rehabilitation can be challenging due to concurrent degenerative or acute rotator cuff tears, sarcopenia, osteoarthritis, and glenohumeral joint stiffness.

The dynamic understanding of the biomechanics of the shoulder is not new. In the Italian Renaissance, Leonardo da Vinci's anatomic sketches of about 1510 demonstrate a profound understanding of the muscles involved in shoulder movement [1]. After dissecting the deep muscles of the human shoulder, Leonardo added wire diagrams to explain the insertions and forces acting on the humeral head, creating precise surface anatomy drawings. From a superior view of the scapula, he was able to visualize the deep muscle on the anterior side (m. subscapularis) together with deep muscles on the posterior side (mm. supraspinatus, infraspinatus, and teres minor) (Fig. 4.4).

More recently, Ernest Codman (1869–1940), a surgeon who contributed substantially to the biomechanical understanding of the shoulder and fracture morphology, proposed a *soft tissue approach* to shoulder pathology. Codman focused on the subacromial bursa and the internal rotators, later known as the rotator cuff. Codman's four-part approach to shoulder fractures formed the basis of the Neer classification (Chap. 9). Codman, who was also one of the pioneers of skeletal radiology in the late nineteenth century (Chap. 7), surprisingly regarded the fracture pattern as a soft tissue pathology with bony involvement.

3.2 Patterns of Displacement

Shoulder fractures can be displaced due to muscular forces acting on the four anatomical parts. The displacements seen in radiographs represent a continuum rather than distinct categories. When we define fractures as *displaced* or *minimally displaced*, we create arbitrary cutoffs in this range of displacements and turn them into binary categories. This cognitive process is discussed in more detail in Chap. 8. The proximal humerus has several axes of displacement. Fracture patterns differ

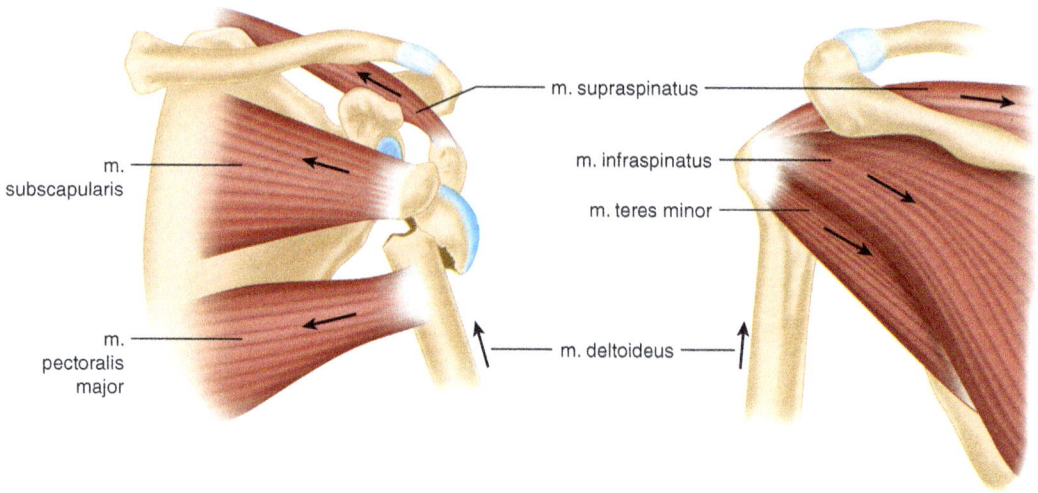

Fig. 3.1 The muscular forces acting on the proximal humerus. Left shoulder, anterior, and posterior view

between humeral neck fractures and tuberosity fractures. All deforming forces are combined in fractures involving both the humeral neck and the tuberosities.

Figure 3.1 illustrates the external forces acting on the proximal humerus. The pectoralis major muscle pulls the humeral shaft medially and anteriorly, while the supraspinatus muscle pulls the greater tuberosity toward the subacromial space. The subscapularis muscle pulls the lesser tuberosity medially, while the infraspinatus, teres minor, and supraspinatus muscles tend to draw the greater tuberosity posteriorly. Lastly, the deltoideus muscle tends to pull the humeral shaft superiorly. Closed reduction of displaced shoulder fractures is rarely successful due to the multiple muscular forces. This also explains why immobilizing displaced shoulder fractures by bandaging the shoulder and upper arm has been unsuccessful for centuries (Chap. 6).

3.3 Anatomical Neck Fractures

Fractures of the humeral neck in adults can occur between the articular part of the proximal humerus and at the tuberosities (*anatomical neck*) or between the anatomical neck and the lower bound of the proximal humerus (*surgical neck*). Fractures of the anatomical neck are intracapsular but often associated with fractures of the tuberosities.

Anatomical neck fractures are often considered severe due to limited blood supply from the anterior and posterior circumflex arteries. Arcuate arteries from the circumflex arteries may cross the fracture lines, and lesions may compromise the nutrition of the articular part. Anatomical neck fractures, although rare, have been known and described since antiquity. When the articular surface completely slips, it has a poor potential for healing. However, slightly displaced lesions may have good healing potential (Fig. 3.2).

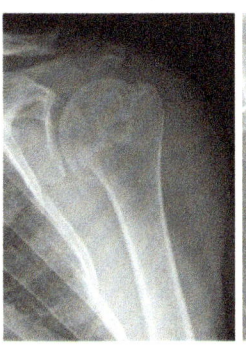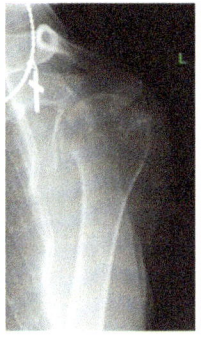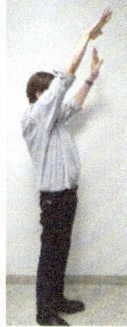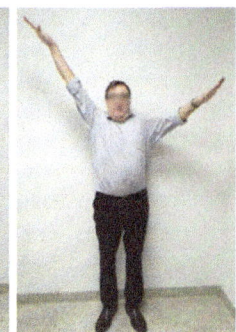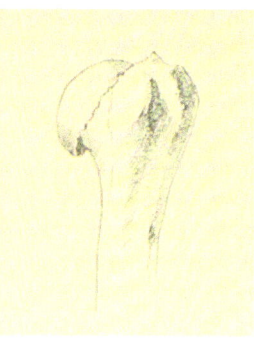

Fig. 3.2 Slightly displaced anatomical neck fracture. Radiographs at admission and 6 months. Photos at 6 months. The patient was pain-free after 3 months. Comparable fracture pattern from Theodor Kocher [2]. (With permission from Wellcome Collection)

3.4 Translated Surgical Neck Fractures

The surgical neck fracture is the most common displaced fracture pattern of the proximal humerus, comprising 28% of all proximal humeral fractures and more than half of displaced fractures [3]. Surgical neck fractures are extracapsular and can be categorized into two main types: translated and impacted.

Albert Hoffa's illustration in Fig. 3.3 shows the deforming forces and the surface anatomy alterations in a medially translated surgical neck fracture. The pectoralis major muscle pulls the humeral shaft medially and anteriorly, while the deltoid muscle pulls the shaft superiorly and rotates the shaft fragment. In the drawing, the lower part illustrates the typical surface anatomy. It includes the concavity formed by the medial translation of the humeral shaft, which may be mistakenly identified as a shoulder dislocation. The rotator cuff has a limited role in the displacement of these fractures.

The medial and anterior displacement of the humeral shaft can be described as a continuum of displacement ranging from slight displacement (Fig. 3.4) to no contact between the head and shaft (Fig. 3.5). Poor alignment and malunion after a fracture do not necessarily indicate a poor outcome for the patient [4]. Even marked malunion seems well tolerated in older people [5], and no correlation between final radiographic alignment and patient outcome has been reported. Attempts to restore the anatomy have yet to be demonstrated as being superior to natural healing, regardless of the degree of displacement [6, 7].

The pectoralis major muscle can cause substantial anterior displacement of the humeral shaft, which may require surgical intervention. In addition, the superior pull from the deltoid muscle can cause the shaft fragment to penetrate the skin, resulting in a need for acute surgery (Fig. 3.6). However, despite persistent angular deformity, most patients with anterior displacement of the humeral shaft can achieve healing and good shoulder function without surgery. In thin individuals, the upper end of the shaft can be felt through the skin.

Fig. 3.3 The surface anatomy and the deforming muscular forces acting on a medially translated surgical neck fracture. Illustration from Albert Hoffa [8]. (With permission from Wellcome Collection. Clinical photo of a comparable fracture pattern)

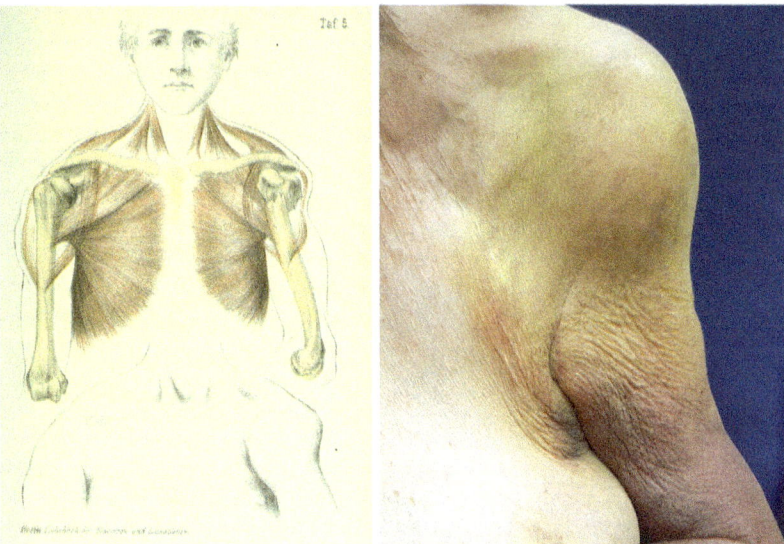

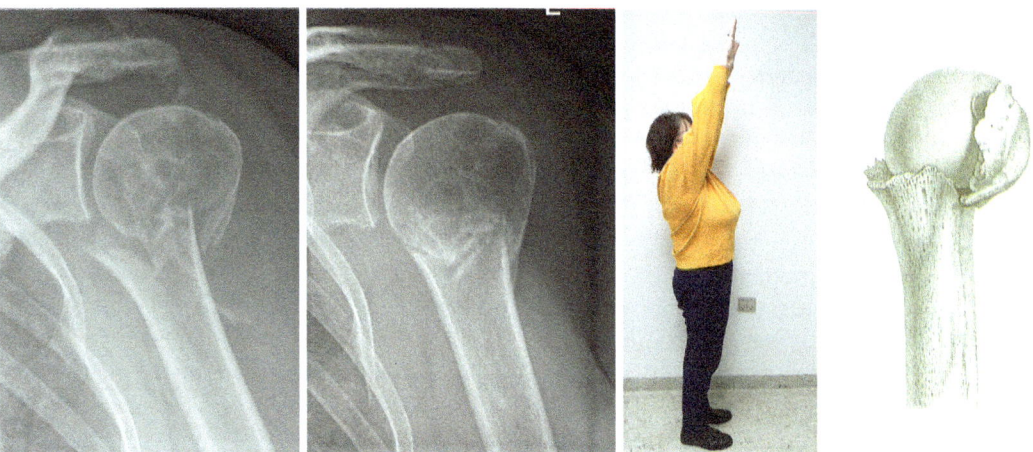

Fig. 3.4 A slightly medially translated surgical neck fracture. The displacement was remodeled, and the patient regained pre-injury shoulder function. Radiographs at admission and 6 months. Clinical photo at 6 months. Engraving of a comparable fracture pattern from Joseph-François Malgaigne [9]. (With permission from Wellcome Collection)

In Fig. 3.7, a severe anterior and medial displacement in a surgical neck fracture is illustrated. The humeral shaft is protruding under the skin. The patient was admitted 6 weeks after the injury. The three-dimensional CT reconstruction reveals early signs of callus bridging. The patient was treated operatively with a hemiarthroplasty to protect the skin and the neurovascular structures. A humeral mega-head was chosen to ensure maximum stability in a noncompliant patient.

Occasionally, lateral displacement of the humerus shaft occurs. The skin can be threatened by perforation from the proximal part of the humeral shaft. A partial resection of the shaft can be performed as a salvage procedure (Fig. 3.8).

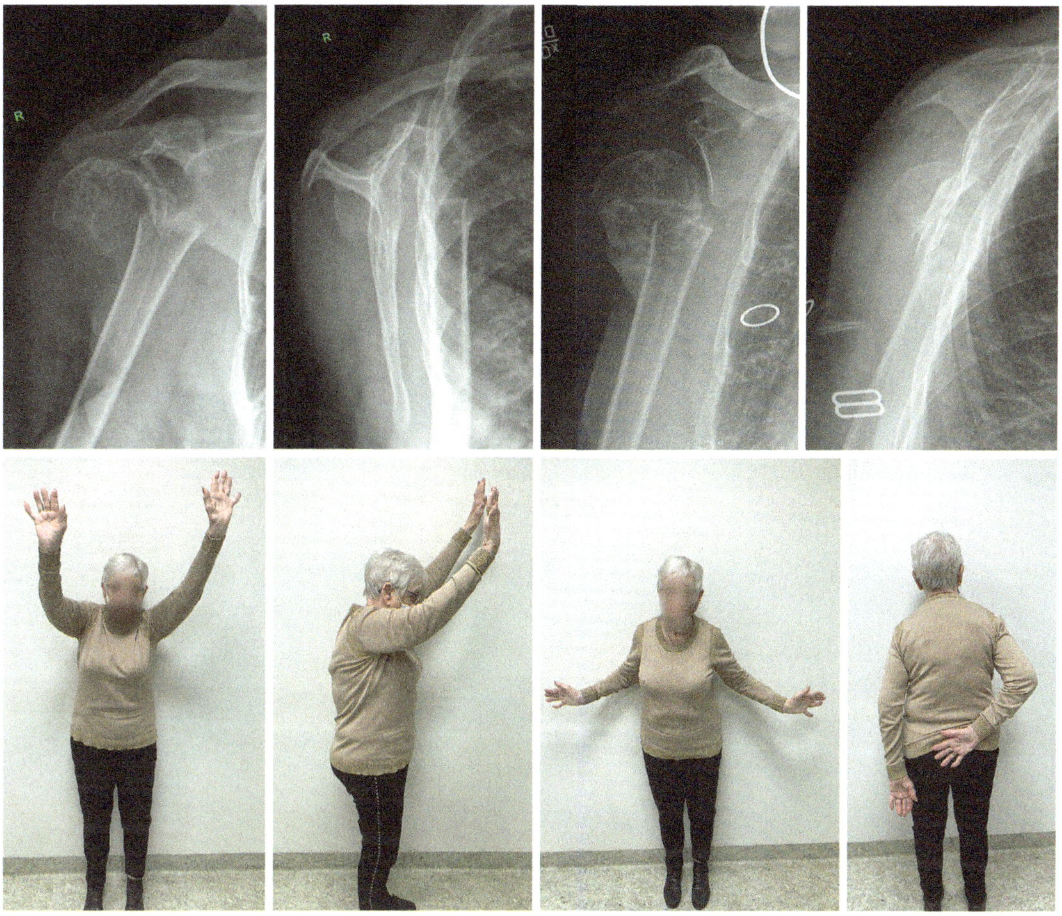

3.4 Translated Surgical Neck Fractures

Fig. 3.5 A surgical neck fracture without bony contact in an 82-year-old osteoporotic female. After 3 months, a massive lateral bone bridge was formed, and the head and shaft were better realigned on both views. The patient regained pre-injury shoulder function. Radiographs at admission and 6 months. Clinical photos at 6 months

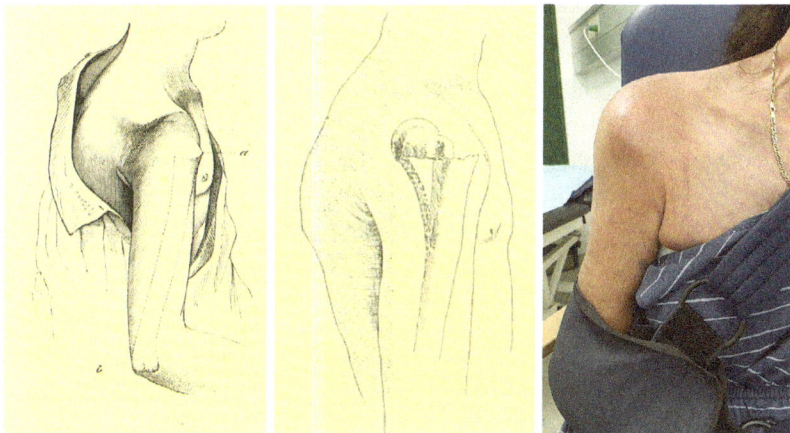

Fig. 3.6 Anterior displacement with bony prominence of the humeral shaft under the skin. Illustration from Benjamin Anger (left) [10] and Theodor Kocher [2]. (With permission from Wellcome Collection. Clinical photo of a comparable pattern of displacement)

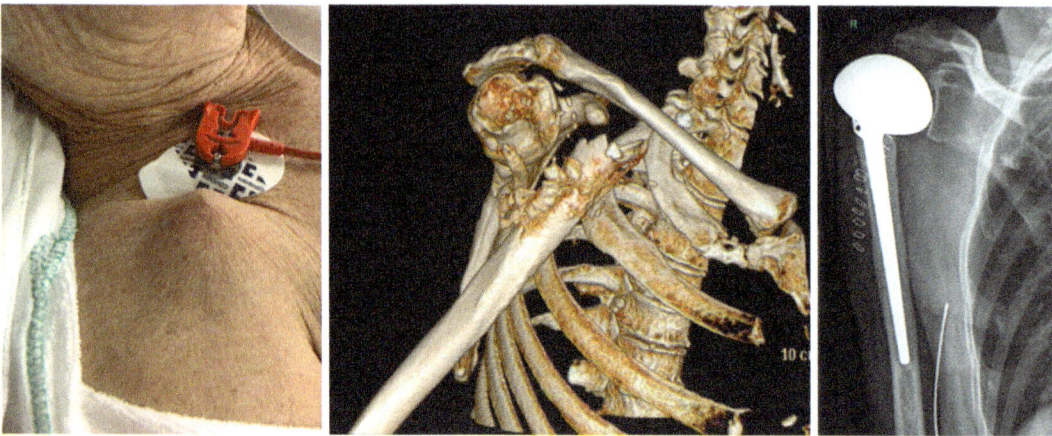

Fig. 3.7 Protrusion of the proximal end of the humeral shaft under the skin in a 76-year-old nursing home resident suffering severe dementia. Clinical photo, three-dimensional CT scan, and postoperative radiograph at 6 weeks

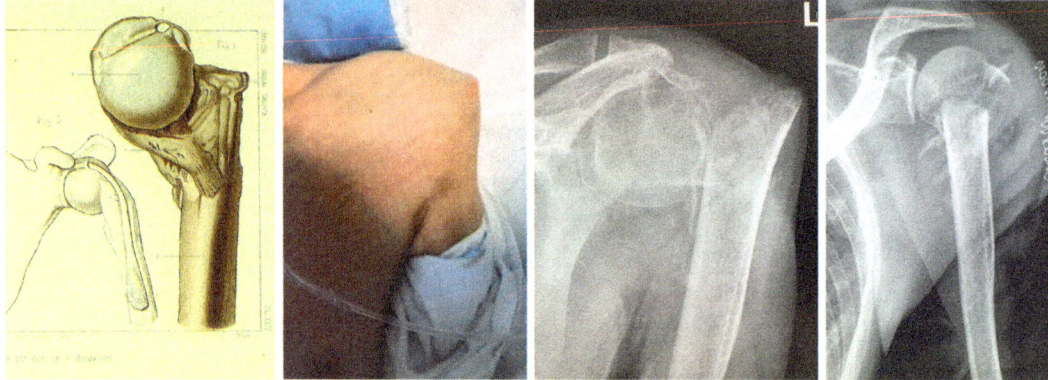

Fig. 3.8 Surgical neck fracture with lateralization of the humeral shaft. Drawing from Benjamin Anger [10]. (With permission from Wellcome Collection. Clinical photo of a terminally ill patient. The proximal end of the humeral shaft was removed for pain relief and skin protection. Pre- and postoperative radiographs)

Most older people with shoulder fractures are likely to have decreased bone mineral density, which may cause some degree of humeral head collapse, whether or not attempts are made to reconstruct the anatomy. If the greater tuberosity remains attached to the humeral head, proximal fractures tend to rotate into a varus deformity while being impacted into the shaft (Fig. 3.9). The greater tuberosity, still attached to the articular part, will point toward the acromion. Formation and consolidation of a lateral bone bridge alleviates pain and improves shoulder function.

3.5 Impacted Surgical Neck Fractures

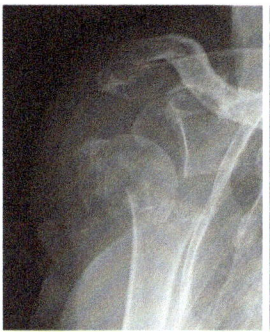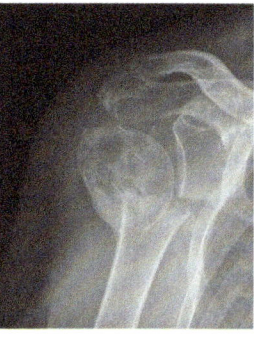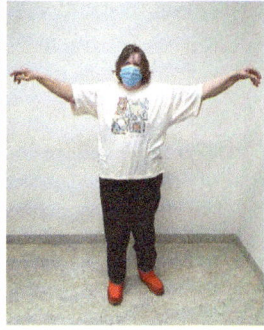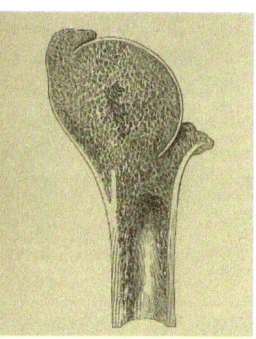

Fig. 3.9 Surgical neck fracture in a 77-year-old female. Radiographs were taken at admission and 4 months after injury. Photo at 4 months. During rehabilitation, the humeral head became better centered. The morphology is comparable to Robert William Smith's specimen [11]. Note the endosteal callus formation. (With permission from Wellcome Collection)

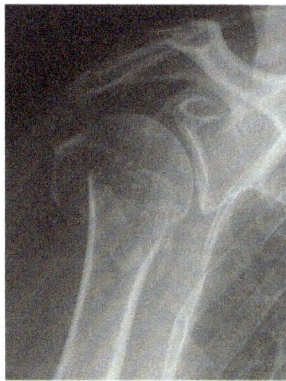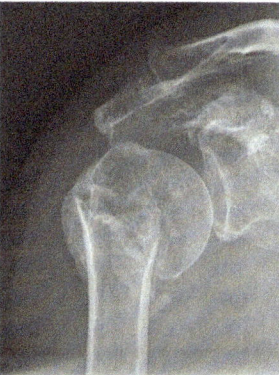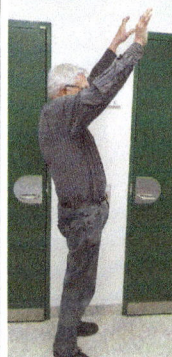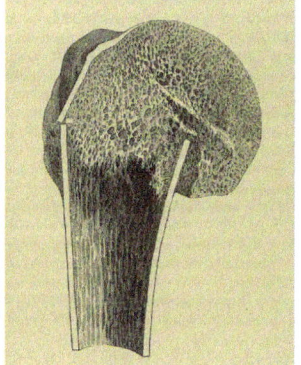

Fig. 3.10 Secondary varus collapse of a surgical neck fracture in a 73-year-old male. Radiographs at admission and 6 months. Clinical photo at 6 months. Comparable pathoanatomical specimen from Robert William Smith [11]. A stabilizing lateral bone bridge and endosteal callus were formed. (With permission from Wellcome Collection)

3.5 Impacted Surgical Neck Fractures

Surgical neck fractures occurring in osteoporotic bone frequently lead to the collapse of the medial cortex, resulting in the displacement of the humeral head into varus. This displacement can occur during or within the first weeks after the injury. This is the expected course of displacement in osteoporotic bone. Suppose the natural healing process is not disturbed. In that case, the pain usually declines; the fracture complex settles, and a lateral bone bridge is formed (Fig. 3.10). Inevitably, these patients have varying degrees of radiographic malunion.

Robert William Smith described in detail the natural healing process of a surgical neck fracture with varus collapse, illustrating it in an engraving from 1847 (Fig. 3.10). The figure shows a cross-sectional view of a healed two-part surgical neck fracture with varus impaction of the humeral head. Smith's pathological description is still remarkably fresh today:

> The inner and posterior portion of the head of the humerus has been driven downwards, and the compact tissue lining the concavity of the neck of the bone has penetrated the reticular structure of the head to the distance of half an inch, and here consolidation has taken place by the direct union of the surfaces opposed to one another… [11] (p. 187)

In patients with surgical neck fractures and low bone mineral density, humeral head collapse with central impaction can be seen (Fig. 3.11). The deltoid muscle pulls the shaft toward the articular part of the humeral head. The cancellous bone provides limited resistance; most of the humeral head can be excavated in severe cases.

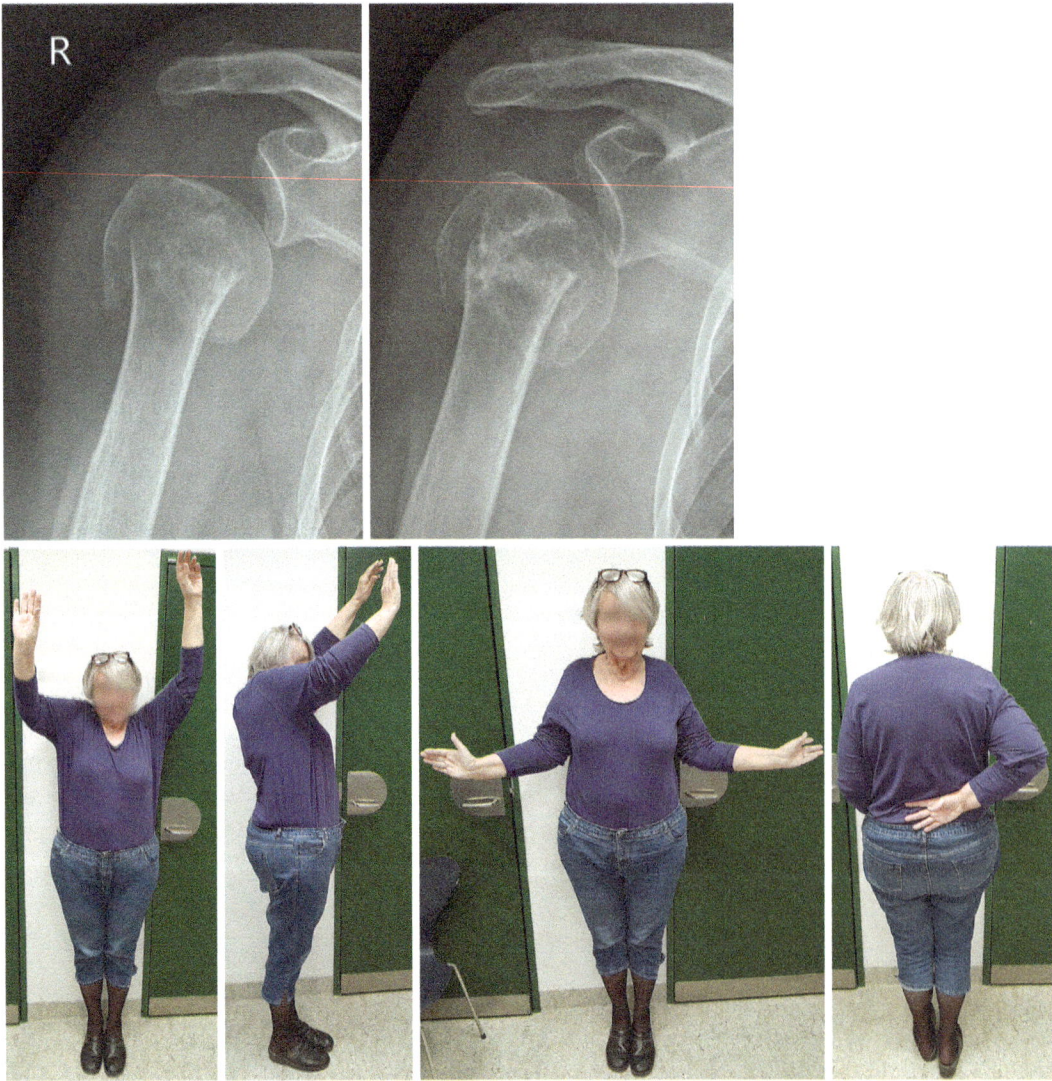

Fig. 3.11 Central impaction of the humeral shaft into an osteoporotic humeral head in a 78-year-old female. Radiographs at 2 weeks and 6 months. Photos at 6 months

3.6 Tuberosity Fractures

Tuberosity fractures can occur alone or in combination with humeral neck fractures. In cases where tuberosity fractures occur alone, they can be considered a total rotator cuff tear accompanied by a bony fragment. This fracture type is more common in younger individuals than combined fracture patterns. Regardless of the treatment approach, regaining rotator cuff function and integrity is vital for restoring functionality.

Numerous efforts have been made to reconstruct the anatomy of the greater tuberosity as viewed from an anterior-posterior radiograph. The indication for surgery in older people is often to restore the anatomy and function or to prevent subacromial impingement. However, results from rotator cuff repair in younger patients cannot be applied to an elderly fracture population. First, procedures involving anchors, cerclage, sutures, screws, and plates may not be successful in older people with poor bone and tendon quality. Second, there is an increased risk of an inferior outcome in cases of later replacement surgery [12, 13]. Third, subacromial pain cannot be predicted from radiographic appearance. The subacromial space is quite broad, and the humeral head rotates during abduction. A narrow acromion-humeral distance does not necessarily mirror the patient's pain level or function. Subacromial impingement remains a clinical diagnosis (Fig. 3.15).

In younger patients with good bone stock, osteosynthesis restoring the greater tuberosity can be an option. It is important to note that before surgery can be considered, the horizontal deforming forces acting on the tuberosities should be considered, regardless of the patient's age and bone quality (Fig. 3.1). The most functionally important displacement of the greater tuberosity is posterior. Biomechanical studies on internal fixation implants tend to focus on axial forces (Chap. 13). Successful tuberosity ingrowth, with or without surgery, is crucial for maintaining shoulder function. In cases where tuberosity ingrowth to an implant is not successful, patients can expect poor shoulder function. If tuberosity fixation and healing to a reverse arthroplasty are not obtained, limited or absent rotational motion can be expected.

3.7 Fractures of the Humeral Neck and the Greater Tuberosity

Two typical morphological patterns can be described. The shaft can be medially and anteriorly translated as in two-part fractures, or the articular part of the humeral head can be impacted in valgus position (Fig. 3.12). Translation of the humeral shaft follows the biomechanics described for two-part fractures. There are different directions of greater tuberosity displacement, with posterior displacement being the most important from a clinical perspective. Internal and external rotation of the arm is essential for daily activities such as washing hair, putting on a bra, and using the toilet.

Valgus-impacted fractures are tempting to reconstruct surgically because the anatomy can often be restored. However, fixing the bones in place does not always result in a good outcome, especially in older people. Bone loss of the humeral head is common, regardless of the treatment provided, and it may lead to failure of reconstructive procedures. Although many alterations of locking plates with augmentations, additional stabilizing implants, and fibular struts have been proposed, they have not been demonstrated to be superior to non-surgical treatment (Chap. 13). Valgus-impacted fractures have an excellent healing potential even without surgery and can lead to a good patient-reported outcome despite malunion. Surgical and non-surgical management share the clinical importance of tuberosity healing.

In fractures with the lesser tuberosity still attached to the humeral head, the subscapular muscle can cause substantial displacement. Reducing and stabilizing the fracture can be challenging, especially in osteoporotic bone. Non-surgical treatment is an option, even in fractures with considerable displacement (Fig. 3.13).

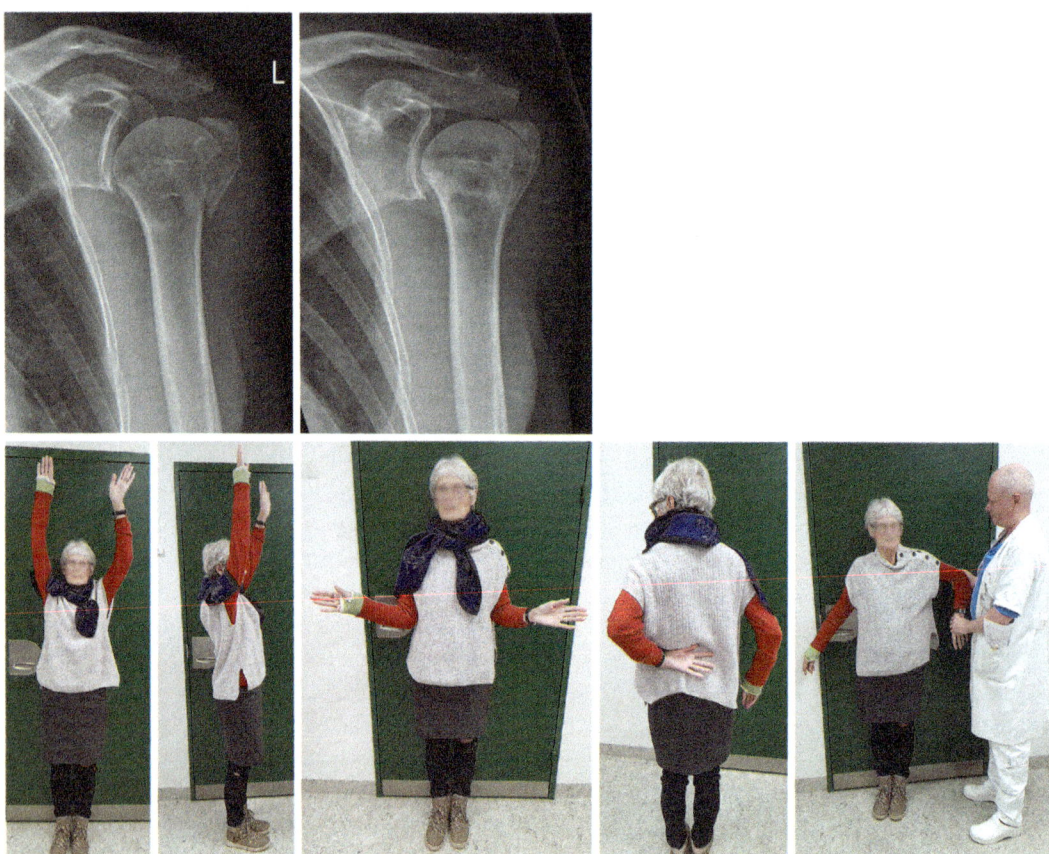

Fig. 3.12 Valgus-impacted humeral neck and greater tuberosity fracture in a 76-year-old female. The initial displacement healed in situ, and pain-free shoulder function was obtained. Radiographs at admission and 6 months. Clinical photos at 6 months

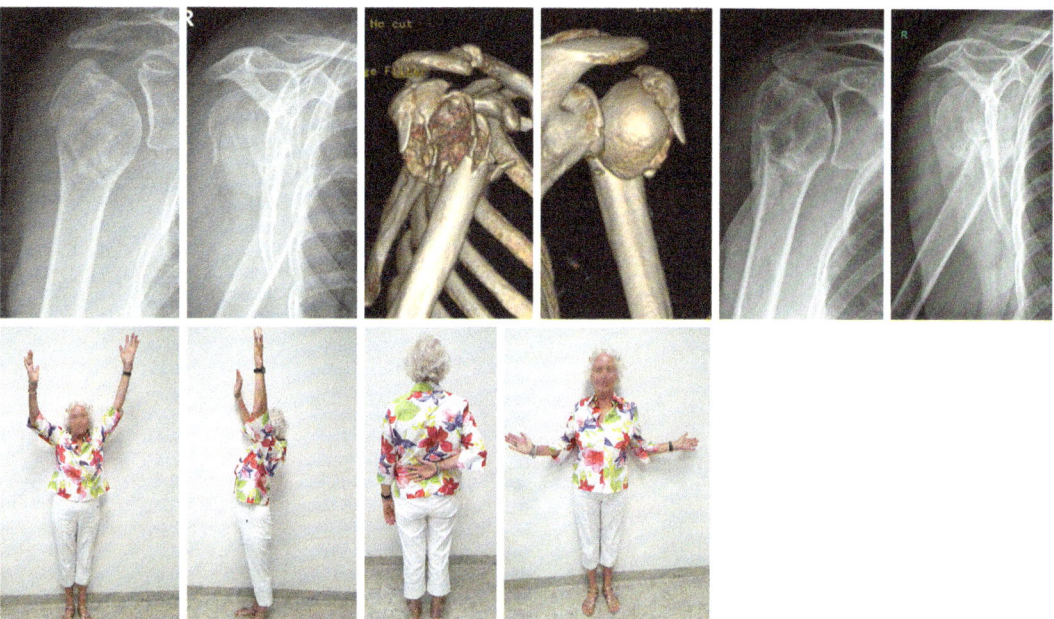

Fig. 3.13 Severely displaced fracture of the humeral neck and greater tuberosity in an 80-year-old female. The shaft was anteriorly translated. The articular part of the humeral head was rotated and displaced posteriorly. The fracture healed with partial collapse of the humeral head and a massive posterior bone bridge. Radiographs and three-dimensional CT reconstruction at admission. Radiographs and clinical photos at 6 months

3.8 Fractures of the Humeral Neck and Both Tuberosities

Fractures that affect the tuberosities, the shaft, and the articular part of the humeral head can range from minimally displaced fractures to fracture-dislocations (Chap. 8). However, limited data is available on these types of fractures outside control groups in randomized trials, so clinical decisions and prognostic predictions must be made cautiously.

Even severe malunion can be tolerated in older people, and it can be realistic to expect pain-free shoulder function at shoulder level (Fig. 3.14). Although the primary reverse shoulder arthroplasty has gained popularity, the evidence is still scanty (Chap. 13). Ongoing and future studies may provide more evidence-based guidance for decision-making.

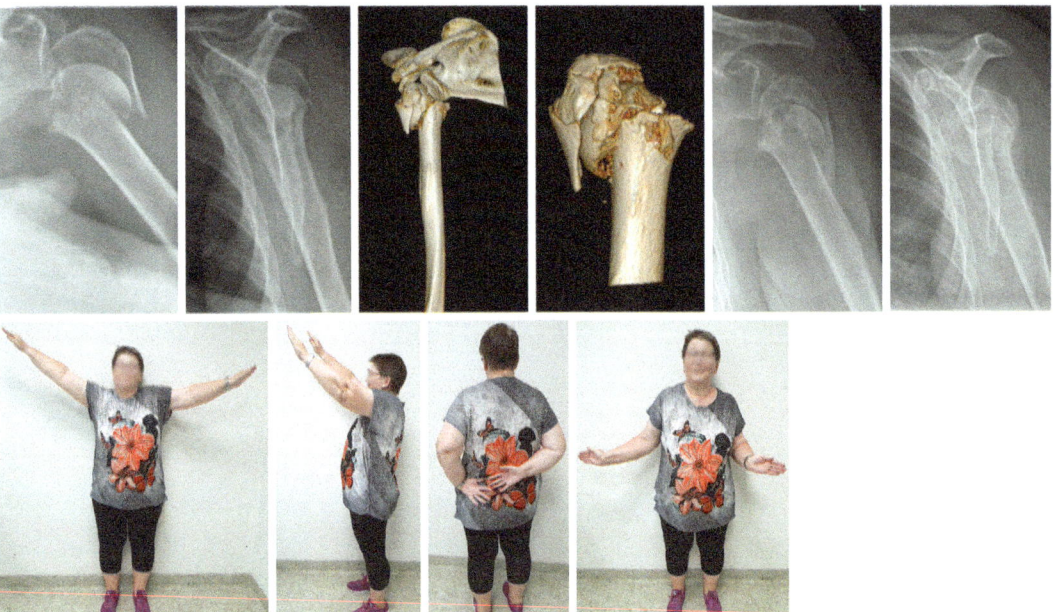

Fig. 3.14 Fracture of the humeral neck and both tuberosities in a 70-year-old female. The fracture healed with a massive lateral bone bridge, including most of the articular surface. Pain-free shoulder function above shoulder level was achieved after 3 months. Internal and external rotation remained restricted. Radiographs and three-dimensional CT at admission. Radiographs and clinical photos at 6 months

3.9 Fracture-Dislocations

Fracture-dislocations are rare but important fracture patterns. In older people, an anterior humeral head displacement is usually accompanied by a greater tuberosity avulsion or a cuff tear (Fig. 3.15). An occult fracture of the humeral neck in older people is often present or may appear during reduction. Neurovascular injuries or glenoid injuries are more common in cases of fracture-dislocations, even after low-energy trauma. Fracture-dislocations require immediate surgical intervention. Ideally, the reduction should be done by a shoulder surgeon who can convert it to a reverse arthroplasty if necessary. Fracture-dislocations were the original indication for joint replacement with monoblock hemiarthroplasty in Charles Neer's 1953 paper [14].

3.10 Articular Surface Fractures

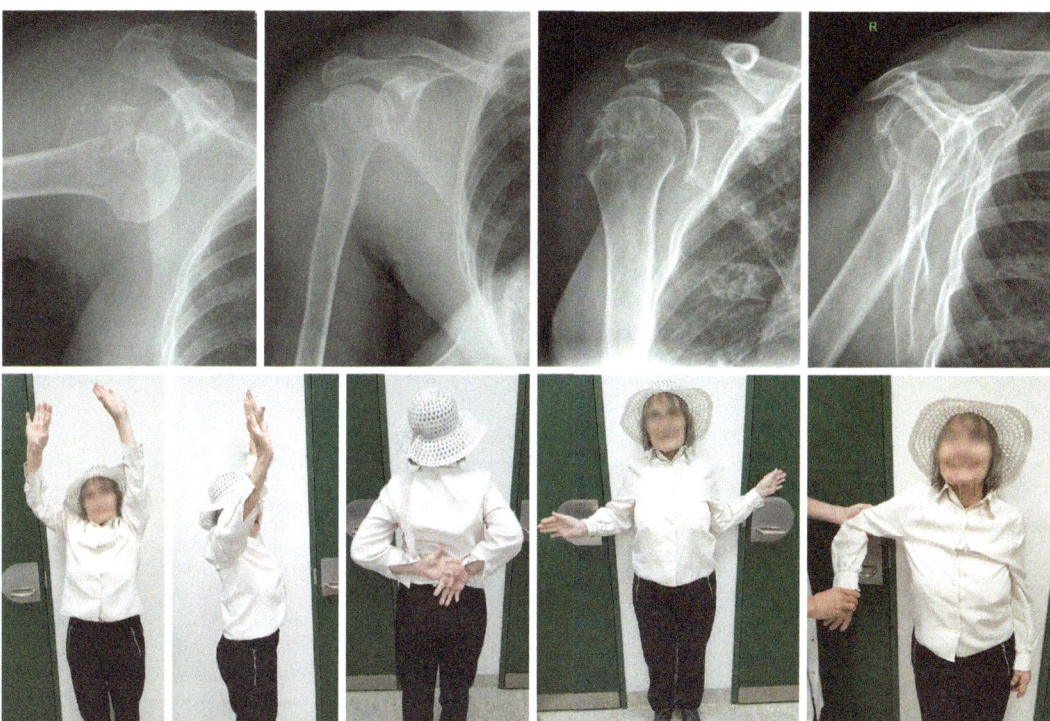

Fig. 3.15 Anterior fracture-dislocation in an 84-year-old female. The dislocation was reduced to an almost anatomical position by closed reduction under anesthesia (radiographs before and after reduction). Subacromial retraction and partial resorption of the greater tuberosity followed. The greater tuberosity was located in the subacromial space on both radiographic views. The patient regained pain-free shoulder function and had no clinical symptoms of subacromial impingement. Radiographs and clinical photos 6 months post-injury

3.10 Articular Surface Fractures

Articular surface fractures encompass a wide range of fracture types, extending from low-energy trauma in older people with a minor step-off in the articular surface to high-velocity injuries with deep cleavages of the humeral head, as shown in Fig. 3.16. The condition of the surrounding soft tissue, the extent of energy transferred to the tissue, and the patient's level of activity must be weighed besides the patient's preferences and the limited clinical evidence available. The dogma that any incongruency in the articular surface leads to post-injury osteoarthritis and should be treated by primary joint replacement is weakly supported by evidence and may originate from analogies from weight-bearing joints like the knee and ankle. Post-traumatic osteoarthritis can indeed develop in some cases, and if symptoms arise, it can be managed with a secondary reverse shoulder arthroplasty.

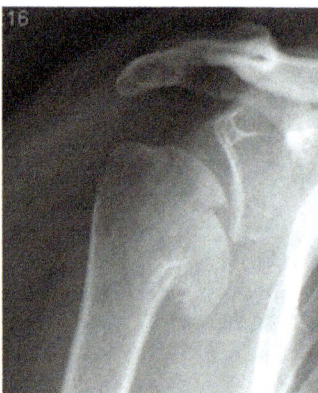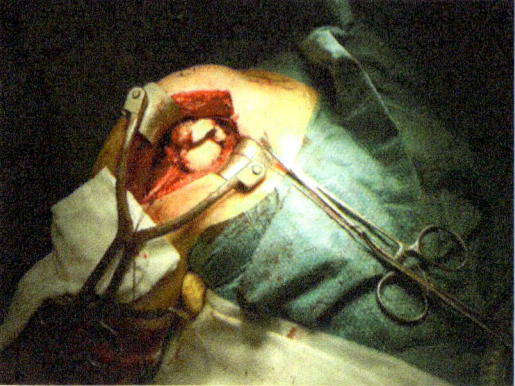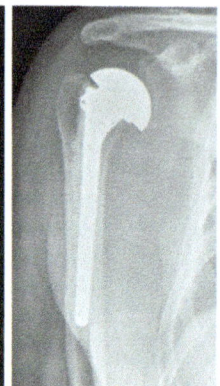

Fig. 3.16 Articular surface fracture in a 26-year-old craftsman who fell from scaffolding. The peroperative photo illustrates that the humeral head had several deep articular fractures and could not be reconstructed. The tuberosities were still attached to the humeral shaft, and the rotator cuff was intact. Replacement of the humeral head with a hemiarthroplasty was feasible, and the patient was able to return to work

3.11 Perspectives

Fracture morphology and displacement are dynamic processes determined by the rotator cuff, the deforming forces acting on the fractured parts, and the quality of the bone. Understanding soft tissue pathology is crucial for comprehending fracture morphology and its clinical course. The commonly practiced radiological decision-making prioritizes assembling the bony puzzle rather than considering soft tissue status, the best evidence, and the patient's preferences. Proximal humerus fractures in poor bone often lead to severe displacement, which worries many orthopedic surgeons; even severe medial translation, impaction, or partial collapse of the humeral neck may not hinder healing, shoulder function, and patient satisfaction, however, even if the radiographs are disappointing from an upper limb reconstruction perspective.

It is an established dogma in orthopedics that increasing fracture displacement leads to a poorer outcome and represents an independent indication for surgery. Following the principles for anatomical reduction and stable fixation has undeniably brought great benefits to fracture patients. However, 65 years after the groundbreaking work of the AO group, it is time to revisit the principles and align the treatment of shoulder fractures with contemporary evidence. The first step could be distinguishing the humerus from the femur and the shoulder from the hip. The weight-bearing properties of the upper arm and shoulder changed with the evolution of *Homo erectus*.

I have outlined some of the most common displacements and their healing potential in this chapter. In Chap. 11, I will discuss the evidence base for non-surgical treatment. Improving patient management by reducing iatrogenic damage and limiting unnecessary surgery requires the application of best evidence and systematic follow-up on all fracture patients—regardless of their treatment (Chap. 16).

References

1. Vinci L da. Atlas der anatomischen Studien in der Sammlung Ihrer Majestät Queen Elizabeth II in Windsor Castle. Gütersloh: Prisma Verlag; 1978.
2. Kocher ET. Beiträge zur Kenntniss einiger praktisch wichtiger Fracturformen. Basel; 1896. Available from: https://wellcomecollection.org/works/mkh547es
3. Court-Brown CM, Garg A, McQueen MM. The epidemiology of proximal humeral fractures. Acta Orthop Scand. 2001;72(4):365–71. Available from: https://actaorthop.org/actao/article/view/20079

References

4. Court-Brown CM, Garg A, McQueen MM. The translated two-part fracture of the proximal humerus. Epidemiology and outcome in the older patient. J Bone Joint Surg Br. 2001;83(6):799–804.
5. Lambert S, Brorson S, Joeris A, Durchholz H, Moro F, Audigé L. International consensus for a core radiological monitoring protocol of proximal humerus fractures. Injury. 2022;53(10):3326–31. Available from: https://www.sciencedirect.com/science/article/pii/S0020138322005010
6. Launonen AP, Sumrein BO, Reito A, Lepola V, Paloneva J, Jonsson KB, et al. Operative versus nonoperative treatment for 2-part proximal humerus fracture: a multicenter randomized controlled trial. PLoS Med. 2019;16(7):e1002855. Available from: https://www.ncbi.nlm.nih.gov/pmc/articles/PMC6638737/
7. Court-Brown CM, McQueen MM. Two-part fractures and fracture dislocations. Hand Clin. 2007;23(4):397–414. v. Available from: https://www.sciencedirect.com/science/article/abs/pii/S0749071207000856?via%3Dihub
8. Hoffa A. Lehrbuch der fracturen und luxationen für ärzte und studierende. Würzburg; 1888. Available from: https://wellcomecollection.org/works/ph3ywwbh
9. Malgaigne J-F. Traité des fractures et des luxations [Internet]. Paris: J.-B. Baillière; 1847. Available from: https://wellcomecollection.org/works/jkwjptc2
10. Anger B. Traité iconographique des maladies chirurgicales. Paris: Germer-Baillière. 1865. Available from: https://wellcomecollection.org/works/j9sn4h7r
11. Smith RW. A treatise on fractures in the vicinity of joints and on certain forms of accidental and congenital dislocations [Internet]. Dublin: Hodges and Smith; 1847. Available from: https://wellcomecollection.org/works/msz6zwcq
12. Kristensen MR, Rasmussen JV, Elmengaard B, Jensen SL, Olsen BS, Brorson S. High risk for revision after shoulder arthroplasty for failed osteosynthesis of proximal humeral fractures. Acta Orthop. 2018;89(3):345–50. Available from: https://actaorthop.org/actao/article/view/7206
13. Jensen ML, Jensen SL, Bolder M, Hanisch KWJ, Sørensen AKB, Olsen BS, et al. Previous rotator cuff repair increases the risk of revision surgery for periprosthetic joint infection after reverse shoulder arthroplasty. J Shoulder Elb Surg. 2023;32(1):111–20.
14. Neer CS, Brown TH, McLauglin HL. Fracture of the neck of the humerus with dislocation of the head fragment. Am J Surg. 1953;85(3):252–8.

Open Access This chapter is licensed under the terms of the Creative Commons Attribution 4.0 International License (http://creativecommons.org/licenses/by/4.0/), which permits use, sharing, adaptation, distribution and reproduction in any medium or format, as long as you give appropriate credit to the original author(s) and the source, provide a link to the Creative Commons license and indicate if changes were made.

The images or other third party material in this chapter are included in the chapter's Creative Commons license, unless indicated otherwise in a credit line to the material. If material is not included in the chapter's Creative Commons license and your intended use is not permitted by statutory regulation or exceeds the permitted use, you will need to obtain permission directly from the copyright holder.

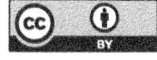

Part II

History: Shoulder Fractures from Ancient Egypt to the Early Twentieth Century

Pre-radiological Diagnostics and Classification of Shoulder Fractures

4.1 Introduction

Medical texts have included descriptions for diagnosing and classifying upper arm fractures since antiquity [1]. Historical sources are scarce, however, especially for ancient times. Providing an overview of how these fractures have been described and classified by different cultures in different periods is a daunting task. Little is known about the development of medical traditions or whether works from a particular culture or region have influenced others. Parts of the overview presented below should be read as an episodic history offering a series of snapshots showing the many ways upper arm fractures have been understood through the ages, rather than as an uninterrupted causal history of how these understandings have developed chronologically.

4.2 Ancient Egypt

The first example of diagnostics and classification of upper arm fractures can be found in the oldest known surgical text, the *Edwin Smith Papyrus*, named after the American Egyptologist who bought it from an Egyptian merchant in 1862. The provenance of the papyrus is unclear; it may have been taken from the grave of a physician buried in the Theban necropolis. Today held at the New York Academy of Medicine, it was displayed at the Metropolitan Museum of Art in New York in 2005 accompanied by a new translation [2].

The papyrus's date is controversial. Based on its classical Middle Egyptian grammar, the consensus is that it is a scribal copy made around 1600 BCE (Fig. 4.1); several archaic words, however, have led some scholars to suggest that it derives from a much older text of the Old Kingdom period (2584–2117 BCE) [3]. If this is correct, it would have been composed in the time of the great pyramids, which may indicate possible trauma mechanisms—but a more recent date is supported by the presence of writing errors and the fact that archaic words and phrases were commonly used in ancient Egyptian texts to make them appear older [4].

The papyrus is 4.68 meters long, written with black and red ink (Fig. 4.2), and consists of 17 columns on the front and 5 on the back. The text is hieratic, a cursive form of hieroglyphic script; consequently, translation begins with transliteration from hieratic to hieroglyphic script and from hieroglyphic to English. This chapter relies on the translation by Allen [2]; dating of Egyptian dynasties follows Kemp [5].

The papyrus text survives from a complete manual for traumatic conditions, now lost. The front face describes 48 surgical cases covering soft tissue injuries, sprains, closed fractures, and compound fractures. The cases are topologically ordered and deal with injuries of the skull (cases 1–9), the eyebrow (case 10), the nose (cases 11–14), the cheek (cases 15–17), the temporal region (cases 18–22), the ear (case 23), the jaw (cases 24–25), the lip (case 26), the chin (case

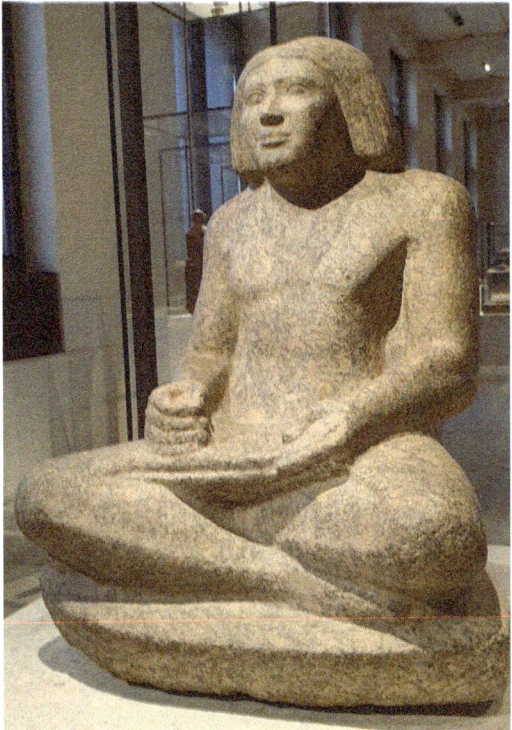

Fig. 4.1 Scribe (twenty-fourth century BCE). Rose granite. Neues Museum, Berlin

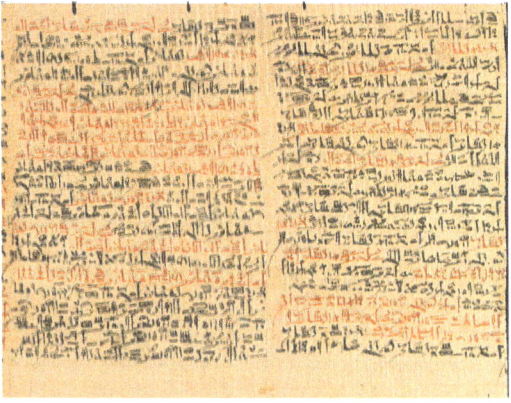

Fig. 4.2 Columns XII and XIII of the *Edwin Smith Papyrus* (copied circa 1600 BCE) with the three cases dealing with humerus fractures [2]. (With permission from the New York Academy of Medicine)

and is interrupted in the middle of case 48. In this chapter, I will discuss the three cases of fractures of the upper arm (cases 36–38) with a focus on diagnostics and classification. In the chapter that follows, I will interpret and discuss the recommended treatments.

The *Edwin Smith Papyrus* is systematically structured, with each case containing four elements: title, examination, prognosis, and treatment. Titles include the anatomical region and the structures involved—"practices for a break in his upper arm with a wound on it," for example (case 37). The examination contains a repetition of the title, the clinical signs, and the procedures the practitioner should perform to reach the diagnosis, ending with a prognostic statement by the practitioner. These can be favorable ("an ailment I will handle"), challenging ("an ailment I will fight with"), or hopeless ("an ailment for which nothing can be done"). All three verdicts are found in the three cases dealing with humerus fractures. While there are no explicit instructions for classifying injuries in the papyrus, the uniform structure of the cases allows us to deduce some principles for classification. The ancient writer classifies injuries according to the anatomical location, the tissue involved, and the prognosis.

Close reading of written historical surgical cases relies on reliable topographical identification of anatomical landmarks. Before interpreting the text, the upper arm should be distinguished from the adjacent structures; the title of all three cases included the term "upper arm"—but we have yet to determine precisely which part. Conceptions and boundaries of ancient anatomical terms and definitions should be interpreted carefully; we cannot assume we are dealing with the same structures and pathologies we accept today. From ancient Egyptian sources, we have a rich vocabulary of about 250 anatomical terms [6, 7]. Various hieroglyphic signs represent the internal organs of mammals, and the terminology of the gross anatomy of the body is rich. The scapula was known as the "razor bone" because of its similarity to an ancient Egyptian razor. The word appeared in a case with a gaping wound above the shoulder blade (case 47). The spina

27), the throat and neck (cases 28–33), the collarbone (cases 34–35), the upper arm (cases 36–38), the chest (cases 38–41 and 45–46), the ribs (cases 42–44), the shoulder (case 47), and the vertebra (case 48). The papyrus is incomplete

scapula and the coracoid process were known as "the fork of the shoulder" or "the two-toed claw." Surprisingly, these structures were not considered part of the scapula. References to the knowledge of nerves, vessels, or tendons have not been found, and we cannot be certain that the term translated as "the upper arm" does not, in fact, designate both the upper arm and the forearm. Because the text has not been preserved in full, we cannot know how the upper arm was distinguished from the elbow or forearm. It is possible that the term translated as "wound" referred to the entire injury, including the underlying fracture [3]. The preserved text shows that the upper arm was at least distinguished from the collarbone (cases 34–35) and the chest (cases 38–41 and 45–46).

Several diagnostic signs of fractures in the upper arm are mentioned. In a broken upper arm: "You find his arm dangling away from him and out of alignment with respect to its companion" [2] (case 36).

The sensation under the fingers of the practitioner examining a broken upper arm is described: "You find that break wiggling under your fingers" [2] (case 37).

The ancient word translated as "wiggling" is *nekhebkheb*, possibly an onomatopoeia for crepitus.

A swelling over a closed injury of the humerus is described as "a swelling risen on the back of that split that is in his upper arm" [2] (case 38).

Ancient Egyptian understandings of pathology are likely to differ from our own and should be mapped on to those of our own with caution. While we find some simple anatomical distinctions to be lacking, at least four technical terms for fractures can be found in ancient Egyptian texts [3]. Two are found in cases involving the upper arm. A *heseb* is described as a simple, closed fracture (case 36). The prognosis of this injury was considered good. If there was a wound over a *heseb*, however, the prognosis was less favorable (case 37). In cases with a "wound that is on the break with blood coming out of it and obstructed on the inside of his wound," the prognosis was hopeless, and nothing could be done [2] (case 37).

A *peshen* was a simple closed fracture. It was considered easy to handle and promised a favorable outcome (case 38).

While the exact meanings of anatomical and pathological terms in ancient Egyptian texts are still to be determined, the three verdicts were used consistently throughout the text, allowing us to classify the injuries into one of three prognostic categories (Table 4.1). A favorable prognosis was found in 30 cases, a less favorable prognosis in 8 cases, and a hopeless prognosis in 14 cases. Some cases described several possible scenarios and more than one verdict.

A modern reader familiar with trauma manuals and applications may be impressed by the rational nature of the ancient text. But it is essential to underscore that religious and magical content heavily influenced ancient Egyptian medicine. On the papyrus's rear face, the scribe who copied the surgical cases also wrote eight magical spells and five prescriptions, including a prescription for turning an old man into a youth. In cases of trauma, the cause was usually apparent, which made it easier to give a prognosis. However, in internal diseases where the causes were often less clear, the condition was sometimes attributed to supernatural forces. We may theorize that this led people to seek supernatural cures instead of rational medicine. We may easily infer that ancient Egyptian medicine, as a field of study, was more informed by ideas of the supernatural than those of today, and the boundaries between rational medicine and magic were not clearly defined [4].

Table 4.1 Classification items for fractures of the upper arm reconstructed from the *Edwin Smith Papyrus* (c. 1600 BC)

Anatomy		Upper arm (not collarbone; the distal boundary is unknown)
Pathology	Bone	*heseb* fracture
		peshen fracture
	Concomitant injury	Superficial wound
		Deep wound
Prognosis	Favorable	"An ailment I will handle"
	Less favorable	"An ailment I will fight with"
	Hopeless	"An ailment for which nothing can be done"

4.3 Ancient Greece

Several surgical texts from Greek antiquity dealing with upper arm fractures, more than a thousand years more recent than the Egyptian papyrus, survived. The most notable of these is the *Corpus Hippocraticum*, a collection of 60–70 books written in the fifth and fourth centuries BCE. Although this collection is associated with Hippocrates and his medical school, it is unknown how many books were written by Hippocrates himself, who lived from around 460 to 377 BCE. Compiled circa 250 BCE in the library of the Museion of Alexandria, only a tiny portion of the texts have survived. Those we know today were translated and copied by Arab authors during the Middle Ages. Most doctors are familiar with Hippocrates's mode of reducing a shoulder dislocation, still used in clinical practice today. This section will discuss the Hippocratic approach to diagnosing and classifying fractures of the humerus, widely used for over 2000 years and studied and debated by medical writers until the nineteenth century. Fractures of the humerus are dealt with in the book *De Fracturis*, parts VIII, XXXV, and XLVI (c. 415 BCE). This chapter relies on the translation by Withington [8].

The Hippocratic School of Medicine considered prognosis to be crucial; the classification of diseases and recommendations for treatment were based on prognostic statements and taxonomy structured from a prognostic perspective. The ancient writer did not aim to create an exhaustive division of clinical phenomena into categories but to state some convenient prognostic categories for the benefit of the practitioner. The rough anatomical division of humerus fractures can be used to illustrate this point: "Sometimes the actual head of the humerus is fractured at the epiphysis, but this, though apparently a very grave lesion, is much milder than injuries of the elbow joint" [8] (*De Fracturis*, XLVI).

The Hippocratic writer distinguished between fractures and dislocations, which may appeal to the modern reader. It should be noted that fracture cases are found in the book *De Articulationes* and dislocation cases in the book *De Fracturis*. Although the exact anatomical location of the injuries described is not entirely clear, the ancient author mentions some anatomical characteristics of the humerus. He notes that "the head of the humerus would be seen to have a strongly marked projection forwards, though not dislocated. For the head of the humerus is naturally inclined forwards, while the rest of the bone is curved outwards" [8] (*De Articulationes*, I) and that "the humerus is naturally convex outwards, and is therefore apt to get distorted in this direction when improperly treated" [8] (*De Fracturis*, VIII).

Although Hippocrates did not discuss fracture-dislocations of the shoulder, such cases may have posed a diagnostic challenge to ancient practitioners.

As in the more ancient Egyptian source, a significant portion of the text is devoted to compound fractures of the humerus. The Hippocratic author similarly notes that cases where the upper arm protrudes indicate a poor prognosis [8] (*De Fracturis*, XXXV).

The practitioner is faced with a dilemma: "If you reduce the fracture, convulsions are liable to supervene, while in cases not reduced there are bilious fevers with hiccough and mortification" [8] (*De Fracturis*, XXXV). A prognostic distinction within compound fractures is made according to whether the bone protrudes to the outer side or the inner side of the arm: "For many important blood vessels stretch along the inner side, and lesions of some of them are fatal; there are also some on the outside, but fewer" [8] (*De Fracturis*, XXXV). The overall prognosis after compound fractures was poor: "There may be survival even in cases where reduction is made, but it is rare indeed" [8] (*De Fracturis*, XXXV).

We have only incomplete and secondary written remains from the famous Alexandrian School of Medicine, which existed in the third century BCE. Unfortunately, many irreplaceable medical documents were lost in a great fire in the library of the Museion of Alexandria in about 272 CE. However, we have an important secondary source of Alexandrian medicine in the Byzantine medical writer Oribasius (325–397 CE). A compiler and mediator of ancient medical writers, he authored 70 books, of which only 25 have survived; his work is nevertheless particularly valuable for researchers and scholars. In *Oribasii Collectionum Medicarum Reliqviae*, XLIX, 14, Oribasius relates a discussion between Pasicrates and Aristion, two doctors from Alexandria, about the treatment of shoulder fracture-dislocations [9]. The discussed fracture was described as a combination of a glenohumeral dislocation and a humeral shaft fracture. The injury was described in detail, and the appropriate management was discussed, pointing toward an ability to differentiate a dislocation from a fracture of the shaft. In cases where crepitus could not be felt, it may have been challenging for the ancient practitioner to distinguish a simple shoulder dislocation from a fracture-dislocation of the proximal humerus.

4.4 Ancient Rome

References to the Alexandrian School of Medicine can also be found in the Roman encyclopedist Celsus (25 BCE–50 CE), who referred to the performance of human dissections by Erasistratus and Herophilus in the third century BCE.

Celsus, a learned Roman medical writer during the reigns of Augustus (27 BCE–14 CE) and Tiberius (14–37 CE), authored the eighth book of *De Medicina* [10], which summarized and expanded on the practice of Roman medicine. The books were published during the early age of printing (1478) and remained influential until the nineteenth century. Celsus was the first to clearly differentiate fractures of the proximal humerus from distal and shaft fractures. Fractures near the ends of bones were considered more painful and difficult to treat; in contrast, fractures of the shaft were deemed less dangerous based on prognostic considerations, as outlined in Hippocrates's writings (*De Medicina*, VIII, 10) [10]. Celsus identified different types of upper arm fractures, with transverse fractures being the least problematic. Multiple and oblique fractures were considered more severe, with fractures causing pointed fragments having the worst prognosis (Table 4.2).

Table 4.2 Classification of upper arm fractures reconstructed from Celsus

Anatomy	"Upper arm" or "humerus"	Prognosis
Gross anatomy	Upper end	Less favorable
	Middle part	Favorable
	Lower end	Less favorable
Fracture anatomy	Transverse	Favorable
	Multiple	Less favorable
	Oblique	Less favorable
	Overriding	Less favorable
	"Pointed"	Worst

Celsus's notion of pathological bone anatomy should be interpreted with caution, as we have no sources supporting studies on human extremities—he broadly used the Latin *nervus*, for example, to designate nerves, tendons, fasciae, and ligaments without specification.

The Alexandrian School of Medicine was known for prioritizing the interpretation of ancient texts over practical medical applications. According to the Greek philosopher Philo of Alexandria (c. 10 BCE–40 CE), medical science in Alexandria was not very capable:

> In medical science, some practitioners who know how to cure almost every complaint, and disease, and infirmity, can nevertheless give no true or even probable account of any of them; and on the other hand, others are very clever, as far as giving an account of the diseases goes, and in explaining their symptoms and causes, and the modes of cure, and are the most excellent interpreters possible of the principles of which their art is made up, but are utterly useless in the matter of attending the bodies of the sick, to the cure of which they are not able to contribute even the slightest assistance [11]. (*Quod Deterius Potiori Insidiari Soleat*, XIII, 43)

The Greek physician Galen (129–215) studied in Alexandria for at least 4 years in the 150 s, a few centuries after the Alexandrian School of Medicine. There are no mentions of the famous Alexandrian dissections in Galen's work. Alexandria offered organized instruction in anatomy during Galen's time, however. The prevailing approach was to combine the study of the surface anatomy of an enslaved person with the dissection of an animal, preferably an ape. When a dissection could not be performed, Galen recommended studies of bones found in dilapidated graves or from accidental findings of decomposed bodies with the bones in situ [12] (*Opera Omnia*, II, 221–2). In later years, he had the privilege of becoming the doctor of the gladiators, which gave him access to casualties.

Galen's works, of which only 20 books escaped the great fire in Alexandria, included a comprehensive interpretation and commentary on the Hippocratic writings, *Hippocrates de fracturis liber et Galeni in eum commentaries*. Around 180 CE, Galen wrote a short introduction to bone anatomy, *De ossibus ad tirones* (Bones for Beginners) [13], with a description of the humerus:

> The humerus – the largest bone except the femur – diarthroses at both ends. At the shoulder end, it has an epiphysis, which swells into a head on a smaller neck. And there is a broad incised hollow in the front, dividing the whole head into two as though [both were] condyles. ... [The] humerus is bowed, yet not sharply or uniformly but convex anteriorly and outwardly, and concave in the reverse. [13] (*De ossibus ad tirones*, 16)

In his commentaries on the Hippocratic account of humerus fractures, Galen is critical of the inconsistent classification he finds: while names and ideas differ, he points out, the treatment of the condition remains unaffected. He also emphasizes that disagreement concerning names is neither helpful nor harmful [12] (*Opera Omnia* XVIII, 419).

The Byzantine medical writer Paul of Aegina (c. 625–690) incorporated the works of Galen and Hippocrates into his medical encyclopedia *Epitome medicae libri septem* [14]. Paul classified traumatic fractures into five types (Table 4.3).

Table 4.3 Classification of fractures reconstructed from Paul of Aegina [14]

Latin terms for fractures	English translation
Raphanatim	Complete, transverse fracture
Scandulatim	Longitudinal fracture
In ungiuem	One part straight, the other lunated
Polentatim	A bone in small pieces
Caulatim	A fracture with complete separation

4.5 Medieval Sources

During the Middle Ages and the Renaissance, the works of Paul of Aegina sustained Galen's legacy. The Arabs dominated medicine from the seventh to the thirteenth centuries; scholars translated and reinterpreted the written inheritance of Greek and Roman antiquity, preserving them for posterity. In the ninth century, the Hippocratic corpus and Paul of Aegina's *Epitome* were translated into Arabic. The Arab writers who compiled the ancient Greek and Roman surgical texts made minor changes to the diagnosis and classification of shoulder fractures; the Arab surgical writer Albucasis (936–1013), for example, believed that each bone had a distinct fracture and that each bone fracture had further variations: "Each kind has its own special technique for setting which will be mentioned in detail, each in its place" [15] (p. 680).

From the twelfth to the fifteenth century, a period coinciding with the flourishing of northern Italian universities, technical surgical books became increasingly widespread. In the late Middle Ages, human dissections resumed, as those conducted in 1315 by the physician and anatomist Mondino de Luzzi (c. 1270–1326) confirm; de Luzzi's textbook of 1316 was eventually printed in 1478 [16]. During the late Medieval period, dissections were mainly used to confirm the theories of Galen, which were not based on naturalistic principles as we understand them today. Contemporary textbooks often featured illustrations of skeletal figures, created from dissections and aligned with Galenic philosophy. It is essential to note that this understanding is theory-dependent and would not satisfy modern standards of osteology (Fig. 4.3). Although they may appear inaccurate to contemporary readers, these illustrations represented state-of-the-art medical knowledge until the mid-sixteenth century.

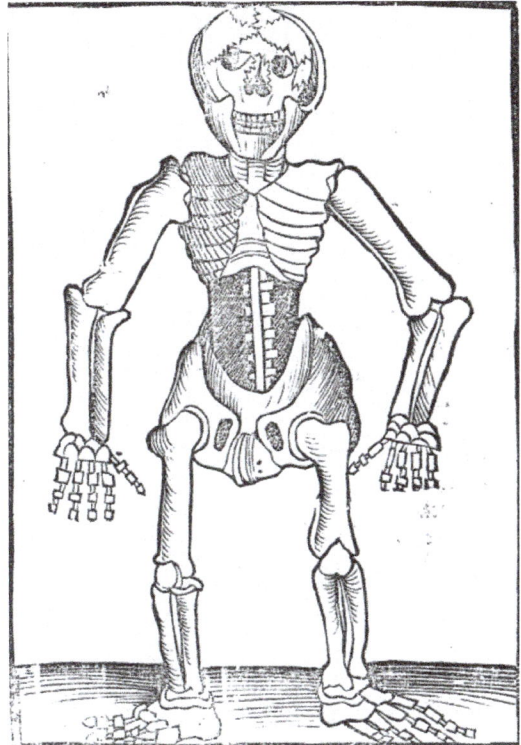

Fig. 4.3 Late Medieval conception of the skeleton. Mondino de Luzzi [16]

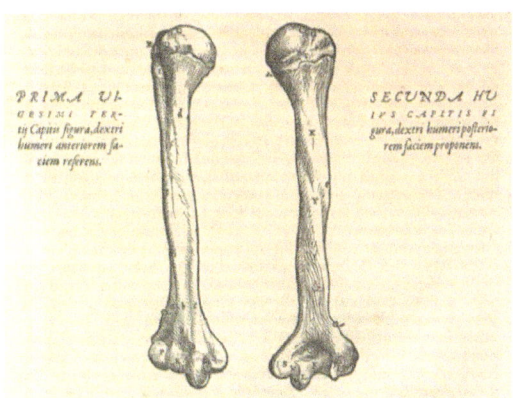

Fig. 4.4 The humerus. Anterior and posterior view. Andreas Vesalius [19]

4.6 Renaissance Sources

Leonardo da Vinci, for whom anatomy was a distinct area of research, took up dissection with the specific aim of improving his artistic work. Although the influence of his anatomical sketches in his lifetime is unclear since his anatomical drawings were not published until almost three centuries later, he had a keen interest in the study of surface anatomy and myology and conducted in-depth research on the functional anatomy of the shoulder. In his initial drawings, the humerus was depicted as curved, echoing Galen in indicating the dissection of apes [17]. Through his preparation of the deep muscles of the shoulder, Leonardo gained an understanding of the biomechanics of the four muscles that constitute the rotator cuff. In a drawing held by the Royal Collection Trust at Windsor Castle [18] (Plate 50, Fig. 5) the glenohumeral joint has been distended to clearly illustrate the insertion of the long head of the biceps, the rotator cuff, and the coracoid process, along with the insertion of the pectoralis minor, the short head of the biceps, and the coracobrachialis muscle. Understanding the biomechanics of the four deep muscles is crucial in comprehending the displacement in proximal humerus fractures. However, in medieval times, only the superficial muscles were considered, leading to the belief that heavy traction to counteract them was the best treatment.

The introduction of printing with movable type in about 1450 substantially improved the dissemination of medical knowledge and provided useful pictorial material for learned practitioners. Andreas Vesalius (1514–1564), the great reformer of anatomy, began his studies with the works of Galen and wrote several books on Galenic anatomy. During his time, access to human corpses for study improved from the time of Mondino. Vivisection of pigs was used to study the internal organs, particularly the heart. Vesalius published his most notable work, *De humani corporis fabrica libri septem*, containing studies on bone anatomy, in 1543 [19]. Vesalius's description of the humerus remains appealing to a modern reader, although the illustration of the bone appears a little short in Fig. 4.4. Although Vesalius did not discuss patho-anatomical matters, his accurate descriptions and illustrations of the musculoskeletal system were crucial for later works on surgery and surgical anatomy. Systematic studies of pathological anatomy did not appear until the eighteenth century.

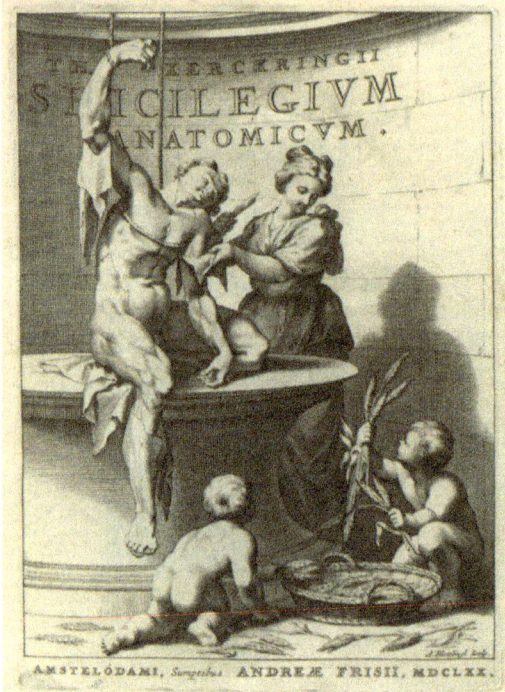

Fig. 4.5 Frontispiece from Theodor Kerckring's anatomical textbook from 1670 [20]. Engraving by Abraham Blooteling (1634–1690). The book's title, *Spicilegium anatomicum* (Latin: *Spica*), refers to the collection of the grain left behind after the harvest. The two children depicted in the engraving symbolize the humble anatomist's collection of observations and the hope of providing minor amendments to the work of the great masters. The corpse is positioned with ropes around the chest and the wrist. The dissection begins with the upper arm

Vesalius's influence was decisive in the Early Modern era, as demonstrated in an anatomical textbook by Theodor Kerckring (1638–1693) (Fig. 4.5) [20].

4.7 French Hospital Surgery in the Eighteenth Century

Comparisons of clinical observations with patho-anatomical findings at dissections can be found in the works of the French hospital anatomist and surgeon Joseph Duverney (1648–1730). Duverney, one of the first academic surgeons with a medical degree conferred by the University of Avignon in 1667, proposed a pathoanatomical and biomechanical classification for shoulder fractures, clearly distinguishing the different parts of the humerus in his *The Diseases of the Bones* [21]. Duverney discussed difficulties differentiating between a proximal fracture and a glenohumeral dislocation. The contusion, ecchymoses, and swelling could mimic a dislocation. If crepitation was present, it was indicative of a fracture; if the humeral head could not be felt in the glenoid cavity, however, it was a dislocation. Duverney classified the muscles that affect a fracture into flexors and extensors. In a fracture close to the joint, the bone fragment located farther from the joint could be moved and pulled upward by both the flexor and extensor muscles. The deltoid muscle played an essential role in Duvernay's account of the displacement of the fracture; there was no mention of the deep muscles, however. In impacted proximal fractures "we may be deceived, for the Deltoid may in a Fracture, by its Contraction, keep the broken Part in such Subjection, that it is very difficult to be assured of it" [21] (p. 116).

Table 4.4 The four species of fractures of the proximal humerus reconstructed from Duverney [21]

Transverse fractures
Oblique fractures
Fractures with splinters
Fractures with bone shivered to pieces

Duverney classified proximal humerus fractures into four distinct *species* based on their characteristics (Table 4.4). Transverse fractures were those where the arms were of equal length, but the patient could not move the affected limb. Depending on the nature of the trauma, the displacement may be forward, backward, or lateral; oblique fractures were prone to displacement and overlapping. Although fractures with splinters or those where the bone was shattered were not described in detail, these may refer to injuries caused by gunshot wounds.

Duverney summarized the prognostics in this balanced statement:

> "The Prognostic of the Fractures of the Arm is taken from their Species, Situation, Largeness, the present Symptoms, and those to be apprehended" [21] (p. 117).

The surgeon was further advised to share with the patient the expected prognosis in terms of a stiff shoulder:

> "The Surgeon should not hesitate to forewarn, that the Ancylosis of the Joint will succeed a Cure, notwithstanding all his Care" [21] (p. 117)

During the eighteenth century, the traditional Hippocratic and Galenic approach to proximal humerus fractures was challenged by the French surgeon Pierre-Joseph Desault (1744–1795). Unlike his colleagues, Desault, who had worked as an assistant for a local barber-surgeon, came from a humble background. He gained knowledge in anatomy at the military hospital in Belfort before moving to Paris in 1766 to establish his anatomy school. In 1786, Desault was appointed as the chief surgeon at l'Hôtel Dieu. As an active surgeon, he performed public operations and introduced bedside teaching and rounds for didactic purposes. In 1779, he published a surgical textbook with Francois Chopart (1743–1785), but he generally preferred bedside teaching over anatomy textbooks. Several of Desault's pupils published his merits, including Xavier Bichat (1771–1802), Guillaume Dupuytren (1777–1835), and Dominique Jean Larrey (1768–1842). Bichat published Desault's lectures in 1801 [22] and the monograph *A Treatise on Fractures, Luxations and Other Affections of the Bones* in 1805 [23]. Desault classified proximal humerus fractures by anatomical level, mechanism of injury, involvement of soft tissue, morphology, displacement, and complicating factors (Table 4.5) [22].

Table 4.5 Classification of proximal humerus fractures reconstructed from Desault [22]

Anatomical level	The upper, middle, or lower part of the humerus
Trauma mechanism	Indirect, direct, or counterstroke
State of the soft parts	Natural or distended
Fracture morphology	Transverse or oblique
Displacement of fragments	In contact or separated, upwards or inwards
Complications	Fracture-dislocations, compound, splinters, infection

The diagnosis was made based on the patient's medical history and clinical examination. A history of falls, pain, and inability to move the arm was typical. The space under the acromion was inspected and palpated to rule out dislocation; extending the arm with an assistant moving the humeral head against the shaft confirmed the diagnosis by the lack of movement of the humeral head and the presence of crepitus. The deltoid muscle pulled toward the natural curve of the humerus, while the pectoralis major, latissimus dorsi, and teres major muscles tended to move the shaft inward. The prognosis was considered good unless the fracture was very close to the humeral head; healing was estimated to take between 26 and 30 days.

While Desault broke from the Hippocratic and Galenic beliefs, his fracture treatments still involved blood-letting and a strict diet [23]. And although he died in 1795, his pathological anatomy of bone and joint injuries continued to be influential until the latter half of the nineteenth century. Chapter 6 will present the work on shoulder fractures of Desault's pupils.

4.8 Perspectives

In this chapter, I have reviewed a collection of historical sources on the diagnosis and treatment of upper arm fractures. One of the most striking features for the modern medical reader is the enduring influence of the ancient Greek and Roman masters Hippocrates and Galen. Even with the rise of empiricism in the seventeenth and eighteenth centuries, the influence of Hippocrates and Galen strongly impacted most aspects of medical thinking. Bloodletting of fracture patients was still practiced in the nineteenth century. While the anatomical knowledge necessary for understanding the biomechanical forces acting on a fractured shoulder was present as far back as the Renaissance, this knowledge was not integrated into these patients' diagnosis, classification, and treatment until the eighteenth century, mainly through French hospital surgery. Figures such as Duverney and later

Desault played important transitional roles, paving the way for the flourishing studies of fracture morphology from the late eighteenth century, as discussed in Chap. 6. It may be challenging for modern readers to imagine how ancient writers understood fracture diagnostics, classification, and treatment, given the profound influence of our differing sociocultural contexts on the practice of medicine. The relationship between ancient authors and practitioners may remain unclear—but it is clear that practitioners have observed, interpreted, and treated shoulder fractures throughout history.

References

1. Brorson S. Management of fractures of the humerus in Ancient Egypt, Greece, and Rome: an historical review. Clin Orthop Relat Res. 2009 Jul;467(7):1907–14. Available from: https://doi.org/10.1007/s11999-008-0612-x
2. Allen JP. The art of medicine in ancient Egypt. New York: Metropolitan Museum of Art; 2005. Available from: https://www.metmuseum.org/art/metpublications/The_Art_of_Medicine_in_Ancient_Egypt
3. Breasted JH, Smith E. The Edwin Smith surgical papyrus. Chicago: University of Chicago. Oriental Institute publications; 1930. Available from: https://isac.uchicago.edu/sites/default/files/uploads/shared/docs/oip4.pdf
4. Nunn JF. Ancient Egyptian medicine. Norman: University of Oklahoma Press; 1996.
5. Kemp BJ. Ancient Egypt: anatomy of a civilization. 3rd ed. Boca Raton: Routledge, Taylor and Francis; 2018.
6. Walker JH. Studies in ancient Egyptian anatomical terminology. Warmintser: Aris & Phillips; 1996.
7. Grapow H. Grundriss der Medizin der Alten Ägypter. In: Deines HV, Grapow H, Westendorf W, editors. Anatomie und Physiologie. Berlin: Akademie Verlag; 1954.
8. Hippocrates, Withington ET (Edward T). Hippocrates. Volume III: On wounds in the head. In the surgery. On fractures. On joints. Mochlicon. Cambridge, MA: Harvard University Press; 1928. (Loeb classical library;149). Available from: https://www.loebclassics.com/view/LCL149/1928/volume.xml
9. Raeder J. Oribasii collectionum medicarum reliqviae. Lipsiae; 1928.
10. Celsus AC. De medicina. In: Spencer WG, editor. De medicina. London: Heinemann; 1935. Available from: https://www.loebclassics.com/view/LCL292/1935/volume.xml.
11. Philo. The works of Philo: complete and unabridged. New update. Peabody: Hendrickson; 1993.
12. Claudius Galenus C. In: Kühn CG, editor. Galeni opera omnia (II). Lipsiae; 1821.
13. Galen. De ossibus ad tirones. Singer C, editor. Available from: https://europepmc.org/backend/ptpmcrender.fcgi?accid=PMC1987542&blobtype=pdf
14. Paulus A. The seven books of Paulus Ægineta (translated by Francis Adams); 1844. Available from: https://archive.org/details/sevenbooksofpaul02pauluoft/page/n15/mode/2up
15. Spink MS, Lewis GL. Albucasis. On surgery and instruments. Berkeley: University of California Press; 1973.
16. Luzzi M de. De omnibus humani corporis interioribus membris Anathomia. Strassburg: M. Flach; 1513.
17. Brorson S. Medieval and early modern approaches to fractures of the proximal humerus: an historical review. Minerva Ortop e Traumatol. 2010;61(5):449–62.
18. Vinci L da. Atlas der anatomischen Studien in der Sammlung Ihrer Majestät Queen Elizabeth II in Windsor Castle. Gütersloh: Prisma Verlag; 1978.
19. Vesalius A, Calcar JS van, Oporinus J. Andreae Vesalii Bruxellensis, Scholae Medicorum Patavinae Professoris, De humani corporis fabrica libri septem. ex officina Ioannis Oporini; 1543. Available from: https://archive.org/details/gri_33125008502920/page/n1/mode/2up
20. Kerckring T. Spicilegium anatomicum, continens observationum anatomicarum rariorum centuriam unam: nec non osteogeniam foetuum in qua quid cuique ossiculo singulis accedat mensibus, quidve decedat et in es per varia immutetur tempora, accuratissime oculis subjicitur. Amstelodami; 1670. Available from: https://archive.org/details/theodorikerckrin1670kerc/mode/thumb
21. Duverney M. Diseases of the bones (translated by Samuel Ingham). London: printed for Tho. Osborne, in Gray's-Inn, Holborne; 1762.
22. Desault P-J. Oeuvres chirurgicales ou, Exposé de la doctrine et de la pratique de P.J. Desault Mequignon l'ainé; 1801. Available from: https://wellcomecollection.org/works/s9u22ekd
23. Desault P-J. A treatise on fractures, Luxations, and other affections of the bones; 1805. Available from: https://wellcomecollection.org/works/pa6vyz7y

Open Access This chapter is licensed under the terms of the Creative Commons Attribution 4.0 International License (http://creativecommons.org/licenses/by/4.0/), which permits use, sharing, adaptation, distribution and reproduction in any medium or format, as long as you give appropriate credit to the original author(s) and the source, provide a link to the Creative Commons license and indicate if changes were made.

The images or other third party material in this chapter are included in the chapter's Creative Commons license, unless indicated otherwise in a credit line to the material. If material is not included in the chapter's Creative Commons license and your intended use is not permitted by statutory regulation or exceeds the permitted use, you will need to obtain permission directly from the copyright holder.

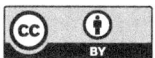

Interventions for Shoulder Fractures from Ancient Egypt to the Eighteenth Century

5.1 Introduction

There are two ways to learn about ancient fracture treatments. We can examine written texts to find passages that mention them, and we can study human remains to determine if fractures occurred, how they healed, and whether they were treated. Written sources are rare; human remains are useful for the reconstruction of a comprehensive understanding of ancient fracture treatments, equally so—and both are subject to inherent biases.

Ancient writers often describe complex procedures that may have been exaggerated or even impossible, while the texts themselves are subject to errors of translation, copying, and interpretation throughout history; moreover, it is essential to be cautious when interpreting anatomical terms, as the concept of naturalistic anatomy as we know it today did not exist until the sixteenth century. Human remains, meanwhile, are usually found in places with good conservation conditions, more typical of burials of the privileged. However, these only afford small samples from different periods.

In Chap. 4, I reviewed historical sources related to diagnostics and classification; in this chapter, I will provide an overview of texts discussing the management of shoulder fractures and present a selection of human remains. The chapter covers sources from ancient Egypt to the late eighteenth century.

5.2 The Edwin Smith Papyrus

The *Edwin Smith Papyrus*, copied around 1600 BCE, is the earliest known text dealing with humerus fractures [1, 2]. According to this ancient document, the general treatment for closed fractures of the humerus involved reducing the fracture by traction and then bandaging it. To reduce the fracture, the patient was placed supine with a roller between their shoulder blades. The fracture was then reduced by simple traction, and a bandage was subsequently applied to stabilize it. A bandage of two strips of cloth with alum and honey, changed daily until the bone was healed, was used to treat a humerus fracture. The recommended method of reducing the fracture and applying the bandage was the same as for a broken collarbone. In the case of a compound humerus fracture, oil was added to the bandage.

The *Hearst Papyrus*, a medical document dating back to around 1450 BCE [3], provides information about the components of adjuvant substances. In the section titled "A prescription to knit a broken bone on the first day," various prescriptions for casts can be found. These casts were created using different starch pastes from flour derived from glutinous sources mixed with honey or cream. By adding cloth to the mixture, a cast that was both moldable and rigid could be formed. While several mummies and skeletons have been found in ancient Egypt with splints still attached, no humerus fracture with the

© The Author(s) 2025
S. Brorson, *Shoulder Fractures in Context*, https://doi.org/10.1007/978-3-031-93604-3_5

bandages in situ has been found, permitting further studies of techniques. Information about ancient Egyptian splinting techniques can be obtained from mummies that have undergone postmortem splinting. One of the most illustrative is the mummy of King Siptah (reign 1197–1191 BCE), in custody of the Egyptian Museum in Cairo, with postmortem splinting of the forearm. Tomb looters broke the forearms of a mummy to remove jewelry, and the mummy was left with fractures, which was unacceptable; priests carefully splinted the forearms to ensure the mummy could make its journey to eternity intact [4].

5.3 Human Remains

In 1908, several specimens with splints in situ were excavated north of Luxor. One of the specimens of particular interest is an open forearm fracture from the fifth dynasty (c. 2450–2325 BCE), with the bandage still in place. It was published in *British Medical Journal* in 1908 [5]. Bloodstains were found on the date palm fibers adhered to the ulna; bundles of coarse grass and straw covered the inside of the bandage. The stiffness of the bandage was secured by a tube made of three pieces of rough acacia bark. There were no signs of healing, which suggests that the patient probably died shortly after the injury.

It is unclear who provided treatment for fractures in ancient Egypt. The medical papyri describe various medical specialties, such as ophthalmologists, proctologists, and dentists. However, it is unknown whether trauma treatment was overseen by priests or performed by local bonesetters; nor can we be certain whether the written prescriptions were available to all practitioners or limited to a learned elite.

The *Edwin Smith Papyrus* refers to three cases of humerus fractures, most likely caused by traumatic injury (Chap. 4). The description of compound fractures and soft tissue damage in the shoulder area could indicate combat injuries or work accidents that occurred during major building projects. At the time the *Edwin Smith Papyrus* was copied, battle axes with copper alloy heads, swords, and various tools were commonly used. Impact weapons such as clubs, sticks, and maces have also been used throughout dynastic times. While the paleopathological literature describes most fractures as traumatic rather than caused by bone weakness, bone weakness was apparently widespread in ancient Egypt; it is a paradox that the early onset of bone loss does not appear to be accompanied by osteoporotic fractures [6].

Our understanding of the prevalence and incidence of humerus fractures in ancient Egypt is based on a limited number of human remains from different periods. These remains are diverse, so no statistically safe estimates can be made about the prevalence of the fractures. Before the flooding caused by the further raising of the Aswan Dam between 1907 and 1912, around 5–6000 bodies and skeletons were excavated from prehistoric to Roman times (4000 BCE to the sixth century CE). Among these excavations, united fractures were found in 2% of the skeletons. Out of these, 7% of individuals had suffered a humerus fracture. Twelve humerus fractures were reported: four surgical neck fractures, one neck and shaft fracture, five fractures of the humerus shaft, one fracture of the distal humerus, and one fracture with severe arthritis interpreted as fracture sequelae [7]. The most common fracture involved the shaft of the ulna. An excavation of 204 adult skeletons from the Giza Necropolis (Old Kingdom, c. 2584–2117 BCE) reported fractures in 18% of the skeletons, but no fractures of the humerus were identified. Eighty percent of the fractures involved the radius or ulna [8]. An excavation from Saqqara covering skeletons from the Old Kingdom to the Ptolemaic period (2686–330 BCE) reported 2 fractures in 181 humeral bones [9].

The population demographics of ancient Egypt differ substantially from those of our time. During dynastic times, the average lifespan was 36 years, and there were relatively few elderly people [10]. There is some debate over whether osteoporosis was present in ancient Egypt. Females experienced bone loss as in modern

5.4 The Hippocratic Corpus

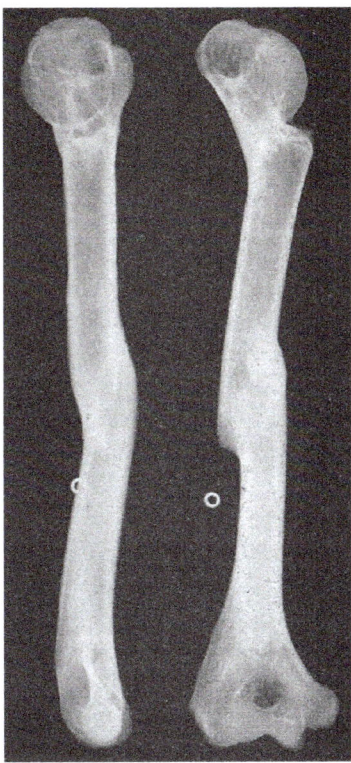

Fig. 5.1 Segmental fracture of a right humerus. Qua, Egypt (c. 1400 BCE). Age and gender unknown. (Reprinted from [12] with permission from Elsevier)

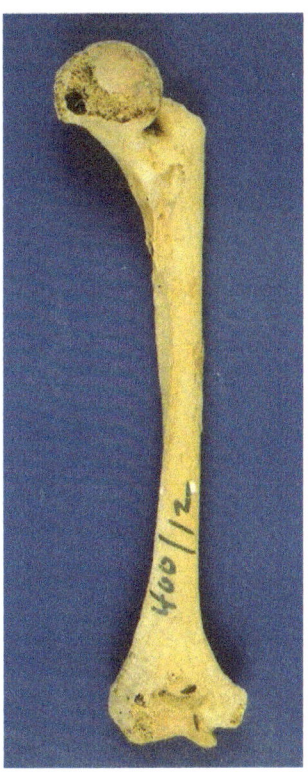

Fig. 5.2 Posterior view of a left humerus from a young female from Egyptian Nubia (c. 1549–1069 BCE). (With permission from ArchaeoScience, Globe Institute, University of Copenhagen)

times, but at an earlier age. A study of compact femoral bones from Sudanese Nubia (CE 350–550) found evidence of early-onset osteoporosis. Factors contributing to this condition may include nutritional stress, heavy workload, pregnancy, and lactation [11]. Several healed fractures of the humerus have survived. Figure 5.1 shows a healed segmental fracture of the humerus. Medial translation of the humeral shaft has caused a marked valgus deformity of the humeral neck. The shaft fracture has healed with good alignment. Both fractures show complete union and remodeling, suggesting long survival. Figure 5.2 is a healed two-part fracture of the surgical neck. Medial translation of the humeral shaft has caused a severe valgus deformity. The completely consolidated fracture complex suggests the patient survived long after the injury. We have no archaeological evidence of the treatment provided.

5.4 The Hippocratic Corpus

The primary source for managing shoulder fractures in ancient Greece was the book *De Fracturis* (c. 415 BCE) in the Hippocratic corpus [13]. The book provided a thorough description of the reduction maneuver, bandaging, and subsequent splinting—an approach recommended with only minor modifications for over 2000 years. The effectiveness of the Hippocratic method was not questioned until the late eighteenth century (at least not by the learned medical community). During the Renaissance, surgical books included illustrations of the Hippocratic reduction maneuver. These illustrations remained consistent, changing only in the clothing depicted and the graphic style [14, 15].

The basic principle was forceful traction and countertraction (Fig. 5.3). The patient was seated on a high stool with a wooden rod like a spade

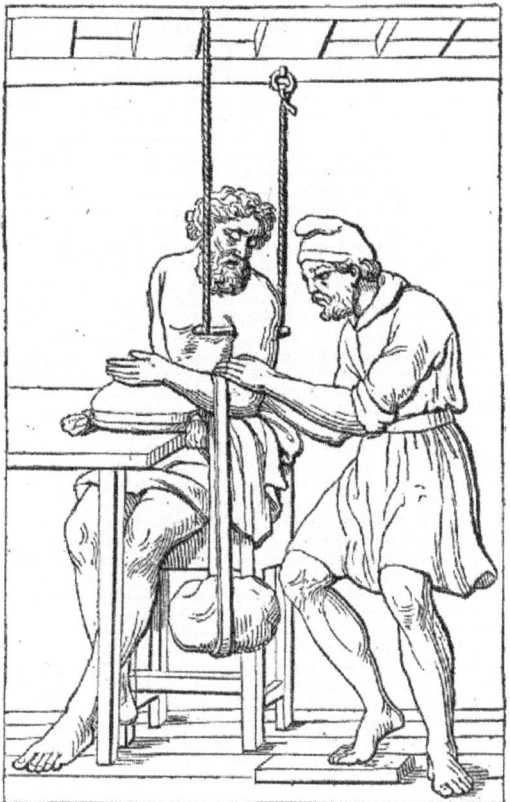

Fig. 5.3 The Hippocratic maneuver to reduce fractures of the humerus. (Reprinted from Littré [16])

handle under the armpit. The rod was fastened on both ends to the roof. One or two leather pillows were placed under the forearm with the arm bent at a right angle in the elbow. A broad shawl with a heavy weight was placed around the proximal forearm; alternatively, a strong assistant could apply the traction. The upper arm was extended forcefully during the procedure, and the practitioner used their palms to reduce the fracture. After the reduction, a moderately tight bandage was applied; the bandage was to be changed every 3 days. Instead of tightening the bandage, the practitioner should increase the number of bandages to obtain fixation. On the seventh day, wooden splints were applied to the affected area (Fig. 5.4) [17]. The splints were adjusted every third day until union was achieved in the bones. With the arm resting in a sling, the expected healing time was 40 days. At this point, the tightness and the number of bandages were reduced.

The success of the Hippocratic treatment was evaluated based on residual swelling and strength. If the treatment was successful, the natural outward inclination of the humerus was restored. In case the bone was not returned to its natural shape, compresses with multiple folds were to be placed on the inner side of the humerus, and moderate pressure was applied by a shawl around the chest and upper arm. It was essential to avoid inclining too far inward, however [13] (*De Fracturis,* VIII). The bandages were fastened with a wax known as cerate, which also helped to harden the cloth covering the entire upper arm. After 3 days, when the swelling had reduced, the arm was to be soaked in hot water before a new bandage was applied. After 7 days, the process was repeated, this time with the inclusion of wooden splints (Fig. 5.4). If the practitioner suspected re-displacement halfway through the healing period, the fracture could be re-reduced and the splints reapplied. A strict diet was prescribed, including abstinence from solid food [13] (*De Fracturis*, XXXVI). Compound fractures of the humerus had a poor prognosis, regardless of whether they were reduced or not. If reduction by extension was attempted, and there was no overriding bone or retracted muscles, a lever combined with extension could be considered a treatment option [13] (*De Fracturis*, XXXV).

Oribasius (CE 325–397) discussed the management of an injury with a dislocated shoulder and a concomitant humerus shaft fracture. His approach to this challenging injury differed to those of the physicians Pasicrates and Aristion of the Alexandrian School of Medicine (third century BCE). Where Oribasius was worried about the status of the soft tissue around the fracture, Pasicrates focused on the joint and reduced the dislocation first; Aristion preferred to treat both injuries using the same procedure. Oribasius, concerned about the re-dislocation of the humeral head during the fracture treatment, recommended reducing the dislocation before setting the fracture by traction with a handle in the armpit to apply countertraction. The fracture treatment was subsequently conducted while the reduced shoulder was held in place [18] (*Oribasii collectionum medicarum*, XLIX). It was practically impossible

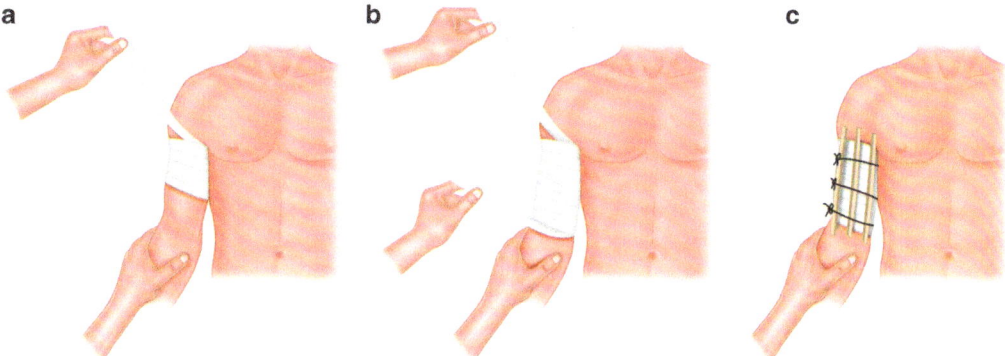

Fig. 5.4 Application of bandages and splints in a fracture of the humerus, according to Hippocrates; (**a**, **b**) the upper arm and shoulder were prepared with wax, and a moderately tight bandage of linen was applied; (**c**) wooden splints were applied on the seventh day [13]

for the ancient practitioner to distinguish a simple dislocation complicated by a shaft fracture from a proximal humeral fracture-dislocation complicated by a shaft fracture. In current clinical practice, humerus shaft fractures with accompanying fracture-dislocations are treated surgically and can be technically challenging (Fig. 5.5).

Celsus (25 BCE–50 CE) slightly modified the Hippocratic method of reduction. He observed that humerus fractures were often displaced, with no contact between the fragments. Crepitus occurs when the broken bones move against each other. When the fragments were in contact, they produced a sound, and a stabbing sensation could be felt under the fingers [19] (*De Medicina*, VIII). Reduction by extension was performed according to Hippocrates, although six bandages were recommended instead of three. In cases with shortening of the humerus, Celsus recommended immediate extension to prevent inflammation, contraction, and swelling of the muscles; the same treatment was applicable for neglected cases. If the reduction and bandaging were successful, the pain disappeared, and the two upper arms became equal in length. Six bandages soaked in liquid cerate should be applied after reduction. An extra layer of wool soaked in wine and oil should be used in compound fractures—although nothing should be tight if gangrene were to be successfully prevented. On the third day, the bandages were changed. On every occasion the skin was uncovered, it was to be fomented with hot water. After 7 or 9 days, the fracture was to be manipulated again if there was deviation in the upper arm. Wooden splints were applied over the bandage; the strongest splints were to be

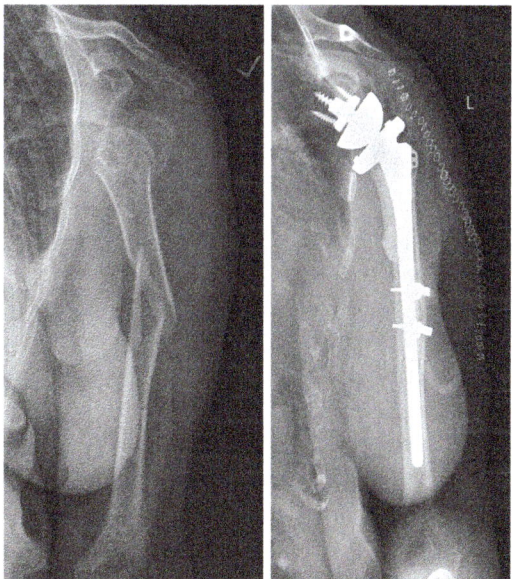

Fig. 5.5 A fracture-dislocation with a concomitant humerus shaft fracture in an 84-year-old female. The handling of this injury has been discussed since the Alexandrian School of Medicine in the third century BCE. Example of modern operative treatment with a cemented total reverse shoulder arthroplasty with a long stem. Cerclage wires have been added to ensure the reduction of the shaft fracture. The patient obtained pain-free shoulder function below shoulder level. Pre- and postoperative radiographs

arranged over the side that tends to deviate, usually on the lateral side; the shortest splint was used in the armpit, and every third day, the straps holding the splints were to be tightened. In proximal humerus fractures, the bandages were to be long enough to stretch under the opposite armpit. The forearm was rested in a sling to immobilize the extremity.

5.5 Galen's Commentaries to Hippocrates

Galen (129–c. 215) provided extensive commentaries and amendments to the Hippocratic book on fractures. Galen's writings offer valuable insight into the ancient thinking concerning the treatment of proximal humerus fractures, which aimed to achieve the correct (Latin: *justum*) position of the extremity. This was achieved when the elbow was at a right angle. When performing the reduction maneuver (Fig. 5.3), Galen commented on the position of the patient and practitioner, with a focus on the practitioner's convenience: the patient should be placed, he suggested, so that they could hardly sit, permitting greater counter extension. Galen recommended the use of iron, bronze, or lead as weights fastened to broad straps around the distal part of the humerus. The procedure involved extending (Latin: *extensio*) and reducing (Latin: *compositio*) to bring the broken and displaced bones together. The muscles surrounding the broken humerus would decrease in size during bandaging. When atrophy was observed, the arm was ready for splinting. Galen repeated the Hippocratic healing time of 40 days, adding that it was expected to be slower in a large humerus. In cases where the outward convexity needed correction, broad strips should be applied around the chest. Pressure should then be applied to restore the natural configuration. A roller was placed between the elbow and the chest to restore the anatomy [20] (*Opera Omnia*, XVIII) (Fig. 5.6).

The Byzantine writer Paul of Aegina (c. 625–690) recommended immediate splinting after applying six bandages on the waxed arm: "After the bandaging, the moderns immediately

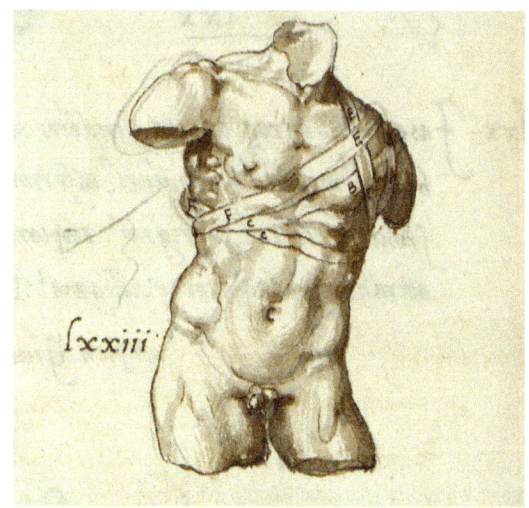

Fig. 5.6 Renaissance interpretation of Galenic bandaging. A valgus pressure was applied to correct the deformity of a broken humerus [21]. (Reproduced with permission of the Bibliothèque nationale de France. Any commercial reuse requires authorization from the Bibliothèque nationale de France)

apply splints, in order to preserve the bones which have been set in their proper place" [22] (*Epitome* VI). The reduction was performed as set out by Hippocrates. If the fracture involved the upper arm, the bandage was to be wrapped around the acromion, scapula, and sternum, extending—not too tightly—down to the elbow. The arm was to be gently secured to the chest. When using splints, it was important to wrap them with wool or flax, and to avoid placing them directly on the joint, to better prevent ulcers and inflammation of the tendons.

5.6 Medieval Treatments

From the fall of the Roman Empire to the late nineteenth century, the Hippocratic mode of reduction remained remarkably consistent. The composition of the adjuvant substances in the bandages and the preparation of the splints were altered slightly. The Andalucian surgeon Albucasis (936–1013) used plasters of egg white and mill dust. He differed from his antecedents by bandaging the hand to the opposite shoulder (Fig. 5.7). If the fracture was "ugly and con-

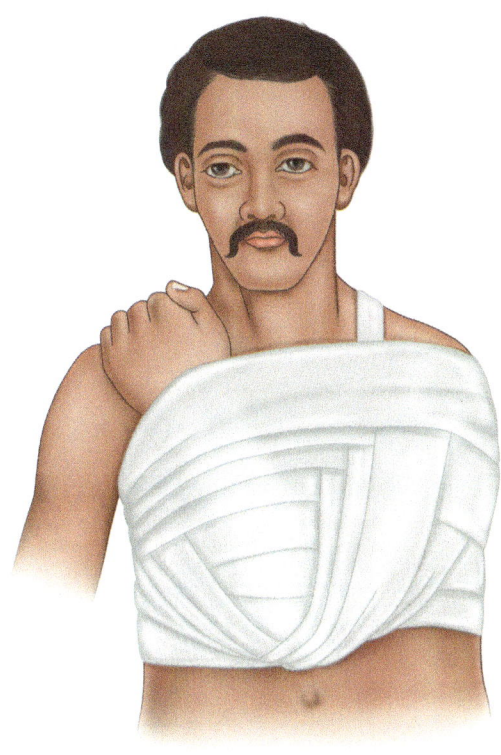

Fig. 5.7 The method of bandaging as described by the Arab medieval writers. Interpreted from Albucasis [24]

tused," up to 2 months in the bandage were required for it to heal. An armamentarium consisting of a saw, osteotome, and bone elevator was recommended by Albucasis for compound fractures when bone fragments needed to be removed. Bloodletting was performed immediately after the injury. The Persian writer Avicenna (980–1037) advised fixing the broken arm to the thorax. The bandages were soaked in water and vinegar; the splints were infused with pomegranate, oleander, and alcanna.

The Arab writers introduced technical surgical literature—but it is unclear whether the operations and instruments described in the literature were ever performed and, if they were, whether any patients survived. In the twelfth century, Roger Frugard of Parma discussed the issue of malunion of the humerus. The humerus should be refractured, he suggested, if the fracture did not heal after 3 or 4 months. Henri de Mondeville (c. 1260–1320), meanwhile, emphasized the comfort of the patient: "Set the bone as gently and as possible with delicate manipulations to minimize the pain" [23].

The Italian surgeon William of Saliceto (1210–1277) proposed bone splinters be removed from compound fractures with the use of probes and fingers, supporting his stance by citing Hippocratic humoral pathology: "Pay no attention to what some surgeons say, that the patient will die or that the fracture will not heal if you remove some marrow. They are wrong. The marrow is formed from the viscous and moist humors, the same as those which participate in the repair of bones, just as flesh forms from blood" [25] (p. 156).

5.7 Renaissance Surgery

Between the thirteenth and eighteenth centuries, a distinction was drawn between surgery and the practice of learned medicine. Doctors were graded by universities, and surgical texts were written in Latin. The practice of surgery, considered less exclusive, was typically performed by barbers. To regulate their practice, guilds of barber surgeons were established, responsible for bloodletting, tooth extraction, cutting boils, and possibly bonesetting (Fig. 5.8).

During the Renaissance period, two pioneers in the field of anatomy, Leonardo da Vinci (1452–1519) and Vesalius (1514–1564), made substantial contributions to the study of normal shoulder anatomy (Chap. 4). Despite their work, however, the traditional Hippocratic method of treating shoulder fractures continued to be used by Renaissance surgeons. Ambroise Paré (1510–1590) recommended forceful traction for such injuries; if the patient had a strong body, he advised, the arm should be extended as much as possible.

An illustrated textbook on ancient surgery, *Chirurgia e Graeco in Latinum conversa* [26], was published by Vidus Vidius (1500–1569) in 1544. Vidius translated the works of Hippocrates, Galen, and Oribasius into Renaissance Latin. He also added his comments to Apollonius of Kitium (first century BCE), Galen, and Oribasius. The illustrations in his translations, probably created by the Renaissance artist Primaticcio

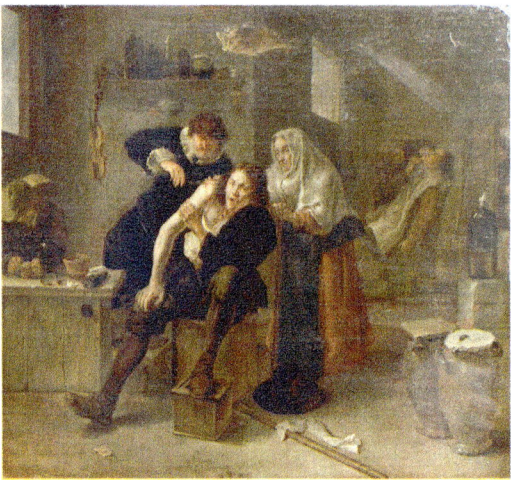

Fig. 5.8 In the barber-surgeon's shop. Gerrit Lundens (1622–1686). Oil on wood. Kunstsammlung der Georg-August-Universität Göttingen, Photo: Birgit Arnu. (Reproduced with permission of the University of Göttingen. Any commercial reuse requires authorization from the University of Göttingen)

(1504–1579), interpreted Hippocrates's machines for reducing fractures and dislocations. Vidius heavily relied on Hippocrates's methods for treating humerus fractures and detailed the steps involved in reduction and bandaging.

During the seventeenth century, the study of human anatomy became part of the university curriculum for physicians and surgeons. While the guilds of barber surgeons remained responsible for handling daily surgical issues, there is limited documentation of their methods. The new anatomical knowledge gained by Renaissance anatomists was not readily integrated into learned medicine. Numerous interpretations of the reduction and bandaging from Hippocrates and Galen suggest that the influence of the anatomists was limited. In the early eighteenth century, humerus fractures were included in the textbooks of several surgeons. Jean-Louis Petit (1674–1750) and Lorenz Heister (1686–1758) differentiated between humeral neck fractures and humerus shaft fractures. Although they provided detailed information on the application of bandages and traction, they did not add much to the Hippocratic reduction [15]. A decisive change in the treatment of humerus fractures arrived with the works of Pierre-Joseph Desault (1744–1795).

5.8 The End of the Hippocratic Legacy

Desault questioned the Hippocratic method of extension, claiming it to be inadequate—in fact, he asserted, it led to considerable damage. His argument was based on the biomechanics of the superficial muscles surrounding the shoulder. When the Hippocratic length of wood was placed in the axilla to apply counter-extension, the pectoralis major, latissimus dorsi, and teres major muscles were all pulled upward, resulting in the same direction of movement of the shaft fragment. The extension machines proposed by Hippocrates "were entirely useless, in as much as they were intended only to increase the natural powers of the operator, which are already more than sufficient of themselves" [27] (p. 76).

Desault developed a new and gentler method for reduction. The procedure involved the patient sitting on a chair or on the side of the bed with their arm slightly flexed and abducted. An assistant would pull the arm on the unaffected side while another would extend the semi-flexed forearm to relax the muscles. The surgeon would then apply gentle pressure according to the direction of the displacement to finalize the reduction and ensure the fragments were correctly positioned. Desault proposed applying a three-layer bandage to maintain the reduction (Fig. 5.9). The rationale was that the muscles acted on the fragments: the pectoralis major, latissimus dorsi, and teres major pulled the shaft inward, while the deltoid muscle pulled it outward; when all the muscles contract, they slightly raise the shaft. The weight of the relaxed arm was almost enough to counteract this upward movement.

Desault criticized the ancient practice of applying bandages with bolsters, forcing the lower fragment outward, wondering why his contemporaries were still performing the harmful treatment at all. He developed a bandage consisting of two rollers, three splints, and a small bolster of linen reaching from the armpit to the elbow (Fig. 5.9). A bandage was used to maintain the extension of the arm. The surgeon applied additional rollers from the forearm to the armpit in oblique turns, alternating from one armpit to the other. A sling

Fig. 5.9 Desault's three-layer bandage recommended for proximal humerus fractures [27]. (With permission from Wellcome Collection)

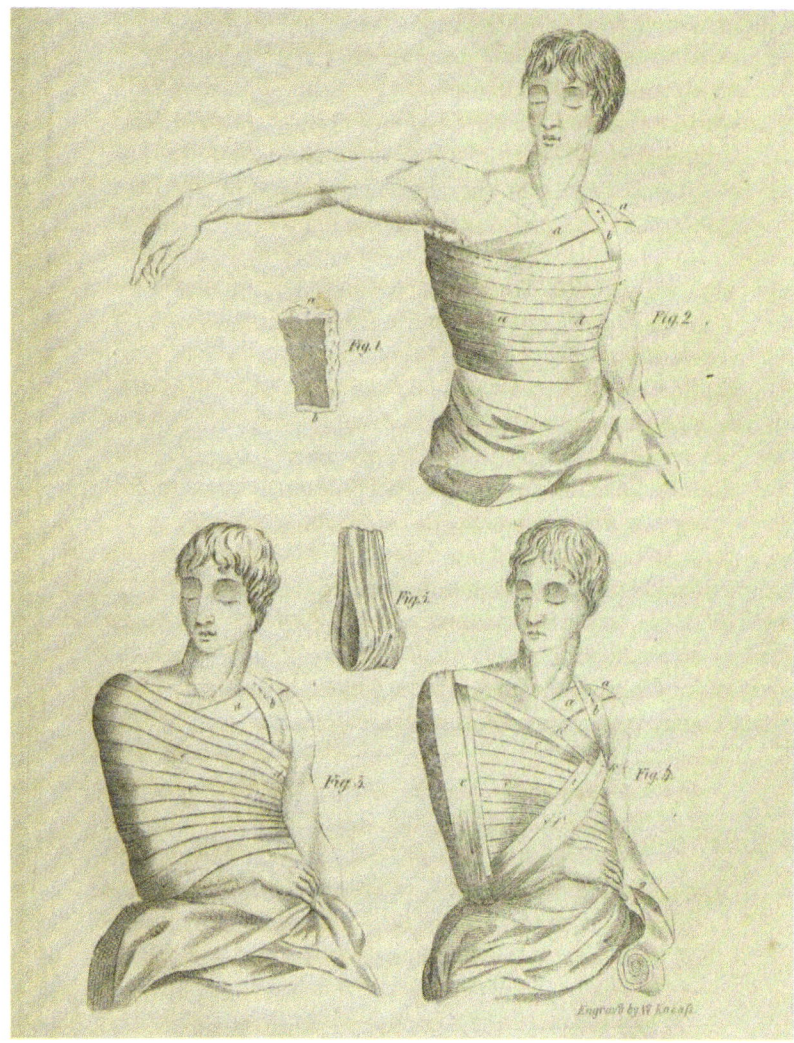

supported the forearm while the arm was pressed toward the trunk and fixed against a bolster serving as a fulcrum to prevent displacement inward. Slightly modified bandages were recommended for cases of external or longitudinal displacement. Desault criticized the ancient writers for seeking a prognosis through the injury's relative proximity to the joint rather than seeking to improve the bandaging: "It is then, from the perfection of the apparatus, and not from the vicinity of the injury to a joint, that the prognosis is to be formed, both as to the consequences and to the duration of the fracture" [27] (p. 74).

The bandage recommended by Desault allowed the patient to get out of bed; returning to work after a shoulder fracture was a concern, even during Desault's time. His pupil, Xavier Bichat (1771–1802) stated: "Desault has cured several patients, but more particularly two, who, being obliged to travel daily, did not, except on the day of the accident, deviate in any measure from their usual mode of life" [27] (p. 84).

5.9 Perspectives

Treatments for shoulder fractures remained largely unchanged for two millennia. The standard treatment involved forceful extension using hands or instruments, followed by bandaging with supportive linen until a stiffer bandage could be applied. It is unclear how much damage the traction treatments have caused the patients. Damage to the neurovascular structures in the axilla was not described until the eighteenth century, but it may have been the consequence of heavy traction. The scarcity of human remains with fractures of the proximal humerus makes any definition of historical fracture populations difficult. High-energy trauma may have been relatively more common due to a younger population and the frequency of war, while nutritional factors and bone weakness may have caused fractures at a younger age. However, the most remarkable finding for a modern reader is the historical persistence of the practices recommended. Like the practice of bloodletting, forceful traction was prescribed and probably used for more than two millennia to conform with the masters from antiquity. Despite the limited treatment options from a modern perspective, there is a rich literature on surgeons blaming each other for misconduct (Chap. 17).

References

1. Allen JP. The art of medicine in ancient Egypt. New York: Metropolitan Museum of Art; 2005. Available from: https://www.metmuseum.org/met-publications/the-art-of-medicine-in-ancient-egypt
2. Breasted JH, Smith E. The Edwin Smith surgical papyrus. Chicago: University of Chicago. Oriental Institute publications; 1930. Available from: https://isac.uchicago.edu/sites/default/files/uploads/shared/docs/oip4.pdf
3. Leake C, Larkey S, Lutz H. The management of fractures according to the Hearst medical papyrus. Oxford University Press; 1953.
4. Smith GE. The royal mummies. Le Caire: L'Institut Francais d'Archéologie Orientale; 1912.
5. Smith GE. The Most ancient splints. BMJ. 1908;1(2465):732–6. Available from: https://www.bmj.com/content/1/2465/732
6. Agarwal SC, Grynpas MD. Bone quantity and quality in past populations. Anat Rec. 1996;246(4):423–32. Available from: https://onlinelibrary.wiley.com/doi/10.1002/(SICI)1097-0185(199612)246:4%3C423::AID-AR1%3E3.0.CO;2-W
7. Smith GE. In: Jones FW, editor. Archeological survey of Nubia: report for 1907–1908. Cairo; 1910.
8. Erfan Zaki M. Success of long bone fracture healing in ancient Egypt: a paleoepidemiological study of the Giza Necropolis skeletons. Acta Med Hist Adriat. 2013;11(2):275–84.
9. Kozieradzka-Ogunmakin I. Patterns and management of fractures of long bones: a study of the Ancient Population of Saqqara, Egypt. Bull John Rylands Libr, Available from: https://doi.org/10.7227/BJRL.89.S.8. 2013;89:133–56.
10. Masali M, Chiarelli B. Demographic data on the remains of ancient Egyptians. J Hum Evol. 1972;1(2):161–9. Available from: https://doi.org/10.1016/0047-2484(72)90017-6
11. Martin DL, Armelagos GJ. Morphometrics of compact bone: an example from Sudanese Nubia. Am J Phys Anthropol. 1979;51(4):571–7. Available from: https://doi.org/10.1002/ajpa.1330510409
12. Bourke JB. Trauma and degenerative diseases in ancient Egypt and Nubia. J Hum Evol. 1972 [cited 2023 Jun 19];1(2):225–32. Available from: https://doi.org/10.1016/0047-2484(72)90023-1
13. Hippocrates, Withington ET (Edward T. Hippocrates. Volume III: On wounds in the head. In the surgery. On fractures. On joints. Mochlicon. Cambridge, MA: Harvard University Press; 1928. (Loeb classical library;149). Available from: https://www.loebclassics.com/view/LCL149/1928/volume.xml
14. Brorson S. Management of fractures of the humerus in ancient Egypt, Greece, and Rome: an historical review. Clin Orthop Relat Res. 2009;467(7):1907–14. Available from: https://doi.org/10.1007/s11999-008-0612-x
15. Brorson S. Medieval and early modern approaches to fractures of the proximal humerus: an historical review. Minerva Ortop e Traumatol. 2010;61(5):449–62.
16. Hippocrates. Oeuvres complètes d'Hippocrate (French translation by Emile Littré). Amsterdam: Adolf M. Hakkert; 1841. Available from: https://archive.org/details/oeuvrescomplte01hippuoft/mode/2up
17. Milne JS. The apparatus used by the Greeks and romans in the setting of fractures and the reduction of dislocations. Interstate Med J. 1909;16:48–60.
18. Raeder J. Oribasii collectionum medicarum reliqviae. Lipsiae; 1928.
19. Celsus AC. De medicina. In: Spencer WG, editor. De medicina. London: Heinemann; 1935. Available from: https://www.loebclassics.com/view/LCL292/1935/volume.xml.
20. Claudius Galenus C. In: Kühn CG, editor. Galeni opera omnia (II). Lipsiae; 1821.
21. Fransesco Primaticcio. Collection de chirurgiens grecs avec dessins attribués au Primatice: reproduction réduite des 200 dessins du manuscrit latin 6866 de la

References

Bibliotheque Nationale. Paris; 1930. Available from: https://archive.org/details/collectiondechir00bibl_0/mode/1up

22. Paulus A. The seven books of Paulus Ægineta (translated by Francis Adams); 1844. Available from: https://archive.org/details/sevenbooksofpaul02pauluoft/page/n15/mode/2up

23. Mondeville H De. The surgery of master Henry de Mondeville: surgeon of Philip the fair, king of France: written from 1306 to 1320. Philadelphia: XLibris Corporation; 2003.

24. Albucasis. On surgery and instruments. Berkeley: University of California Press; 1973.

25. Pifteau P, Salicetti G, Rosenman LD, editors. The surgery of William of Saliceto. Xlibris: Bridgeport; 2002.

26. Vidius V. Chirurgia è Graeco in Latinum conversa, Vido Vidio Florentino interprete. Paris: Pierre Gaultier; 1544.

27. Desault P-J. A treatise on fractures, Luxations, and other affections of the bones; 1805. Available from: https://wellcomecollection.org/works/pa6vyz7y

Open Access This chapter is licensed under the terms of the Creative Commons Attribution 4.0 International License (http://creativecommons.org/licenses/by/4.0/), which permits use, sharing, adaptation, distribution and reproduction in any medium or format, as long as you give appropriate credit to the original author(s) and the source, provide a link to the Creative Commons license and indicate if changes were made.

The images or other third party material in this chapter are included in the chapter's Creative Commons license, unless indicated otherwise in a credit line to the material. If material is not included in the chapter's Creative Commons license and your intended use is not permitted by statutory regulation or exceeds the permitted use, you will need to obtain permission directly from the copyright holder.

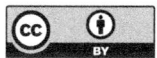

Pathoanatomical Conceptions of Shoulder Fractures in the Nineteenth Century

6.1 Introduction

Much of the pathoanatomical knowledge of shoulder fractures acknowledged today was established some two centuries ago, almost a hundred years before radiological imaging [1]. From a modern orthopedic perspective, it would be unthinkable that fracture morphology might be determined from the surface anatomy, swelling, ecchymoses, crepitus, range of motion, pain localization, impaired function, and simple clinical tests. In the early nineteenth century, it became possible to perform careful dissections and compare autopsy findings with clinical history. The corpses available were either patients who died from other causes with fracture sequelae or acute fractures from lethal injuries. A small number of fracture specimens with specific fracture patterns were available for didactic purposes and were carefully referenced with respect to their owners. The most thorough studies on shoulder pathology were performed in the first part of the nineteenth century, before major surgery was an option [2, 3].

6.2 The French Pathoanatomical School

Paris was the center of pathological anatomy at the end of the eighteenth century. New knowledge of injuries to bones and joints was obtained thanks to a reliable flow of corpses into the city's hospitals. In some cases, the patient's history or medical record was available; in others, the surgeon had treated the patient, who had agreed to donate the shoulder for scientific purposes on their decease. Most of the prominent pathological anatomists in the nineteenth century were also surgeons. It was common to publish case reports, including autopsy records and illustrations of the pathology. The images were often of high pathoanatomical accuracy and artistic value.

Among the prominent surgeons in Paris were pupils of Pierre-Joseph Desault (Chap. 5): Alexis Boyer (1757–1833) and Guillaume Dupuytren (1777–1835). Like his master, Boyer gained his first surgical training with a local barber-surgeon. The author of an anatomical textbook in four volumes and two books on surgical technique was appointed surgeon to Napoleon and the imperial family. His lectures *Leçons sur les maladies des os* were translated into English and published in 1807 [4]. Boyer, relying on Desault's biomechanical reasoning, gave this thorough account of displacement in surgical neck fractures:

> Fractures of the neck of the humerus are always attended with derangement, which is produced by the action of the pectoralis major, latissimus dorsi, and teres major, which being attached to the lower portion near its superior extremity, draw it first inward and upward, in which last direction it is powerfully aided by the biceps, coraco-brachialis, and long portion of the biceps. The superior portion itself is, in this case, directed a little outward by the action of the infraspinatus, supraspinatus, and teres minor, which make the head of the humerus perform a rotatory motion in the glenoid cavity [4]. (pp. 148–9)

For Boyer, the poor prognosis for fractures near the joint resulted from false anchylosis—a particular risk in cases with swelling or insufficient bandaging. Therefore, the shoulder and elbow should be frequently moved during healing [4].

Surgeons of the early nineteenth century revived the ancient Alexandrian discussion on distinguishing shoulder dislocations from fracture-dislocations (Chap. 4). In his *Leçons orales de clinique chirurgicale faites à l'Hôtel-Dieu de Paris* [5], Dupuytren distinguished the two injuries by trauma mechanism: if the arm was in a position of flexion or abduction in a fall, it would cause a dislocation. If the arm was close to the body, with the hand kept in the pocket, for example, a fall would cause a fracture. Dirt on the hand suggested a dislocation; if ecchymoses and excoriations were present, it pointed toward a fracture. In the rare cases of fracture-dislocations, nothing could be done. Although reduction could be provided, the correct diagnosis was still essential for applying the proper bandage. If the surface anatomy could be restored, but the patient had a very swollen shoulder, it was likely a fracture rather than a dislocation [5]—but if there was any uncertainty, a reduction could be attempted.

6.3 Sir Astley Cooper

The nineteenth century saw several authors espousing therapeutic nihilism concerning treating fracture-dislocations. In *A Treatise on Dislocations and on Fractures of the Joints* from 1842, the British surgeon Sir Astley Cooper (1768–1841) stated with resignation: "But let the surgeon do what he will, the head of the bone will probably remain in the axilla, and the upper motions of the arm will be in a considerable degree lost" [6] (p. 427).

Astley Cooper described his dissection of several shoulders with fracture-dislocations. An anterior view of a right shoulder with sequelae from a fracture-dislocation is shown in Fig. 6.1. The patient had promised Cooper the dissection of his arm. An extract from the report illustrates his rigorous dissection and observation:

> The supra-spinatus was somewhat lessened, as was the teres minor, which has lost much of its natural colour; the infra-spinatus was stretched; the sub-scapularis, diminished and rounded by the projection of the head of the os humeri, adhered to its cartilaginous surface…the head of the os humeri had been thrown forwards on the inner side of the coracoid process, and had united by bone to the scapula…a new and very useful joint had been formed…The greater tubercle of the os humeri was

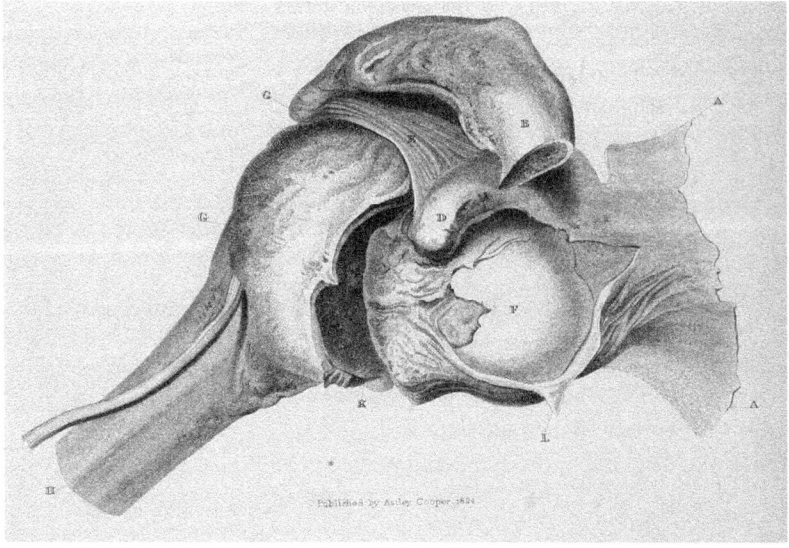

Fig. 6.1 Dissection of a chronic fracture-dislocation with retention of the humeral head in the axilla [6]. (With permission from Wellcome Collection)

exceedingly increased, and the tendon of the biceps passed through the bone. The tubercles were separated with the body of the bone, and not with the head [6]. (p. 419)

In another case of a fracture-dislocation, the tuberosities were fractured. The broken shaft was in contact with the glenoid cavity, and the head was firmly united with the scapula:

> The tubercles of the neck of the os humeri were broken off with the head of the bone; and the fractured extremity of the neck of the os humeri was placed in the glenoid cavity of the scapula. The underhand motion of the shoulder was restored; but the elevation of the bone, beyond a right angle, was strongly resisted and even with difficulty could be accomplished in the dead body [7]. (p. 275)

Astley Cooper suggested a classification of proximal humerus fractures based on autopsy findings [7] (p. 272). Three *species* of fractures were distinguished:

1. Fracture-dislocations.
2. Fractures of the anatomical neck and the tuberosities. It includes breaks in the epiphysis in young people.
3. Fractures below the articulation but above the insertion of the pectoralis major, latissimus dorsi, teres major, coracobrachialis, and deltoid muscles. This is called the surgical neck.

Astley Cooper further proposed a simple clinical test to distinguish fractures from dislocations (Fig. 6.2) [7]. The surgeon firmly grasped the head of the humerus with the fingers and rotated the humerus by the elbow. If the head followed the shaft, it was a dislocation. If the head did not move with the shaft, it was a fracture. While it has been challenging to diagnose fracture-dislocations or impacted fractures by this method, it may nevertheless have been helpful in distinguishing a humeral neck fracture from a simple shoulder dislocation.

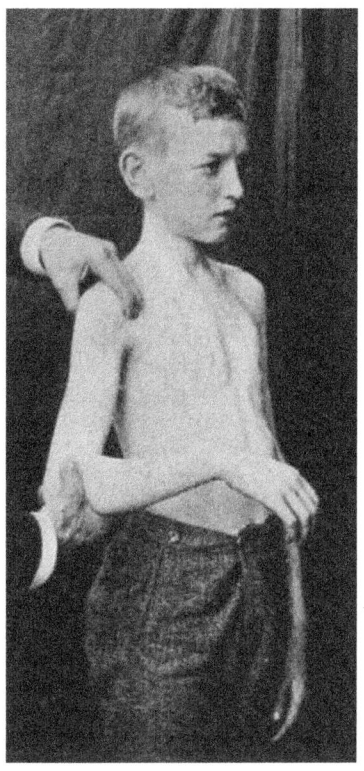

Fig. 6.2 Astley Cooper's test to distinguish fractures from dislocations [8]. (With permission from Wellcome Collection)

6.4 Robert William Smith

The Irish surgeon and anatomist Robert William Smith (1807–1873) is best known for describing the eponymous fracture of the distal radius with volar displacement. Smith undertook a substantial number of autopsies and preserved specimens for didactic purposes. His work *A treatise on fractures in the vicinity of joints and on certain forms of accidental and congenital dislocations* was published in 1847 and contained several dissections of shoulder fracture sequelae [9]. Smith was especially concerned with the deforming forces acting on different fracture patterns. He opposed

Cooper's assumption of a common pathology of the anatomical neck and the tuberosities:

> The anatomist, however, is aware that the tubercles do not constitute any part of the anatomical neck of the humerus, a fracture through which, as already stated, is intracapsular and is characterized by symptoms totally different from those which attend fractures through the tuberosities, or through the line of the junction of the epiphysis with the shaft of the bone. In the latter, the deformity is considerable, in consequence of the lower fragment being drawn inwards by the muscles which constitute the fold of the axilla…counteracted by the supra-spinatus, infra-spinatus, and teres minor attached to the greater tubercle; the bone being thus placed between two opposing factors… [9] (p. 185)

Smith discussed the various patterns of impaction in humeral neck fractures, highlighting the challenges in accurately diagnosing injuries of this kind. The length of the humerus did not change in impacted fractures. During clinical examination, the humeral head moved in line with the shaft; crepitus was not usually detectable, and there were no protruding bones or palpable bone fragments in the axilla. Given that the fractures would heal with a certain amount of deformity, "the prudent surgeon will never omit to announce to the patient that a certain degree of impairment of the motions of the joint will be a permanent result of the injury" [9] (p. 191).

For Smith, the lack of nutrition to the articular fragment in displaced anatomical neck fractures was predictable given that "the superior fragment is cut off from all connection with surrounding tissue, it has no round ligament to conduct vessels into it from above, it becomes, truly, a foreign body in the articulation, and would be likely to perish from want of nutrition" [9] (p. 189).

Robert William Smith presented a remarkable fracture morphology resembling a glenohumeral dislocation (Fig. 6.3). The acromion was prominent; the deltoid was flattened; the arm was shortened, and the glenoid cavity could not be felt. By dissection,

> …the head of the bone was found to have been separated from the shaft by a fracture, which traversed the anatomical neck of the humerus. It was reversed in the articulation, so that the fractures surface was directed upwards toward the glenoid cavity, and the cartilaginous articulating surface thrown downwards toward the shaft, and having assumed this position, it was driven to a considerable distance into the cancelled structure between the tubercles [9]. (p. 194)

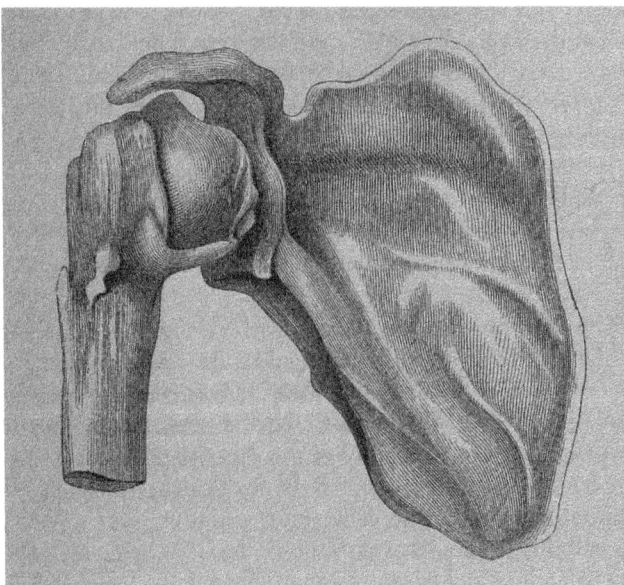
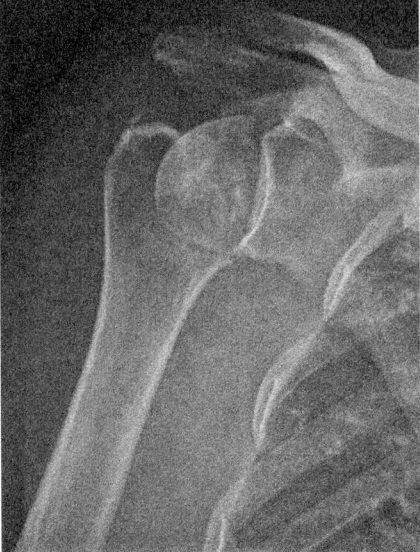

Fig. 6.3 Anatomical neck fracture. The articular surface is reversed and impacted into the shaft. Robert William Smith's specimen from 1847 [9] and a radiograph of a comparable fracture anatomy in a 73-year-old female. The patient received a reverse total shoulder arthroplasty. (With permission from Wellcome Collection)

Smith distinguished the anatomical neck from the epiphyseal lines. Regardless of tuberosity involvement, three levels of neck fractures should be distinguished: (1) fractures of the anatomical neck; (2) fractures at the epiphyseal line; and (3) surgical neck fractures. Impaction could appear within or outside the capsule. Impaction inside the capsule did not produce crepitus. The healing of fractures was supposed to derive from the lower fragment. Cartilage could not be expected to heal to bone [9].

6.5 Joseph-Francois Malgaigne

The French surgeon and anatomist Joseph-Francois Malgaigne (1806–1865) published several specimens of proximal humerus pathology.

In Fig. 6.4, a posterior incision was made through the capsule to demonstrate the pathoanatomy of an intracapsular fracture involving the anatomical neck and both tuberosities. The articular surface points posteriorly due to rotational displacement. Like Astley Cooper, Malgaigne classified fractures into three groups based on anatomical segments and their relation to the capsule, further noting that fractures could present in combinations.

Malgaigne carefully documented the pathological changes in shoulder fractures in patients with poor bone stock. In the surgical neck fracture shown in Fig. 6.5, the diaphysis was impacted into the cancellous bone of the humeral head in varus position. The diaphyseal cortical bone was thin.

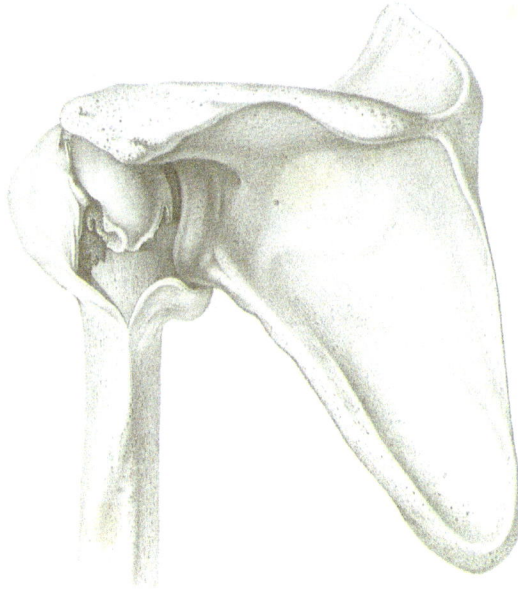

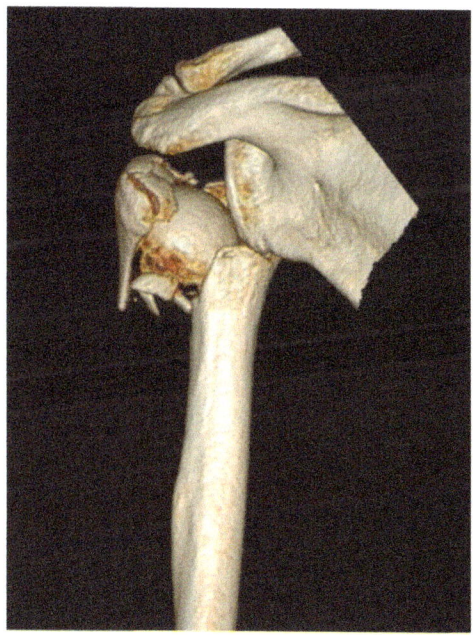

Fig. 6.4 Posterior dissection of a left shoulder. The tuberosities were separated from the head and the shaft. The shaft was in contact with the glenoid cavity [10]. A three-dimensional CT reconstruction of comparable fracture anatomy in a 77-year-old female. (With permission from Wellcome Collection)

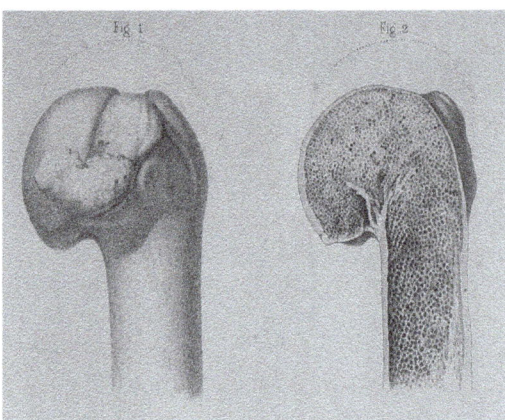

Fig. 6.5 Healed extracapsular fracture (surgical neck) with marked displacement. The head and tuberosities were inclined downward. The dashed lines mark the anatomical position of the head [10]. (With permission from Wellcome Collection)

Table 6.1 Classification of proximal humerus fractures by Ludwig Thudichum. Translated from [11]

1. Anatomical neck fracture
   (a) Intracapsular fracture without impaction
       (i) Intracapsular fracture
       (ii) Intracapsular fracture-dislocation
   (b) Intracapsular fracture with impaction
       (i) Intracapsular fracture with impaction
       (ii) Intracapsular fracture with impaction and complicating tuberosity fracture
2. Fracture of the greater tuberosity
3. Fracture of the lesser tuberosity
4. Separation of the epiphysis from the shaft
   (a) Epiphysiolysis
   (b) Fracture involving the epiphyseal line
5. Surgical neck fracture
   (a) Extracapsular fracture without impaction
       (i) Extracapsular fracture
       (ii) Extracapsular fracture-dislocation
6. Extracapsular fracture with impaction

6.6 Ludwig Thudichum's Pathoanatomical Classification

In 1851, the 22-year-old German physician Ludwig Thudichum (1829–1901) defended his doctoral thesis *Ueber die am oberen Ende des Humerus vorkommenden Knochenbrüche* [11]. In it, he reorganized the classification systems of the first half of the nineteenth century to make them more clinically useful (Table 6.1). Fractures were first classified according to the anatomical segments involved before the presence of impaction or dislocation was specified. Epiphysiolyses were classified separately (Fig. 6.6). From a modern perspective, Thudichum's synthesis of fracture classifications appears remarkably accurate, lacking only a definition of displacement (found in the Neer classification) and a distinction between varus and valgus displacement (found in the AO classification). His dissertation was published almost half a century before radiology enabled the imaging of fractures.

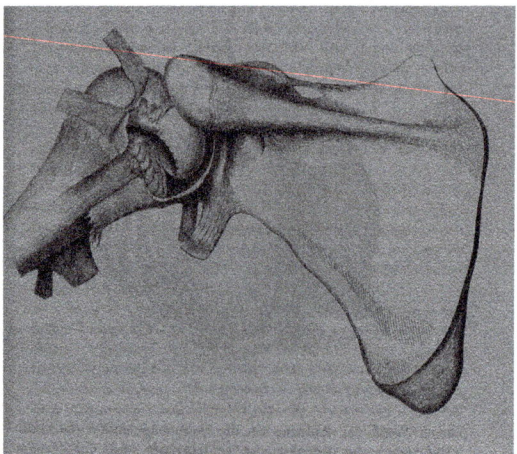

Fig. 6.6 Fracture involving the epiphyseal line in a young person [11]. (With permission from Wellcome Collection)

6.7 Theodor Kocher

The last pre-radiological classification of shoulder fractures was proposed by the Swiss surgeon Emil Theodor Kocher (1841–1917). The first surgeon to receive the Nobel Prize, Kocher gave a comprehensive account of proximal humerus fractures in his *Beiträge zur Kenntniss einiger praktisch wichtiger Fracturformen* [12] of 1896—the same year Röntgen published *On a New Kind of Rays* [1]. Kocher combined the well-known pathoanatomical classification based on the fracture level with the pathophysiological findings from biomechanical studies. Figure 6.7 and Table 6.2 define the most common pathoanatomical patterns presented by analogy with proximal femur fractures.

Kocher performed numerous biomechanical studies by inflicting deforming forces on cadaver bones. Recording the fracture patterns caused by pressure or impact from above, below, outside, inside, abduction, adduction, flexion, and rotation, he accounted for 14 typical patterns of proximal humerus fractures; differences in the force applied, he noted, could bring about other varieties of fracture patterns. Kocher distinguished abduction and adduction fractures according to the direction of displacement viewed from the anterior side. Figure 6.8 and Table 6.3 illustrate and define common patterns of infratubercular fractures.

If necrosis of the humeral head necessitated an operation, Kocher recommended the resection of intraarticular fragments in an aseptic procedure. In infratubercular fractures with severe displacement, closed reduction was recommended. Difficulties in reducing displaced infratubercular fractures may be caused by the interposition of the biceps tendon (Fig. 6.9).

A great number of bandaging methods appeared in the course of the nineteenth century. Some were new; others were modifications of ancient techniques. The insights into pathoanatomy and pathophysiology led to the development of functional bandages such as abduction bandages, bandages with permanent traction, and bandages with varus or valgus pressure. After

Table 6.2 Explanation of Fig. 6.7

Supratubercular fracture
1. Anatomical neck fracture (purely intracapsular)

Infratubercular fracture
2. Pertubercular fracture (including epiphyseal fracture in young people)
3. Subtubercular fracture (surgical neck fracture)

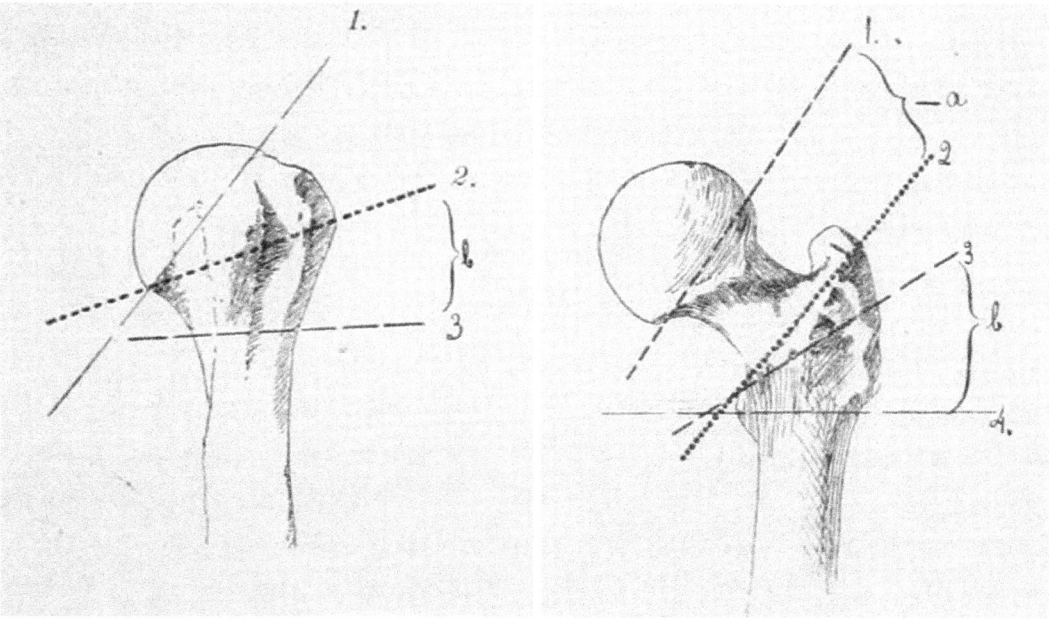

Fig. 6.7 Comparative study of anatomical fracture patterns of the proximal humerus and the proximal femur [12]. (With permission from Wellcome Collection)

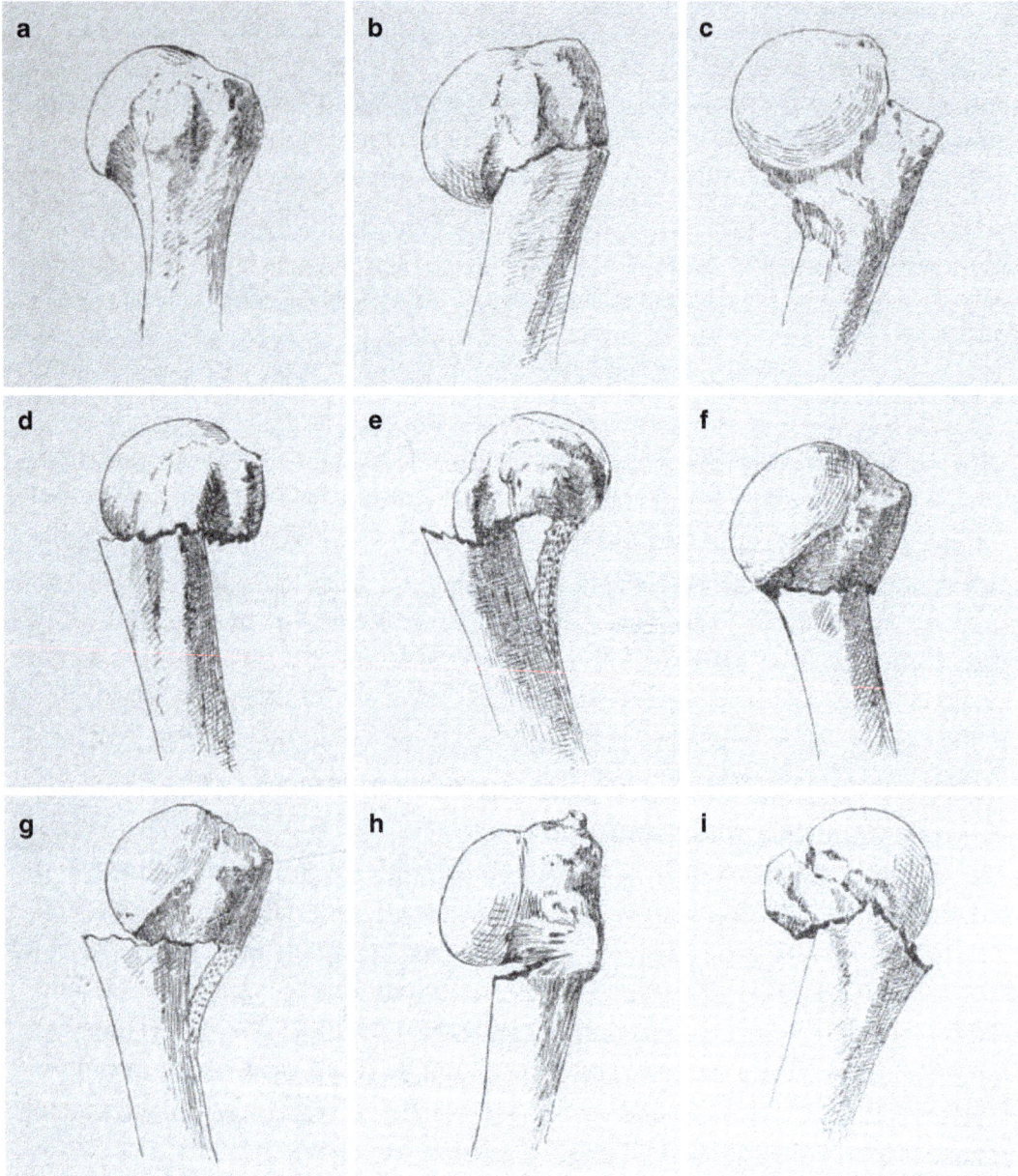

Fig. 6.8 Infratubercular fractures as classified by Kocher. Interpretations by Kocher in Table 6.3. (With permission from Wellcome Collection)

Table 6.3 Explanation of Fig. 6.8

(a) Normal humerus
(b) Pertubercular fracture with impaction of the humeral head in adduction, anterior view
(c) Pertubercular fracture in adduction and extension. Anterior displacement of the shaft, medial view
(d) Pertubercular fracture in abduction. Anterior displacement of the shaft, anterior view
(e) Pertubercular fracture in extension. Anterior displacement of the shaft, lateral view
(f) Subtubercular fracture in abduction. Anterior impaction, anterior view
(g) Subtubercular fracture in abduction. Anterior displacement of the shaft, anterior view
(h) Subtubercular fracture with impaction in adduction, anterior view
(i) Pertubercular Y-fracture with displacement in abduction. The anatomical neck is involved, anterior view

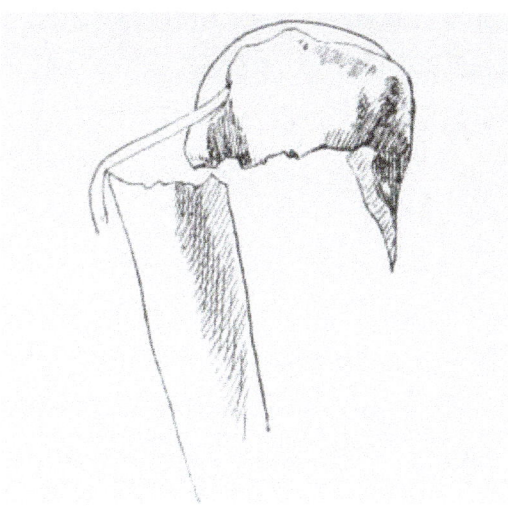

Fig. 6.9 Entrapment of the biceps tendon in a displaced pertubercular fracture [12]. (With permission from Wellcome Collection)

Antonius Mathijsen's introduction of plaster of Paris in 1852 [13], the method was incorporated into bandages such as hanging casts and casts to immobilize both the shoulder and the elbow joints. I have reviewed nineteenth-century bandaging elsewhere [3].

6.8 Perspectives

The pathoanatomical studies conducted in the first half of the nineteenth century brought about a shift in the understanding of bone pathology. These studies allowed for comparing patient history, clinical findings in vivo, and the corresponding pathological changes. The interval between the occurrence of an injury and the appearance of pathological findings explains why most preserved specimens are of healed fractures found in patients who died from other causes. The interpretation of pathoanatomical studies from the nineteenth century has limitations. Many practitioners were illiterate and may not have followed learned medicine, while written sources and human remains documenting actual practice are lacking. Hospital surgery for shoulder fractures was then rare, and admission to the hospital was restricted. Surgeons gained new knowledge of pathological anatomy by dissecting corpses brought into hospitals. By the early twentieth century, the implementation of aseptic procedures and implants reached a level permitting surgery for acute shoulder fractures (Chap. 7).

References

1. Röntgen WC. On a new kind of rays. Science. 1896;3(59):227–31.
2. Brorson S. Cuff tear arthropathy in the nineteenth century: "chronic rheumatic arthritis" with "partial luxation upwards" of the humeral head. Int Orthop. 2019;43(10):2415–23.
3. Brorson S. Management of proximal humeral fractures in the nineteenth century: an historical review of preradiographic sources. Clin Orthop Relat Res. 2011;469(4):1197–206. Available from: https://www.ncbi.nlm.nih.gov/pmc/articles/PMC3048260/
4. Boyer A. The lectures of Boyer, upon diseases of the bones. London: J. Callow; 1807. Available from: https://archive.org/details/b21299304/
5. Dupuytren G. Leçons orales de clinique chirurgicale faites à l'Hôtel-Dieu de Paris. Tome 3. Paris: Germer Bailliére; 1833. Available from: https://gallica.bnf.fr/ark:/12148/bpt6k6347453q/f9.item.texteImage
6. Cooper A. A treatise on dislocations, and on fractures of the joints. Appendix; 1842. Available from: https://wellcomecollection.org/works/spg5dpj4
7. Cooper A. Of the dislocation of the os humeri upon the dorsum scapulæ, and upon fractures near the shoulder joint. Guys Hosp Rep. 1839;IV:265–84.
8. Scudder CL. The treatment of fractures. W.B. Saunders Ltd; 1902. Available from: https://wellcomecollection.org/works/xurkgqfu
9. Smith RW. A treatise on fractures in the vicinity of joints and on certain forms of accidental and congenital dislocations. Dublin: Hodges and Smith; 1847. Available from: https://wellcomecollection.org/works/msz6zwcq
10. Malgaigne J-F. Traité des fractures et des luxations. Paris: J.-B. Baillière; 1847. Available from: https://wellcomecollection.org/works/jkwjptc2
11. Thudichum L. Ueber die am oberen Ende des Humerus vorkommenden Knochenbrüche. Giessen: J. Ricker'sche Buchhandlung; 1851. Available from: https://wellcomecollection.org/works/ebjjuvsd
12. Kocher ET. Beiträge zur Kenntniss einiger praktisch wichtiger Fracturformen. Basel; 1896. Available from: https://wellcomecollection.org/works/mkh547es
13. Mathijsen A. New method for application of plaster-of-Paris bandage. 1852. Clin Orthop Relat Res. 2007;458:59–62. Available from: https://journals.lww.com/clinorthop/fulltext/2007/05000/the_classic__new_method_for_application_of.16.aspx

Open Access This chapter is licensed under the terms of the Creative Commons Attribution 4.0 International License (http://creativecommons.org/licenses/by/4.0/), which permits use, sharing, adaptation, distribution and reproduction in any medium or format, as long as you give appropriate credit to the original author(s) and the source, provide a link to the Creative Commons license and indicate if changes were made.

The images or other third party material in this chapter are included in the chapter's Creative Commons license, unless indicated otherwise in a credit line to the material. If material is not included in the chapter's Creative Commons license and your intended use is not permitted by statutory regulation or exceeds the permitted use, you will need to obtain permission directly from the copyright holder.

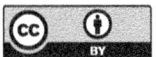

Radiology and the Advent of Surgical Interventions for Shoulder Fractures

7.1 Introduction

The speed at which radiology was adopted for the diagnosis of bone pathology and the planning of operative procedures on bones is astonishing. The new technique was announced in January 1896 by the German physicist Wilhelm Conrad Röntgen (1845–1923) [1]. The first papers on the clinical use of radiographs appeared later in the same year. One of the pioneers in developing and implementing the new technology was the Boston-based physician Ernest Amory Codman (1869–1940). Codman, whose seminal works on the shoulder will occupy a considerable part of this chapter, made an unsurpassed contribution to shoulder surgery—but he was much more than a surgeon who operated on shoulders. He graduated from Harvard Medical School and began to practice in 1895, almost coincident with Röntgen's discovery. Codman was a medical polymath who advocated systematic outcome data collection to improve patient care—the *end result idea*, centered on the proposal that every patient treated at a hospital should have the eventual outcome of their treatment registered and published. It was an idea that made enemies of certain of his colleagues, who feared for their professional integrity. The many facets of Ernest Codman's life and work have been described in the biography *Ernest Amory Codman: The End Result of a Life in Medicine* by Bill Mallon [2]. Codman contributed substantially to medicine in several ways. With Harvey Cushing, he introduced "ether charts" to monitor the anesthetized patient; as a general surgeon, he improved the treatment of duodenal ulcers; he studied bone sarcoma, both proposed classifications, and established the first register of bone sarcoma. He also wrote *The Shoulder*, the first monograph on shoulder surgery. In this chapter, I will focus on the aspects of Codman's work relevant to his rethinking of shoulder fractures.

7.2 Skeletal Radiology

Codman's contribution to skeletal radiology is less known than his contribution to shoulder surgery. The contributions were, however, intertwined. Today, fracture surgery would be unthinkable without preoperative radiographic assessment and planning. From 1896, Codman worked hard to map the skeleton's normal anatomy, performing countless radiographs on cadavers. In 1898, he succeeded in presenting his first work on skeletal radiology [3], which included an atlas of the radiological changes in the wrist in different positions. Radiographs at that time were termed *skiagrams* (shadow writing), referring to the picture created by the shadow of the bone. Codman became one of the first skiagraphers.

Codman contributed the chapter *The Röntgen ray and its relation to Fractures* to Charles Locke Scudder's textbook *The Treatment of Fractures*, first published in 1900 [4]. From it, the reader gains a clear impression of Codman's excitement about the accurate and reliable information to be gained from applying the new technology to shoulder pathology in a clinical setting:

> Fractures of the shoulder joint are often impossible to recognize without the X-ray, particularly in those cases where the swelling and effusion about the joint prevent manipulation. Fractures of the tuberosities of the humerus, of the surgical and anatomical neck, can be differentiated with great certainty. … Separation of the tuberosities we now found is a much more common accident than we supposed [4] (pp. 433–4).

At the turn of the century, the broad implications of the new technology became increasingly clear to surgeons. In 1900, in the preface to the first edition of his textbook, Scudder summarized the unique situation: "The final results after the open incision of closed fractures emphasize the fact that anesthesia, antisepsis, and the Röntgen ray are making the knowledge of fractures more exact, and their treatment less complicated" [4] (p. 9).

Open surgery on closed fractures, this is to say, was now viable. In a paper in *The Johns Hopkins Hospital Bulletin* from 1903, Codman argues for the use of radiography in fracture treatment, referring to the instant benefits to the patient and concluding that: "It is not fair to the patient to learn fracture pathology in the old way" [5] (p. 121).

In preoperative planning, Codman recommended radiography before the application of paddings and splints and adding a second series after the application. Although a pioneer in early radiology, Codman identified himself as a surgeon: "What I am to say to you tonight, [on the use of X-rays in surgery] therefore, I will trust you will take as from a surgeon rather than from an X-ray specialist. I hope that it is because I am a surgeon that I have the honor of speaking to you on the X-ray" [5] (p. 120).

7.3 The Short Rotators and the Subacromial Bursa

From 1896 to 1899, Codman dissected shoulders in the anatomy department, with a particular focus on the subacromial bursa, which had captured his interest during a visit to Vienna in 1892–1893. His first publication on the shoulder pathology appeared in 1904 and discussed the condition of periarthritis, a condition which would likely be termed subacromial pain, subacromial bursitis, or rotator cuff syndrome today. Viewed from the perspective of the subacromial bursa, Codman described four types of bursitis: an acute and a chronic type, a type we would probably call periarthrosis humeroscapularis or frozen shoulder today, and finally, the complete rotator cuff tear. In 1908, Codman elaborated on the clinical condition of subacromial bursitis. He described the clinical finding we term *painful arc* in everyday clinics. He also described the typical 2-year duration of periarthrosis humeroscapularis. Codman reported two cases of rotator cuff repair performed in 1909 and 1911 [6].

Codman defined the role of the subacromial bursa in abduction when the humeral head with the greater tuberosity needs to pass under the acromion process. He described the narrow subacromial space and the role played by the bursa in abduction: "How could this occur unless a joint existed between these two bones, for if there were no joint or bursa there, the greater tuberosity would carry its roof of deltoid muscle in under the acromion and pinch it" [7] (p. 613).

Codman returned to subacromial impingement in 1934, a condition arising in fracture cases where the supraspinatus tendon and the attached bone are pulled into the subacromial space: "In some cases, the fragment having been pulled by the supraspinatus too far under the acromion causes a decided obstacle because in abduction it impinges between the humeral head and the acromion" [8] (p. 320).

Between 1912 and 1926, Codman worked primarily on implementing his *end result idea*. From 1927, he prepared his iconic book *The Shoulder* [8]. The book, privately published in 1934, was a comprehensive collection of Codman's insights into both academic and practical aspects of shoulder surgery. For this chapter, I will concentrate on the sections of his book that discuss proximal humerus fractures.

7.4 Codman on Fractures

Codman's approach to these fractures differed from that found in contemporary textbooks. From the perspective of a modern reader (as it perhaps was in Codman's time), browsing the book may be disappointing; this is not a manual on the diagnosis, treatment, and prognosis of a broken bone. His primary interest was the subacromial bursa and the supraspinatus tendon—a perspective is hinted at by the title *The Shoulder: Rupture of the Supraspinatus Tendon and Other Lesions In or About The Subacromial Bursa*.

> It is remarkable in studying the literature of fractures in the upper end of the humerus to find how little detail is given to the probable relations the muscles and bursae bear to the fragments. Few authors even mention the subacromial bursa in this connection, and many do not even mention the tendons of the short rotators [8] (p. 328).

The fracture anatomy and the displacement of the bony parts were viewed from a soft tissue perspective. Fractures were included if related to the bursae or tendons of the functional unit of the small rotators (the rotator cuff): "I do not intend to describe in detail the diagnosis or treatment of fractures about the shoulder, but to state briefly certain points which are suggested from a study of the bursa and tendons, and their probable relations to the fragments in the various types of bone injury" [8] (p. 313).

Chapter 9 in Codman's book, "The Role of the Supraspinatus in Dislocations and Fractures of the Shoulder Joint," contained an account of the biomechanical mechanism behind dislocations and fractures viewed from the supraspinatus tendon. These occurred from the humeral shaft acting as a lever with the acromion as a fulcrum; a proximal humerus fracture could appear when the fulcrum was stronger than the lever. The mechanism behind anterior dislocations could also lead to lesions of the bony part of the proximal humerus. The lesions included [8] (p. 278):

1. Separation of the humeral epiphysis (in young people)
2. Fracture of the surgical neck
3. Fracture of the tuberosities
4. Fracture of the anatomical neck
5. Comminuted fractures in which the typical form consists of four fragments: the two tuberosities, the anatomical neck, and the shaft

Fractures of the tuberosities or rupture of the tendons could appear as complications to shoulder joint dislocations [8] (p. 286). Codman's definition of a fracture-dislocation was basically: "If the articular head becomes free and remains displaced, the injury is called a fracture-dislocation" [8] (p. 314).

A good outcome was more likely if the articular head were to remain between the tuberosities and the glenoid. Otherwise, the prognosis was uncertain, and the surgeon should be cautious in predicting the result: "...but if it [the humeral head] has escaped from the capsule there should be no delay in deciding between operation and a stiff shoulder. Social and general conditions determine this decision, and the surgeon cannot promise much" [8] (p. 323).

7.5 The Four-Part Classification

Chapter 10, in Codman's book "Fractures in Relation to the Subacromial Bursa," contained Codman's main contribution to proximal humerus fractures. Observing that fracture lines often follow the old lines of the epiphyseal union, he noted that "the epiphyseal line is retained in adult life as a thin wedge-shaped subdivision, marking off the tuberosities and the anatomic head from the diaphysis ... and the head of the bone tends to become divided into four main fragments, of various combinations of these four fragments" (Fig. 7.1) [8] (p. 314).

Codman classified fractures according to the parts involved, proposing possible combinations—notwithstanding his confession that he had limited experience with some of the examples he gave. Fractures of the humerus generally had a good prognosis; he claimed: "There is one very striking thing about fractures, and that is that most cases eventually recover pretty good use of their shoulders in spite of any kind of treatment" [8] (p. 331). The worst prognosis was given to a rupture of the supraspinatus tendon close to the insertion at the greater tuberosity—without osseous involvement, this injury posed a severe problem to the surgeon. The joint fluid could pass freely into the bursa, and the lesion would never heal; disability and pain would persist on account of the friction. Most extracapsular fractures united readily because of the contact between the raw bony parts and the absence of joint fluid.

Codman had a particular interest in depression fractures of the greater tuberosity. These injuries involved the supraspinatus tendon, and the biceps tendon, held toward the shaft by the pectoralis major, was often entrapped (Fig. 7.2). While these injuries look trivial and inconspicuous on radiographs, they are disabling fractures with a worse prognosis than surgical neck fractures: after 3–6 months, it was an injury that "causes incapacity because the callus about the fragment impinges on the acromion as the arm is raised" [8] (p. 327). This fracture pattern was not accessible for surgery: "Even if you could raise the depressed fragment, the callus would impinge even more on the acromion" [8] (p. 327).

According to Codman, the fragments of the tuberosities usually remained in a state reflecting their original continuity. The musculotendinous cuff and the capsule held together the four parts, merging with the periosteum of the proximal humerus. In surgical neck fractures, the intracapsular structures were undamaged except for substantially displaced fractures or in neglected cases of anchylosis. The bursa was directly implicated in intracapsular fractures and might fill with blood [8]. The articular surface could escape, while the tuberosities attached to the short rotators did not tend to escape. In complicated cases, the subdeltoid portion of the bursa was often damaged. Codman stressed that healing of bone and tendons could not be expected with joint fluid present between the healing parts.

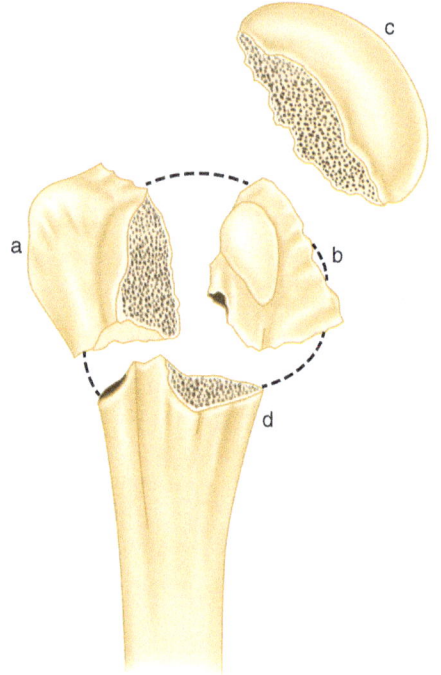

Fig. 7.1 The four parts of the proximal humerus. Anterior view of a right humerus, (a) greater tuberosity, (b) lesser tuberosity, (c) humeral head with articular surface, (d) humeral shaft

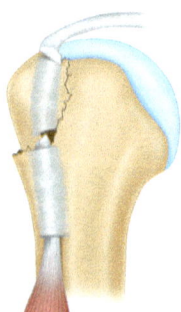 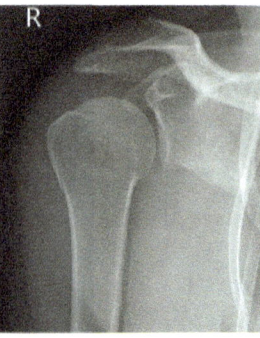 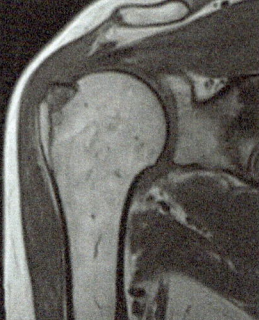 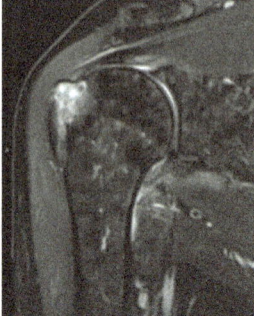

Fig. 7.2 Depression fracture of the greater tuberosity with entrapment of the biceps tendon and leakage of joint fluid [8]. (With permission from Wellcome Collection). Comparable lesion in a 50-year-old female with a hairline fracture of the greater tuberosity but persistent subacromial pain. An MRI scan after 5 months revealed delayed union and bone edema. The rotator cuff was intact

7.6 Early Surgical Interventions

The following section highlights operative interventions for shoulder fractures in the first decade of the twentieth century. Although it is not recorded if Codman operated on bone in shoulder fractures, the scene was certainly set for invasive procedures in closed shoulder fractures. In the 1902 edition of Scudder's textbook, Codman contributed the chapter *On the Röntgen ray and its relation to fractures* [9]. In the same book, Scudder presented a case with a silver wire fixation of a surgical neck fracture (Fig. 7.3).

The Belgian surgeon, instrument maker, and artist Albin Lambotte (1866–1956) was a pioneer in osteosynthesis. The term "osteosynthesis" appears in the title of his book *L'intervention opératoire dans les fractures récentes et anciennes envisagée particulièrement au point de vue de l'ostéo-synthèse avec la description de plusieurs techniques nouvelles in osteosynthesis* [11], which included a collection of fracture cases treated operatively using internal fixation: he worked with various implants, including screws, plates, wires, staples, and nails (Fig. 7.4); in oblique fractures, screw and cerclage were combined (Fig. 7.5). Each case in the book is accompanied by sketches and patient information, attesting to the care with which he planned his surgeries. Fifty of his surgical drawings have been published posthumously [12]. He also performed osteotomy in malunited fractures of the proximal humerus. Lambotte relied on Kocher's classification of shoulder fractures and used Kocher's posterior approach to reduce fracture-dislocations.

The dispute between supporters of surgical and non-surgical treatment is by no means new. Should osteosynthesis only be offered in the event of failed nonoperative treatment, or should it be used as a primary treatment? The president of the British Orthopaedic Society, the Welsh surgeon Sir Robert Jones (1857–1933), commented on the euphoria accompanying the new surgical options in a presidential address in 1912:

> I am, however, very confident that the question is not "Must we prepare ourselves to admit that primary operation is to become the recognized routine?" There are two very real questions – first, "Can we improve our nonoperative technique so as to remove the discrepancies which are in some instances glaringly apparent?" and, secondly, "Can we lay down any laws to guide us when we ought to operate at once?" [14] (p. 1389)

Jones pointed toward the increasing challenge of fracture patients insisting on surgical treatment. Importantly, he stated that the choice of a non-surgical solution was not evidence of neglect on the part of the treating surgeon: "The moment the public is brought to believe that a fracture

Fig. 7.3 Early methods of internal fixation of surgical neck fractures with (**a**) silver wire [4] (p. 10) and (**b**) staples [10] (p. 99). (With permission from Wellcome Collection)

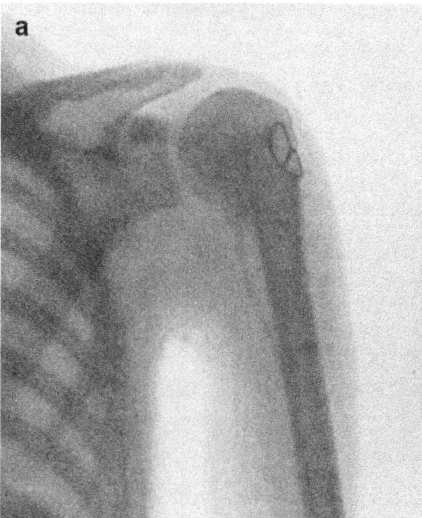 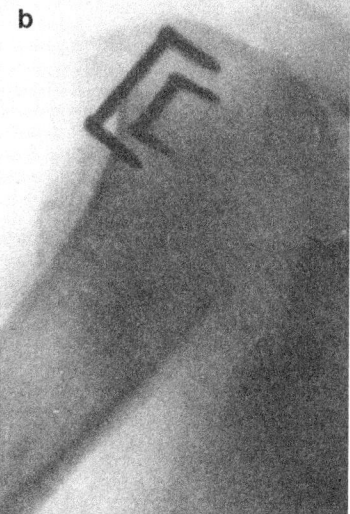

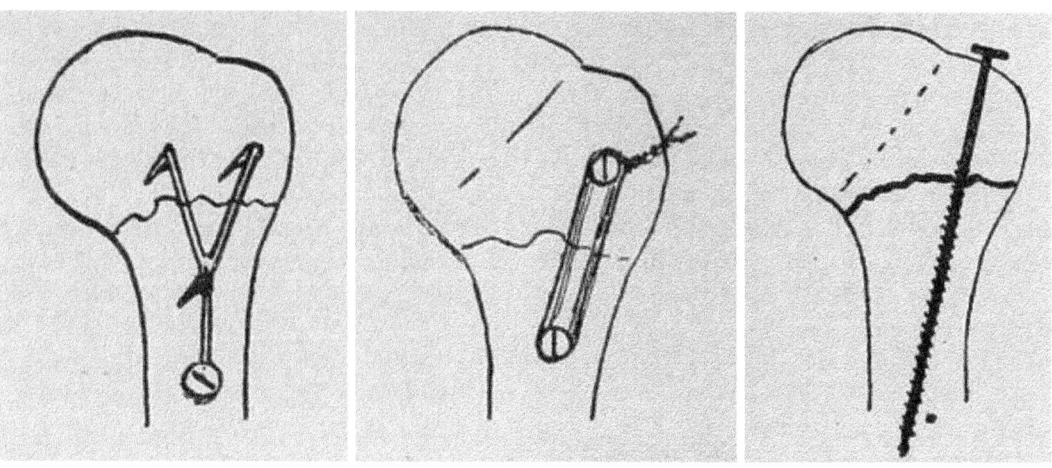

Fig. 7.4 Early fixation methods with crampon, suture, and intramedullary screw [11] (pp. 81–2). (With permission from Wellcome Collection)

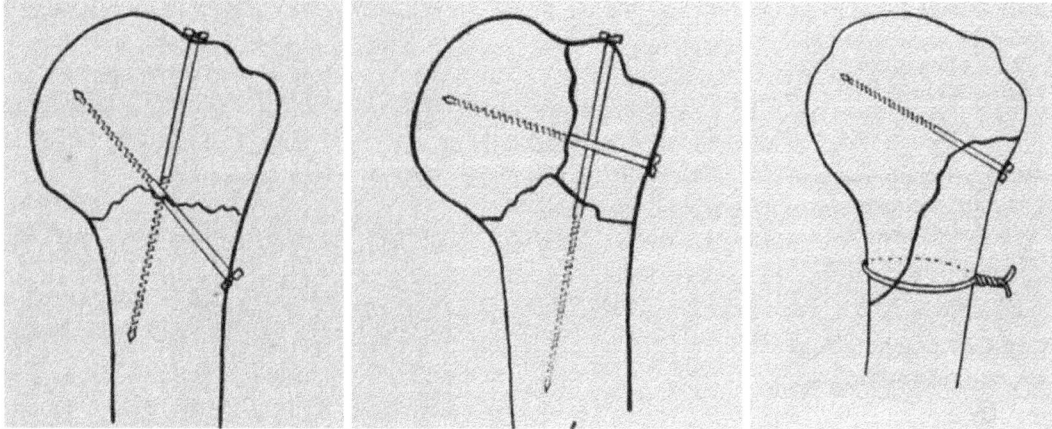

Fig. 7.5 Crossed screw osteosyntheses and combined cerclage and screw osteosynthesis in an oblique fracture [13] (p. 409–10). (With permission from Wellcome Collection)

which is not operated upon is evidence of neglect, the peace of mind of the doctor is at an end" [14] (p. 1394). Non-surgical treatment was recommended unless there was *extreme deformity*:

> In fractures through the anatomical neck it is never necessary to do more than place the wrist in a sling and allow the arm to hang by the side. The same treatment may be employed in fracture of the surgical neck when deformity is not extreme. The abducted position is best, however, when it has been necessary to correct extreme deformity by extension in the abducted plane. Passive movement should not be begun too early-certainly not before the fourth week [14] (p. 1393).

I will conclude this brief overview of the early history of shoulder fracture surgery with Robert Jones's commentary on the debate over whether surgical or non-surgical treatment was appropriate for fractures of the surgical neck. His statement, speaking from the past to the present, is astonishing in its freshness more than a century later: "Statistics do not seem to throw much light on the vexed question whether or not it is better to operate on fractures of the surgical neck of the humerus, for the percentage s of good results are nearly equal by each method" [14] (p. 1393).

7.7 Perspectives

Ernest Codman's contribution to shoulder surgery is not fully acknowledged. He was controversial in his time for emphasizing the importance of systematic follow-up on all patients—a proposal which, were it to be adopted, could lead to the early detection of unnecessary or harmful treatments in shoulder surgery, ultimately benefiting both patients and society. Codman's four-part approach was originally not intended as a fracture classification; it began, rather, as an account of the biomechanics of rotator cuff pathology, including the fractured bony part attached to the tendons of the rotator cuff. His focus on greater tuberosity avulsions and depressions, along with entrapment of the long tendon of the biceps and involvement of bursae and tendons, may lead to a better understanding of the often-poor association between radiographs and clinical symptoms in this patient group. His soft tissue perspective on shoulder fractures may add a more functional approach to the strong focus on bone pathoanatomy in modern traumatology.

References

1. Röntgen WC. On a new kind of rays. Science. 1896;3(59):227–31.
2. Mallon B. Ernst Amory Codman: the end result of a life in medicine. Philadelphia: Saunders; 2000.
3. Codman EA. Experiments on the applications of the roentgen rays to the study of anatomy. J Exp Med. 1898;3(3):383–91.
4. Scudder CL. The treatment of fractures [Internet]. W.B. Saunders Ltd; 1902. Available from: https://wellcomecollection.org/works/xurkgqfu/items.
5. Codman EA. The use of X-ray in surgery. Johns Hopkins Hosp Bull. 1903;14(146):120–4.
6. Codman EA. Complete rupture of the supraspinatus tendon. Operative treatment with report of two successful cases. Boston Med Surg J. 1911;164(20):708–10.
7. Codman EA. On stiff and painful shoulders the anatomy of the subdeltoid or subacromial bursa and its clinical importance: subdeltoid bursitis. Boston Med Surg J. 1906;154:613–20.
8. Codman EA. The shoulder: rupture of the supraspinatus tendon and other lesions in or about the subacromial bursa. Malabar: T. Todd; 1934. Available from: https://wellcomecollection.org/works/k83a3rba.
9. Codman EA. The Röntgen ray and its relation to fractures. In: Scudder CL, editor. The treatment of fractures. 3rd ed. Philadelphia, London: W.B. Saunders; 1902. p. 425–40. Available from: https://wellcomecollection.org/works/xurkgqfu.
10. Lane A. The operative treatment of fractures. London; 1905. Available from: https://wellcomecollection.org/works/hhvtn2t6.
11. Lambotte A. L'intervention opératoire dans les fractures récentes et anciennes envisagée particulièrement au point de vue de l'ostéo-synthèse avec la description de plusieurs techniques nouvelles. Paris: A. Maloine; 1907. Available from: https://wellcomecollection.org/works/ufsrbypb/items.
12. Lambotte A. Les débuts de l'ostéosynthèse en Belgique. Bruxelles; 1971.
13. Lambotte A. L'intervention opératoire dans les fractures récentes et anciennes envisagée particulièrement au point de vue de l'ostéo-synthèse avec la description de plusieurs techniques nouvelles. Paris; 1913. Available from: https://ia801604.us.archive.org/0/items/b21291111/b21291111.pdf.
14. Jones R. Presidential address on the present position of treatment of fractures. BMJ. 1912;2:1589–94. Available from: https://doi.org/10.1136/bmj.2.2710.1589.

Open Access This chapter is licensed under the terms of the Creative Commons Attribution 4.0 International License (http://creativecommons.org/licenses/by/4.0/), which permits use, sharing, adaptation, distribution and reproduction in any medium or format, as long as you give appropriate credit to the original author(s) and the source, provide a link to the Creative Commons license and indicate if changes were made.

The images or other third party material in this chapter are included in the chapter's Creative Commons license, unless indicated otherwise in a credit line to the material. If material is not included in the chapter's Creative Commons license and your intended use is not permitted by statutory regulation or exceeds the permitted use, you will need to obtain permission directly from the copyright holder.

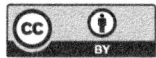

Part III

Classification: Knowing and Telling a Fracture

Why Do We Classify Shoulder Fractures? 8

8.1 Introduction

Naming, describing, and classifying diseases and their symptoms have been integral to medicine since ancient times. Doctors and schools of medicine have debated whether to describe symptoms or seek underlying causes since the Hippocratic writings (fifth and fourth century BCE). In this section, I will briefly present the classical discussion that provides a conceptual framework for understanding aspects of classifying shoulder fractures.

The Cnidian School of Medicine, primarily known from commentaries in the Hippocratic corpus and the works of Galen, was founded in the ancient Greek city of Cnidus, on the west coast of what is today Turkey. It was known for its rivalry with the Coan School of Medicine on the Greek island of Cos, particularly in the field of disease classification. Although the theoretical differences between the two schools are indistinct [1], their approaches to the classification of diseases are relatively clear and demonstrate a tension between the Coan School, which preferred to classify diseases broadly, and the Cnidian School, which preferred to classify them more precisely. For the writers of the Hippocratic texts, the nature of the disease should be understood before any treatment could be considered. The morbid phenomena observed were used to determine the causes of the disease and to predict patient outcomes; the purpose of disease classification was to most accurately determine the correct prognosis. The Cnidian doctors, on the contrary, focused on describing each case in its peculiarity.

In *Regimen in Acute Diseases* (III), the Hippocratic writer states that "though [the Cnidians] wished clearly to set forth the number of each kind of illness their account was incorrect. For the number will be almost incalculable if a patient's disease be diagnosed as different whenever there is a difference in the symptoms, while a mere variety of name is supposed to constitute a variety of the illness" [2].

Galen further referred to the Hippocratic criticism of the Cnidians for their ignorance of the specific and generic differences between diseases [1]. The core question in the ancient discussion was whether morbid phenomena should be given in their specificity, remaining as disparate and individual cases, or grouped according to general principles.

In line with the Cnidian position, a detailed radiographic description can be more accurate than a classification using predefined categories when describing a shoulder fracture. In the context of modern fracture classification, the core question is whether we should describe the individual case thoroughly from imaging material or attempt to classify the fracture in a predefined category. The topic prompts philosophical considerations questioning whether fractures can be held to be discrete categories, *natural kinds* waiting to be discovered, and the possibility of arriving at such categories. Can a human construct like a fracture classification reflect natural kinds to any degree, and do fracture categories have a distinct natural history?

The ensuing epistemological questions include whether we can know if we have arrived at such natural kinds and, if classification fails, whether the failure is due to human perception or inherent weaknesses in the classification. While it is impossible to deeply consider these philosophical questions in this book, they will frame the discussion that follows below on the challenges of classifying shoulder fractures. Focusing on the desired properties of a fracture classification in clinical practice and research, I will advocate for an *instrumentalist* approach to classification, meaning that classifications are more or less useful depending on the specific activities and objectives of their use.

8.2 Morphological Fracture Classification

Technical terms for upper arm fractures are found in the oldest known surgical text (Chap. 4). In the Hippocratic corpus, the author distinguished fractures of the metaphysis, the diaphysis, and the epiphysis of the humerus, aiming at an accurate prognosis. Galen described the gross anatomy of the humeral neck and the epiphysis with the tuberosities as anatomical landmarks. In late Roman sources, distinct morphological patterns, including transverse, oblique, and overriding fractures, were distinguished. Specific prognoses were ascribed to the pathological categories. Pathoanatomical studies in the early nineteenth century brought more detailed fracture morphology into the classifications (Chap. 6). In the mid-nineteenth century, most categories found in the later Neer and AO classifications were already present in Thudichum's pathoanatomical classification [3]. By the end of the nineteenth century, biomechanical studies on cadaver bones brought a variety of new fracture *species* into the classifications [4]. Thus, the imaging-based classification systems we use in clinical practice were established before Röntgen published *On a New Kind of Rays* in 1896 [5] (Chap. 7).

Fracture classification is based on fundamental assumptions about the categories included and their mutual ordering, although these assumptions are not always explicitly stated or reflected upon. *Displacement* can be considered a continuum assessed from imaging or peroperative findings. Fracture classifications convert *continuous* data into *categorical* data. For instance, displacement can be defined as more than 1 cm between two or more of the four anatomical segments of the proximal humerus. The cutoff point used to distinguish between the two categories of displaced versus *minimally displaced* fractures is arbitrary but still clinically useful, as patients in the minimally displaced category are not considered for surgery. The cutoff point of 1 cm of displacement has been used for over 50 years for clinical and academic purposes, notably as a criterion for surgical intervention; in this regard, however, no association with patient outcome has been demonstrated.

Fracture classifications are either *categorical* (*nominal*) or *ordinal*. Categorical classifications name a fracture morphology, while ordinal classifications order categories by severity. Severity can refer to the patient's outcome or the expected difficulties encountered during surgery. The *prognostic distance* between categories may vary within a classification system. This violates the assumption that the classification system represents an *interval* scale with equal prognostic distance between each category. When validating fracture classifications, it is crucial to consider that not all steps between categories have equal clinical significance. As explained in Chap. 10, statistical methods can be used to adjust for the different distances between the categories.

In contrast with classification systems for fractures of other bones, most proximal humerus fracture classifications combine fracture displacement and fracture parts when defining the categories. Classification involves a quantitative assessment of the displacement of fracture lines and a qualitative evaluation of the involvement of the tuberosities or the articular surface.

Our expectations about the prevalence of certain patterns affect our choice of categories. If we assume a particular fracture pattern to be common, we tend to use the category more often. The reported prevalence of displaced fractures has varied widely in the epidemiological literature, ranging from 15% to 85% [6] (Chap. 2). However, the prevalence of 15% displaced fractures, persistently reported in the literature, has not been found in any epidemiological study in the last 50 years. This both calls into question the usefulness of displacement as a criterion for surgical intervention and calls for better studies of prevalences. Despite the lack of evidence-based cutoff values, focusing on the displacement of the four anatomical parts provides a convenient biological and biomechanical frame.

8.3 Clinical Properties of a Fracture Classification System

A classification system for shoulder fractures should ideally meet the criteria outlined in Table 8.1. It should identify clinically meaningful categories, guide treatment, and estimate the prognosis and risk of complications. The goal is to identify different fracture patterns relevant to specific interventions and enable comparison of outcomes of various interventions for each fracture pattern. An ideal fracture classification should provide a unique treatment approach for each category to support clinical decision-making.

A fracture classification system should possess certain internal properties to be clinically useful. The classification should be *exhaustive* in that it should classify all fractures and be *exclusive*—meaning that each fracture can be classified in only one distinct category. Further, it should be logically satisfactory and easy to remember. A comprehensive classification may meet coding and outcome analysis requirements but should not be too complicated to support clinical decision-making.

A classification should further be *validated* according to *therapeutic* and *prognostic* relevance and against other established classification systems. Ideally, it should be possible to *translate* between classifications for clinical and academic

Table 8.1 A non-exhaustive list of desirable properties of a classification of shoulder fractures

Clinical properties	Clinically meaningful
	Guide treatment
	Estimate prognosis
	Predict specific complications
	Logically satisfactory
	Easy to remember
Communication	Precise definitions
	Enhance clinical communication
	Translatable to other systems
	Useful for didactic purposes
	Suitable for databases
	Suitable for research
	Allow comparison between studies
	Allow for pooling of data
	Suitable for clinical audit
	Quality assessment
	Reimbursement
Internal properties	Exhaustive
	Exclusive
	Reliable
	Reproducible
	Validated
"Natural history"	A distinct natural history
	Relate to etiology (mechanism)
	Relate to morphology
	Biomechanical meaningful

purposes (Chap. 10). A classification should be *reliable* in pointing out the relevant categories and be *reproducible* between and within observers using the instrument. It should distinguish fractures that require therapeutic approaches and estimate the patient's prognosis.

8.4 Implications of Radiology-Based Classifications

The Neer classification (Fig. 9.4) [7] combines categorical and continuous data. The extent of displacement is first determined from continuous data and, if displaced, followed by an evaluation of the fracture configuration. This combined process may affect the cognitive process of interpreting an image and assigning it to a specific category. In fracture classification, the extent of long bone displacement is often considered to reflect injury severity and to predict the patient's outcome. This has not been demonstrated for shoulder fractures. The Neer classification was designed as an ordinal system to assign a worse prognosis to higher categories. It was also meant to distinguish between minimally displaced and displaced fractures to identify patients who would benefit from surgery. However, more current studies have shown that displaced fractures are more common than previously expected, which could lead to unnecessary surgical procedures based on the Neer classification.

Older people can usually tolerate considerable displacement of the surgical neck (Fig. 3.5), while a hairline fracture of the greater tuberosity can cause long-lasting subacromial pain in younger individuals (Fig. 7.2). Evaluating a radiograph with a ruler does not necessarily allow us to predict functional outcome or any associated soft tissue injury. In cases of a two-part anterior fracture-dislocation after closed reduction (spontaneous or assisted), the radiographs may show a minimally displaced fracture with greater tuberosity appearing in the near anatomical position. Extensive soft tissue damage, however, is present. The treatment prioritizes regaining stability. This injury can be understood as a glenohumeral dislocation accompanied by a total rotator cuff tear with a bony fragment attached. This view was proposed by Ernest A. Codman (1869–1940), who provided the foundation for the Neer classification (Chap. 7). A shift toward an excessive focus on radiological bone morphology later followed.

The extent to which the criterion of 1 cm of displacement within the Neer classification applies to the tuberosities is still uncertain. This uncertainty may also explain the various indications for surgical intervention for greater tuberosity fractures in the literature. The deforming forces continuously act on the fractured parts, and the initial radiographs are snapshots of the deforming forces and the bone quality. Fracture morphology is subject to change post-injury, which can result in a shift in categories. For instance, a minimally displaced surgical neck fracture in osteoporotic bone can displace into a varus, or the humeral head can collapse, as shown in Fig. 1.3. This change does not necessarily warrant a change in treatment approach, however—rather, a change in the classification category. Open reduction and internal fixation aim to reduce the displaced fracture into an anatomical (non-displaced) position and provide stable fixation. This procedure often fails in osteoporotic bone, resulting in a new pattern of displacement and failure of the osteosynthesis (Fig. 12.6).

The AO classification is another popular imaging-based classification used in clinical practice and research (Chap. 9). Of the system, one of the group's co-founders, Maurice Müller (1918–2009), wrote: "A classification is useful only if it considers the severity of the bone lesion and serves as a basis for treatment and for evaluation of the results" [8].

The AO classification system is an example of an ordinal and *hierarchical* classification. Triads divide the fractures into three *types*, with 9 *groups* and 27 *subgroups*. The severity of the injury is indicated in the diagram in Fig. 8.1. Setting out the ordinal reasoning behind the classification, the authors stated: "In the classification the nine groups are organized in order of increasing sever-

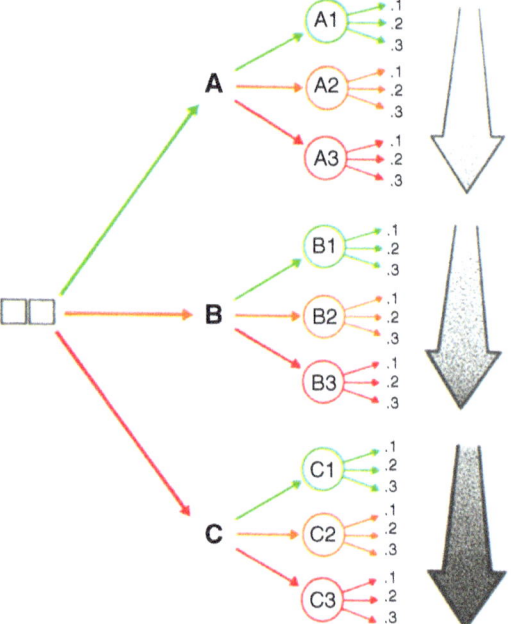

Fig. 8.1 The general principle for classification of long bone fractures. The categories are ordered according to increasing severity [8]. (With permission from Springer Nature)

ity, based on their morphological complexity, the difficulty of treatment and their prognosis. The order of the colors green, orange and red, as well as the increasing darkness of the arrows, indicate the increasing severity" [8].

The AO system classifies long bone fractures according to a generic classification and aims at a standard description for all fractures of the human skeleton. However, it became clear that certain anatomical regions, among them the proximal humerus, required unique and specific descriptions. Some aspects of the generic classification remained, such as the hierarchic triads. As discussed in Chap. 10, introducing advanced imaging technologies like CT, three-dimensional CT, and three-dimensional printing models has resulted in new descriptions and classifications.

The AO classification was developed in the context of fracture management utilizing osteosynthesis. The classification focuses on varus and valgus malalignment, impaction, and metaphyseal comminution, highlighting the expected difficulties of open reduction and internal fixation. In joint replacement, fixation of the tuberosities to the humeral stem is a major concern for postoperative function, and the involvement of the tuberosities is included in the classification. In classifying shoulder fractures, several treatment options may be relevant for a specific category: for example, open reduction and internal fixation or non-surgical treatment in displaced surgical neck fractures. On the other hand, a particular treatment option can be relevant for several categories: non-surgical treatment of two-, three-, and four-part fractures in older people, for example. Some categories only apply to specific surgical practices. Adopting evidence-based practices can necessitate modifications to the classification systems.

The alphanumerical construction of the AO classification with 27 subgroups translated into a five-digit code appears logically satisfactory in data collection, audit, and research but needs an abbreviation for clinical use. Developing a fracture classification that can be used for clinical decision-making and research purposes is challenging. The AO classification system is often simplified to nine groups or three types. This results in losing information from a research perspective and makes comparisons between studies questionable (Chap. 10). Therefore, it has been suggested that every fracture should be classified into two separate systems: one for clinical use and one for research. However, this approach may represent an obstacle for clinicians in performing clinical research.

8.5 Telling a Fracture

A fracture classification system should facilitate communication between clinicians, researchers, and administrators. However, striking a balance between providing detailed information for research purposes, enabling effective communication between clinicians, and supporting the extraction of data for clinical audit or reimbursement are challenging. In this section, I will discuss some didactic aspects of fracture communication.

New residents unfamiliar with the classifications given in textbooks usually learn about them in a clinical setting, where, typically, imaging material is presented during the morning rounds and a senior surgeon decides whether to operate on the patient based on their clinical experience. Afterward, a fracture category is assigned to the radiograph to justify the treatment decision and further guide the treatment and prognostics. Although textbooks and platforms recommended for residents are organized according to fracture categories, treatment decisions are not. Classifications developed to guide treatments are often used to justify a direction already taken. Applying a specific category to a case is a dynamic process that includes, among many factors, the experience and capability of the surgeon, as well as personal preferences, traditions, hardware availability, costs, and industry recommendations. Consider two examples of clinical reasoning with subsequent classification:

Example 1: "This fracture needs a prosthesis. It is severely displaced, and the bone quality is poor. I think it is a four-part fracture."

Example 2: "This is a perfect case for a locking plate. The fracture is unstable. The humeral head is intact, but there is metaphyseal comminution. It is an A3.3. Do we have the long plates in stock and a backup if conversion to a prosthesis is needed? I suspect several fracture lines extending to the humeral head. We may find a head-split."

In a culture of acting, the immediate assignment of a procedure to a radiograph is appreciated. However, the value of senior surgeons' prompt and confident statements about when a shoulder fracture *needs* surgery can be questioned. Current practice often overlooks that most displaced proximal humerus fractures can be treated non-surgically—but this decision requires knowledge of the last decade of clinical research. Surgeons unfamiliar with this evidence may rely on dogmas established half a century ago.

There is a risk of the patient getting lost in the classification. Important patient-related factors can disappear in our attempts to capture all information in an image-based classification. Focusing solely on radiographic appearance and assigning an implant based on a radiographic pattern may not benefit the patient. Recent evidence is often neglected, and patient-related factors, including treatment preferences, are frequently overlooked. In most patients with shoulder fractures, the treatment can wait to allow for shared decision-making in an outpatient setting after 1–2 weeks, when pain has diminished and the patient is ready to receive information about the benefits and harms of the treatment options. At this point, classification can be a valuable tool for treatment planning, whether surgical or non-surgical. Few shoulder fractures need acute intervention, with fracture-dislocations being the most prominent example.

8.6 Philosophical Considerations

Indications for surgery drift with the ever-changing preferences for procedures and implants. This drifting may challenge the assumption of fractures ordered in static categories. For example, the group of fractures *not amenable to surgery* rapidly decreased with the introduction of locking plate technology. Moving from non-locking to locking plates can hardly be ascribed to changes in the properties of the fractures. The similarities and differences in fracture classifications are bound to human abilities in handling morbid phenomena.

Does a classification category have a distinct underlying *natural history*, and how can we determine a match? On his classification, Neer stated in 2002: "A system has scientific validity if the categories within it have their own unique natural history, prognosis, and treatment requirements" [9].

How can we identify a mismatch when a classification is not working? The discussion can be interpreted as a variant of the discussion on *taxonomic realism* regarding morbid phenomena. Does classification of morbid phenomena (in our case, fractures) seek to arrive at distinct entities (natural kinds) that exist regardless of our attempts to capture and classify them? If it does, a classification can be more or less accurate in pointing out any preexisting categories. This position conflicts with the dynamic view on classification as formed by changing surgical communities set out above. It may also clash with arbitrarily set distinctions like converting continuous data (displacement) into binary categories (displaced versus minimally displaced).

Constructivist medical philosophers have questioned the claim that classifications are static and ahistorical. The Polish microbiologist and philosopher of medicine Ludwik Fleck (1896–1961) proposed that we should understand medical taxonomy as a sociocultural phenomenon belonging to a certain period, determining the selective attention and omissions necessary to establish categories [10]. From a constructivist perspective, it is not meaningful to debate whether classifications possess *true* categories with a distinct natural history. As the categories that make up a classification cannot be validated through observation and experimentation, they are better understood by comprehending their historical and sociocultural preconditions. I have argued elsewhere that Fleck was convinced that it was possible to arrive at entirely different classifications based on morbid phenomena [11, 12].

Fracture classifications are shaped by their sociocultural context. But the constructivist position becomes rather radical when applied to classifying broken bones. Our experience and intuitions strongly support the idea that broken bones exist. Although the surgical neck is not a well-defined anatomical landmark, we agree that this is the most common fracture site. It is not a social construct that hits patients who suffer a shoulder fracture—but both their experience and the caregivers' perceptions are tied to a certain context. Irrespective of the circumstances, a patient undergoing surgery based on a classification assignment will experience the result of distinct binary decision-making and the process of an irreversible surgical procedure. A balanced perspective could acknowledge that some unknown categories may exist regardless of our perception or interpretation. However, it is challenging to differentiate between failures due to violating underlying categories and errors caused by observer variability, measurement errors, or other properties bound to the classification system.

8.7 Perspectives

The connection between classification categories and treatment options is dynamic and bound to a particular surgical tradition. Although changes in classification are often linked to changes in treatment options, this does not necessarily guarantee the classification's relevance for the clinical outcome. Identifying pathoanatomical details relevant to operative planning of locking plate osteosynthesis seems less important if locking plates are not superior to non-surgical treatment, or even harmful. The increasing involvement of patient-related factors in clinical decision-making may also diminish the impact of classification as a tool for clinical decision-making. For decades, it was assumed in orthopedic practice that treatment decisions could be meaningfully made exclusively from imaging material. In such a setting, the choice of classification category played a pivotal role. In more recent orthopedic practice, numerous patient and surgeon-related factors are included in the treatment decision.

Implementing evidence-based guidelines for treating shoulder fractures is expected to reduce the number of surgeries required. Consequently, there may be a greater emphasis on identifying the specific categories where surgery is still justified and categorizing cases with different prognoses following non-surgical treatments. The development of new imaging techniques and models should be calibrated with the clinical need for classification, and they should demonstrate value for decision-making and patient outcome before implementation. Imaging-based fracture classification is insufficient for high-quality clinical decision-making because it neglects important patient-related factors, including osteoporosis, comorbidity, history of falls, smoking, sarcopenia, and other factors essential for bone healing and rehabilitation. A decision-making process based solely on imaging fails to integrate the three crucial elements of evidence-based practice: the best evidence, clinical expertise, and patient preferences [13].

References

1. Lonie IM. Cos versus Cnidus and the historians: part I. Hist Sci. 1978;16(1):42–75.
2. Hippocrates. Prognostic. Regimen in acute diseases. The sacred disease. The Art. Breaths. Law. Decorum. Physician. Dentition. Loeb Classical Library. Jones WHS, translator. Cambridge, MA: Harvard University Press; 1923. Available from: https://www.loebclassics.com/view/LCL148/1923/volume.xml.
3. Thudichum L. Ueber die am oberen Ende des Humerus vorkommenden Knochenbrüche. Giessen: J. Ricker'sche Buchhandlung; 1851. Available from: https://wellcomecollection.org/works/ebjjuvsd.
4. Kocher ET. Beiträge zur Kenntniss einiger praktisch wichtiger Fracturformen. Basel: Carl Sallmann; 1896. Available from: https://wellcomecollection.org/works/mkh547es.
5. Röntgen WC. On a new kind of rays. Science. 1896;3(59):227–31.
6. Brorson S. Proximal humeral fractures. In: Court-Brown C, McQueen MM, Swiontkowski MF, Ring D, Friedman SM, Duckworth A, editors. Musculoskeletal

trauma in the elderly. Boca Raton: Taylor & Francis Group; 2017. p. 257–71.
7. Neer CS. Displaced proximal humeral fractures. I. Classification and evaluation. J Bone Joint Surg Am. 1970;52(6):1077–89.
8. Müller ME, Koch P, Nazarian S, Schatzker J. Principles of the classification of fractures. In: The comprehensive classification of fractures of long bones. Berlin, Heidelberg: Springer; 1990. p. 4–7. Available from: http://link.springer.com/10.1007/978-3-642-61261-9_2.
9. Neer CS. Four-segment classification of proximal humeral fractures: purpose and reliable use. J Shoulder Elb Surg. 2002;11(4):389–400.
10. Fleck L. Genesis and development of a scientific fact. Chicago: University of Chicago Press; 1979.
11. Brorson S. Ludwik Fleck on proto-ideas in medicine. Med Health Care Philos. 2000;3(2):147–52. Available from: https://link.springer.com/article/10.1023/A:1009943420053.
12. Brorson S, Andersen H. Stabilizing and changing phenomenal worlds: Ludwik Fleck and Thomas Kuhn on scientific literature. J Gen Philos Sci. 2001;32(1):109–29. Available from: https://link.springer.com/article/10.1023/A:1011236713841.
13. Sackett DL. Evidence-based medicine and treatment choices. Lancet. 1997;349:570.

Open Access This chapter is licensed under the terms of the Creative Commons Attribution 4.0 International License (http://creativecommons.org/licenses/by/4.0/), which permits use, sharing, adaptation, distribution and reproduction in any medium or format, as long as you give appropriate credit to the original author(s) and the source, provide a link to the Creative Commons license and indicate if changes were made.

The images or other third party material in this chapter are included in the chapter's Creative Commons license, unless indicated otherwise in a credit line to the material. If material is not included in the chapter's Creative Commons license and your intended use is not permitted by statutory regulation or exceeds the permitted use, you will need to obtain permission directly from the copyright holder.

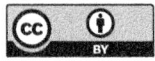

Imaging-Based Shoulder Fracture Classification Systems

9.1 Introduction

Fracture classification systems are closely tied to a specific period and represent the interests and capabilities of the orthopedic community of their time. In the case of shoulder fractures, several classification systems have been developed in an attempt to create a comprehensive and *definitive* classification that surpasses all previous systems. We have learned from orthopedic history that this is unlikely to be achieved. However, some classification systems are more useful in clinical practice and research. This chapter discusses the two most commonly used classification systems, the Neer classification and the AO classification, within their historical contexts and outlines the main concerns associated with these classifications.

9.2 Historical Context

In the 1940s, a notable shift in focus occurred when prominent surgeons began questioning the relevance of anatomical classification to the mechanism of injury. They suggested classifications that directly linked the trauma mechanism to the radiographic appearance. Ernst Dehne (1905–1983) proposed an etiological classification that included three mechanisms of injury, namely, *lateral*, *dorsal*, and *central*, linking the mechanism of injury to pathoanatomy, radiographic appearance, and clinical properties [1].

The mechanisms, thought to have distinct clinical implications, were diagnosed through specified radiographic views. Dehne argued that the anatomical classifications were limited because the cleavage line did not align with the anatomical landmarks. He proposed that cleavage lines were determined by the direction of the traumatizing force, thus permitting a more accurate classification [2]. Reginald Watson-Jones (1902–1972) took this concept further, suggesting that the mechanism of injury could be inferred from the radiographic appearance. Consequently, he believed that anatomical classification had limited value in determining treatment for surgical neck fractures: "The customary subdivision of fractures of the neck of the humerus … bears no relationship to the mechanism on injury, and is of no value in determining treatment" [3]. Watson-Jones distinguished three varieties of surgical neck fractures: *contusion crack fractures*, *impacted adduction fractures*, and *impacted abduction fractures*.

Fig. 9.1 A chest-arm plaster applied with the shoulder in 60° of flexion to counter angular deformity caused by anterior translation of the humeral shaft [4]. (With permission from VISDA)

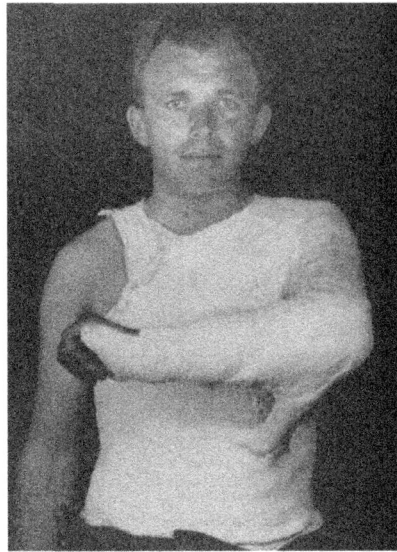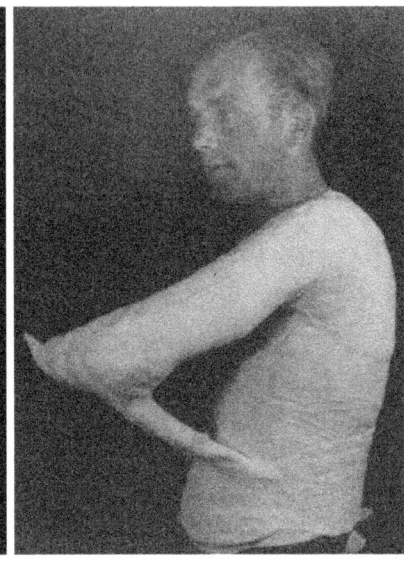

At that time, the treatment options included non-surgical treatment, closed reduction, intramedullary nail, or arthrodesis. Ingenious immobilization regimens were developed to counter the mechanism of injury (Fig. 9.1).

Other classifications directly associated fracture morphology with the direction of the fall [5].

Charles Neer (1917–2011) entered the scholarly discussion on shoulder fracture classification in 1953 by reporting 20 fracture-dislocations treated at the Columbia-Presbyterian Medical Center in New York between 1929 and 1952. He realized that the terminology was unclear, with poorly defined terms like *fracture subluxation*, *abduction fracture-dislocation*, and *fracture with dislocation of the shaft*. He aimed to correlate terminology and pathology before going on to the details of treatment and results [6]. Neer adopted the four anatomical parts defined by Codman to account for the muscular forces acting on the fracture. He explained Codman's framework for the mechanism of injury, where the humeral head was locked in a pivotal position against the acromion (Chap. 7). Depending on the inflicting force and the quality of the bone, this mechanism led to a surgical neck fracture, a simple dislocation, or a fracture-dislocation. He also added that a substantial number of fractures might have been dislocated but spontaneously reduced, leaving a major soft tissue injury.

Neer found humeral head resection to be the best treatment for unimpacted fracture-dislocations. Alternatively, in cases with major injuries of the humeral head, he suggested that "a recently devised articular replacement currently being investigated" later known as the monoblock Neer hemiarthroplasty could be considered. Neer defined fracture-dislocations as fractures with the humeral neck outside the capsule. The dislocation could be anterior (subcoracoid) or posterior (subspinous). Anterior fracture-dislocations were further divided into impacted and unimpacted [6].

In 1955, Neer published a paper on the indications for using his newly designed hemiarthroplasty in fractures. He emphasized that replacement surgery was only indicated in cases where resection was needed intraoperatively. In acute cases, a replacement could be used in only three situations: "fracture dislocation with extrusion of the anatomic head; 'impression' fracture involving more than 50% of the articular surface; and 'head-splitting' fracture" [7].

Between 1953 and 1967, Neer gathered patient cases treated under anesthesia at his institution. He selected 300 cases with two radiographic views available (anterior-posterior and lateral) and correlated them with intraoperative findings. This process revealed distinct anatomical categories, leading to a new classification [8].

9.3 The First Neer Classification (1970)

Neer developed his classification system in response to the inadequacy of existing systems in identifying fractures that required specific treatment. Contemporary literature suffered from confused terminology and a lack of useful guidelines. Neer aimed to combine pathoanatomical patterns with biomechanics; most importantly, he introduced a definition of displacement. Displacement was present, he proposed, if there was more than 1 cm of displacement or 45° of angulation between two or more of Codman's four parts. Interestingly, the arbitrary definition of displacement was not part of Neer's original submission, being suggested by the editor of the *Journal of Bone and Joint Surgery* [9].

Previous anatomical classifications grouped fractures with different treatment requirements. With Neer, fractures were grouped based on displacement. He abandoned terms like *abduction fracture* and *adduction fracture* because different radiological configurations could be obtained by rotating the arm. The displacement criteria allowed all minimally displaced fractures to be grouped together regardless of the fracture lines. Thus, fractures were initially divided into *minimally displaced* and *displaced*.

Neer further considered the humeral head's vascular supply, the articular surface condition, and traction from the muscles attached to the parts. Neer defined six groups in 1970 [8] (horizontal rows I–VI in Fig. 9.2). Group I included all minimally displaced fractures, regardless of the fracture lines. Group II included displaced fractures of the anatomical neck. Group III included displaced fractures of the surgical neck, further divided into angulated, separated, or comminuted. Group IV consisted of displaced fractures of the greater tuberosity without or with a humeral neck fracture, resulting in two-part or three-part fractures. Group V consisted of displaced fractures of the lesser tuberosity with or without a humeral neck fracture, also resulting in two-part or three-part fractures. Groups IV and V merged into the displaced four-part fractures involving the humeral neck and both tuberosities. Group VI included fracture-dislocations further divided into anterior or posterior dislocations. Depending on the parts involved, they could appear as two-, three-, or four-part fractures. Group VI also included fractures of the articular surface, divided into impression or head-splitting fractures (Fig. 9.2).

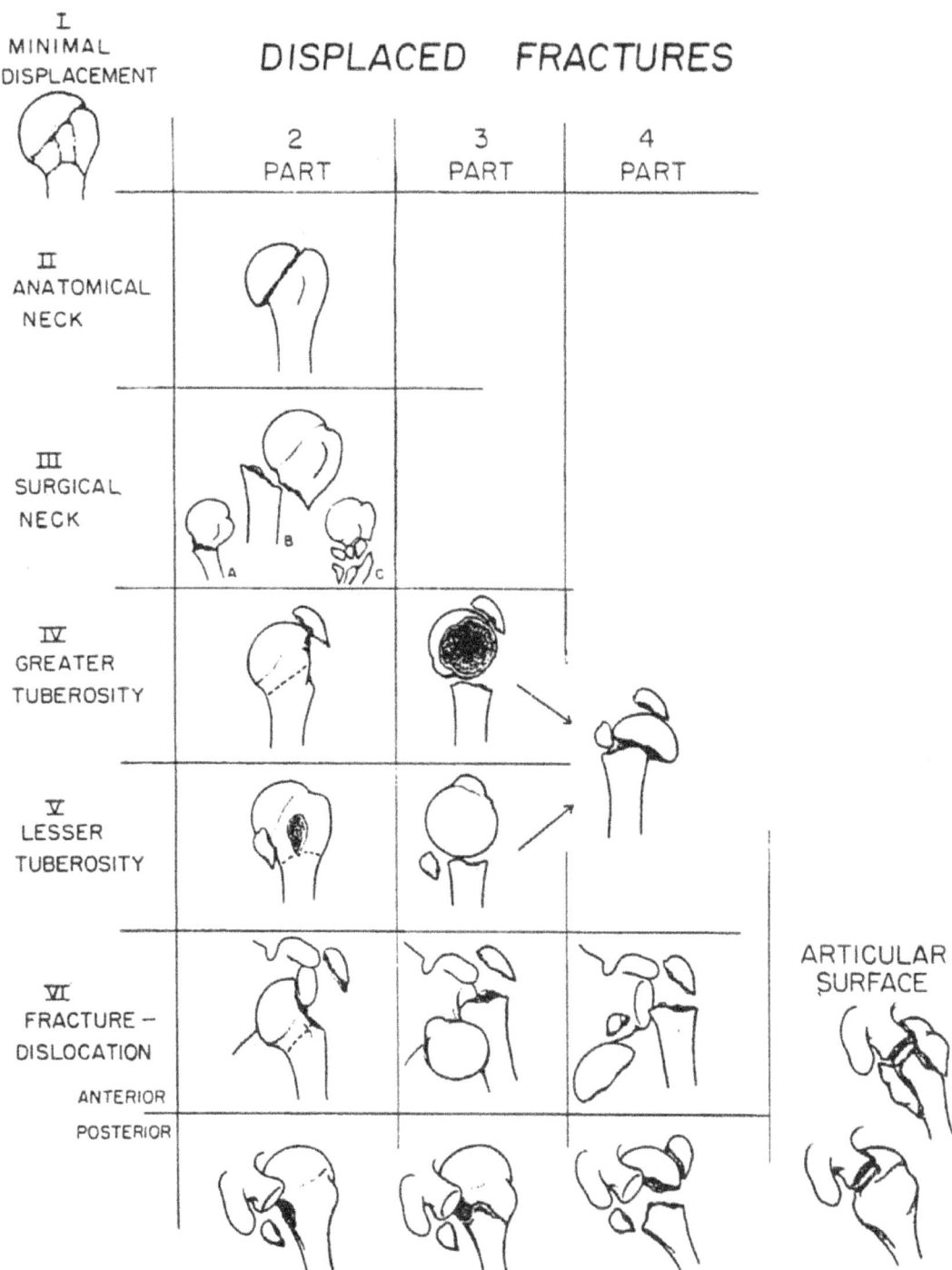

Fig. 9.2 The first Neer classification from 1970 [8]. The groups (Roman numbers) were removed from the classification in 1975 [10]. (With permission from Wolters Kluwer)

9.4 Early Criticism of the Neer Classification (1993)

The original Neer classification had some inherent weaknesses. First, the 16 main fracture patterns in the scheme were based on interpretations of anterior-posterior radiographs. Assessment of fracture angulation, however, includes lateral views. Second, whether the anatomical or surgical neck was involved in three- and four-part fractures was unclear. Third, the groups were not mutually exclusive, as four-part fractures could be classified as both group IV and V. Finally, the six groups were not logical and did not follow a prognostic order. For example, a displaced fracture of the anatomical neck (Group II) was expected to have a worse prognosis than a displaced surgical neck fracture (Group III) due to the risk of vascular compromise. In some cases, two-part anterior fracture-dislocations (Group VI) could be treated using closed methods and had a better prognosis than some four-part fractures (Group IV/V). Neer recognized the limitations of his grouping in his first classification system and simplified it in 1975 [10]. The six Roman numerals were removed, and the category definitions were restated to make the classification easier to understand and remember. In a personal communication, he later emphasized that the classification was not intended for simple reading of radiographs; "the 4-segment classification system has always used interpretative decision making to confirm the category of complex and borderline cases and has not been based on x-rays alone" (C.S. Neer, Personal correspondence with Stig Brorson, 8 May 2003).

It should be mentioned that *groups* have not been part of the Neer classification for 50 years. The continued use of Roman numerals and groups in clinical and research settings adds to the confusion.

A more substantial criticism of the Neer classification appeared in the *Journal of Bone and Joint Surgery* in 1993–1994. Two observer studies had been published demonstrating low agreement between and within observers using the Neer classification [11, 12]. An editorial by Albert H. Burstein raised concerns about the classification, questioning its reliability in guiding treatment and prognostication due to this lack of agreement [13]. The criticism of the Neer classification as a poor tool caused a backlash from the surgical community. Three senior shoulder surgeons argued that the lack of agreement may not always pose a clinical problem; not all fracture categories, they pointed out, were equally important, and therefore failing to distinguish between a two-part and a three-part fracture did not have the same clinical implications as failing to distinguish between a one-part fracture and a four-part fracture [14]. They argued that reliability was not the only measure of the clinical value of a classification, mentioning the delicate balance between a more comprehensive scheme allowing for greater prognostic stratification at the price of more variability. Interestingly, they stated that: "The Neer classification is designed to be somewhat arbitrary, leaving some room for discussion about different fracture patterns and their appropriate treatment" [14].

In his reply to Burstein's editorial, Charles Neer argued that the confusion had arisen due to the bad use of a good tool. He further stated that displacement was a continuum, and there would be situations where the actual condition of the humerus head could only be determined intraoperatively. For Neer and his colleagues, the lack of agreement rose from a want of experience: "However, as to those of us who actually treat these difficult displacements, surgeons who know the anatomy, muscle attachments, and blood supply of the shoulder can interpret the radiographs much better than inexperienced surgeons and most radiologists" [15].

The editor-in-chief backed Albert H. Burstein in replying that if only shoulder experts had the necessary skills to use the classification system, it would diminish its value to the point of uselessness [16].

9.5 Neer's Second Response to His Critics (2002)

In 2002, Neer published the review article "Four-Segment Classification of Proximal Humeral Fractures: Purpose and Reliable Use," summarizing over 30 years of experience with his classification. He addressed criticism, clarified the use of his classification, and made several adjustments to the categories [9]. He justified the scientific validity of the categories by referencing their unique natural history, prognosis, and treatment requirements. The anatomical accuracy was proven through clinical use and *direct observations* in the operating room. He explained inconsistencies in the use of the classification by attributing them to the quality of radiographs and inexperienced observers. It is not necessary to agree on the treatment, he stated; but if progress is to be made, we must agree on the pathoanatomy of the lesion. He maintained the 16 categories because "a classification causes confusion if there are too few or too many categories" [9].

He also mentioned the prognostic distinct subcategory of the *four-part valgus-impacted fracture* pattern described a few years earlier [17], explaining that four-part fractures represent a range of lateral displacement of the articular part of the humeral head, which is separated from the tuberosities and its blood supply. Therefore, the valgus-impacted four-part fracture was seen as a *borderline precursor* to the four-part fracture described in the 1970 classification system. The medial periosteum remains intact in this lesion, leaving the humeral head with a lesser risk of avascular necrosis. In Fig. 9.3, I have interpreted Neer's suggestion on a continuum of lateral displacement. The *four-part family* ranges from minimally displaced hairline fractures between the four anatomical parts to the four-part fracture-dislocation. Neer discussed whether the four-part fracture with lateral displacement should be classified as a fracture-dislocation or a four-part fracture. He stuck to the displaced four-part fracture. A prosthetic replacement was recommended if the head had lost its soft tissue attachments.

Neer further divided the two-part surgical neck fracture into three clinical types: impacted, unimpacted, and comminuted. Closed reduction with percutaneous pinning was the preferred treatment. He did not add to his previous explanation of observer disagreement and ascribed low agreement to inexperienced observers or poor quality of radiographs (C.S. Neer, Personal correspondence with Stig Brorson, 8 May 2003). Both assumptions were later questioned (Chap. 10).

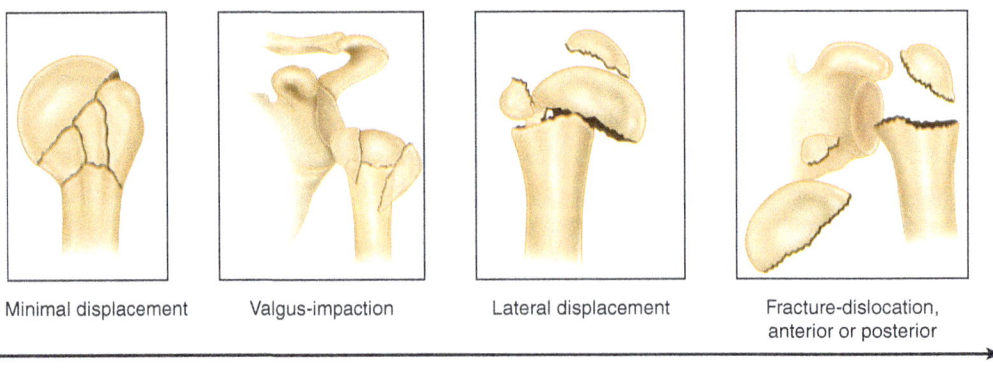

Fig. 9.3 The *four-part family* interpreted from Neer [9]. The categories can be considered as dividing a continuum of displacement into ordinal categories

9.6 The AO Classification System (1990, 2007, and 2018)

A globally accepted parallel to the Neer classification, the AO (Arbeitsgemeinschaft für Osteosynthesefragen) classification was published in French in 1987 [18]. The English version was first published in 1990 [19], with substantial revisions in 2007 [20] and 2018 [21]. The AO classification is a morphological classification that adapted specific pathoanatomical patterns of the proximal humerus to the general AO classification system, which provides standardized definitions for long bone fractures. Fractures of the proximal humerus can be divided into three *types*, with 9 *groups* and 27 *subgroups* (Fig. 9.4). Fractures are classified by combining the part of the bone with

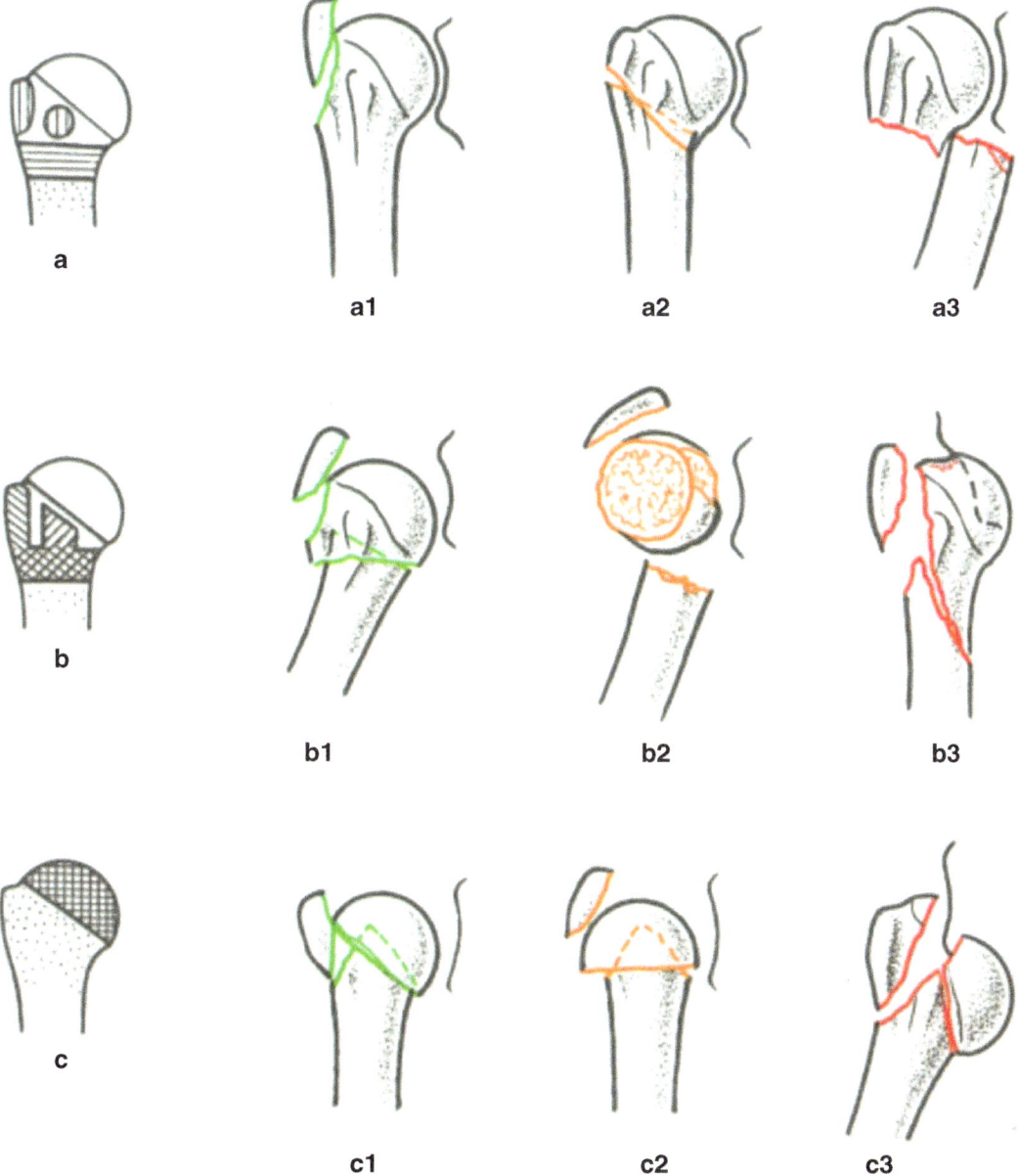

Fig. 9.4 The three types and nine groups of the proximal humerus, including the original description of the groups [19]. (With permission from Springer Nature)

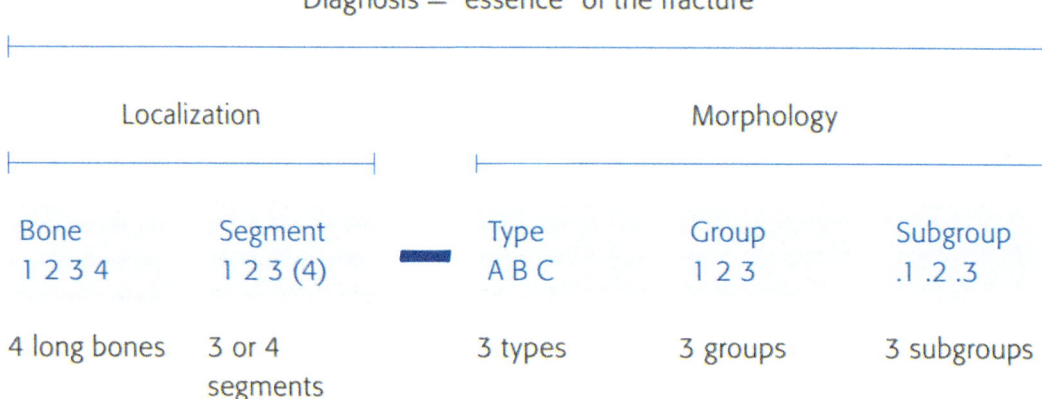

Fig. 9.5 The structure of the five-digit coding within the AO classification system [22]. (Copyright by AO Foundation, Switzerland. With permission)

the specific fracture morphology. The fracture patterns are divided into hierarchical triads. For each fracture, three questions must be answered: which type, which group, and which subgroup. Once these questions are answered, the fracture can be coded according to a five-digit alphanumeric system that includes the name of the bone, part of the bone, type, group, and subgroup. This system is illustrated in Fig. 9.5.

The AO classification was intended to be ordinal, at least at the group level: "In the classification, the 9 groups are organized in order of increasing severity, based on their morphological complexity, the difficulty of treatment, and their prognosis" [19].

The AO group originally developed the system to document cases of surgical treatment in a unified way, starting in 1958. The classification provided a standardized language aiming at translating any verbal description into a five-digit code ready for documentation and research, thus allowing for multicenter collaboration, retrospective assessment of treatment outcome, and complications.

The AO classification, planned to be revised every 10 years, was unique in its capacity to respond to both criticism and continuing clinical research. In 2018, the codes were reviewed for usage and accuracy. The intention was to include the Neer classification in the sense that the fracture designations *two-part*, *three-part*, and *four-part* were applied: "The Neer classification has been integrated into the fracture description for proximal humeral fractures to facilitate the clinician's comprehension of the terms unifocal and bifocal fractures" [21].

One important feature of the Neer classification, the displacement criteria, was explicitly excluded; however, it was considered to be too subjective and served to hinder consistent coding [23]. Displacement became a *universal modifier* but was not defined. The Neer parts were added to AO types A, B, and C. Some categories were removed because they were better described using modifiers and qualifications. This created gaps. The 2018 revision reduced the original 27 subgroup classification into 3 types, 6 groups, and 13 subgroups (Fig. 9.6). The missing categories were merged into other categories and replaced by *universal modifiers* and *qualifications*. Group A3 remained without subgroups.

The changes included in the 2018 revision were not validated because "the validation process was expensive and not practical, so a decision was made to not validate all edits" [23].

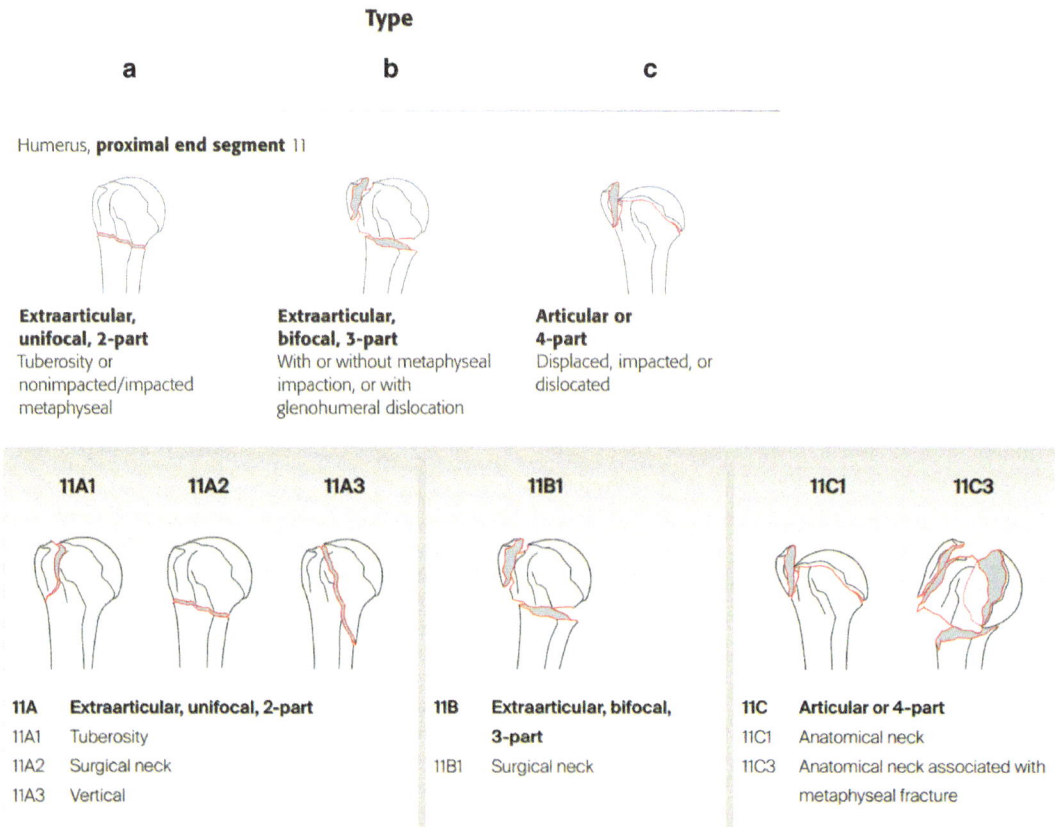

Fig. 9.6 The three types and six groups from the 2018 revision of the AO classification [23]. (Copyright by AO Foundation, Switzerland. With permission)

9.7 Criticism of the AO Classification System

The AO classification was developed and used within a surgical community for whom displaced long bone fractures should be reduced to anatomical position and fixed; in this regard, the shoulder was considered no different from the hip and the humerus no different from the femur. The classification was developed to support surgical decision-making and to predict the risk of challenges during osteosynthesis. The hierarchy of severity was based on the energy of injury and the complexity of treatment. This does not apply to shoulder fractures in older people, where severely displaced or even dislocated fractures can follow a simple fall from standing height.

The AO classification and the Neer classification have some similarities and shortcomings. Both systems try to organize nonhierarchical fracture patterns hierarchically. The AO classification aims to categorize fractures of four anatomical structures into triads. In clinical practice, the intended hierarchical structure may not always be applicable. For instance, while an A1 fracture may require surgery, A2 fractures can typically be treated non-surgically. Not all the numerous subgroups are in use, and not all categories guide treatment. Several categories not found in the Neer classification are present in the AO classification and vice versa (Chap. 10).

Unfortunately, neither classification has successfully demonstrated observer agreement at a clinically acceptable level, creating challenges for communication, coding, and documentation. Certain choices made during the AO five-digit coding process could result in errors being aggregated. It is currently unclear what the 2018 revision has added to clinical decision-making. The changes made to the classification system, including redefining, merging, and omitting categories, may have altered the psychometric properties of the system. Additionally, the clinical relevance of these categories needs to be demonstrated. It is important to note that validation after surgery does not necessarily validate the system for the majority of patients who can be treated without surgery. With a growing trend toward evidence-based and non-surgical approaches for shoulder fractures, the AO classification may need to be revised to better support the management of shoulder fractures in the future.

9.8 Perspectives

Charles Neer's classification reflects his assumptions that 85% of all proximal humerus fractures are minimally displaced, and displaced fractures should be operated. Both assumptions have been questioned (Chap. 2). While the categories in the Neer classification reflected the diagnostic and therapeutic options available at his time, Neer contributed substantially by rethinking previous pathoanatomical classifications and disregarding contemporary etiological classifications. He introduced a definition of displacement that allowed for capturing clinically relevant categories and proposing prognostic groups. The classification improved communication between clinical decision-makers and facilitated the collection and reporting of outcome data.

The main challenge with the Neer and AO classifications has been the lack of agreement within and between observers using them (Chap. 10). The Neer classification includes standard radiographic views in the decision process. The introduction of modern imaging technology such as three-dimensional CT scans has substantially increased the amount of data available for classification. This has not necessarily resulted in improved patient outcome. Most randomized trials on interventions for proximal humerus fractures are based on the Neer classification and exhibit both its advantages and disadvantages.

References

1. Dehne E. Fractures of the upper end of the humerus. A classification based on the etiology of the trauma. Surg Clin North Am. 1945;25:28–47.
2. Dehne E. Grundsätzliches über die Brüche des Oberarmkopfes. Arch Orthop Unfallchir. 1939;39(4):434–64.
3. Watson-Jones R. Fractures and joint injuries. 4th ed. Edinburgh/London: E & S Livingstone; 1955.
4. Madsen E. [Fractura colli humeri]. Nord Med. 1949;41(25):1097–100.
5. Razemon JP, Baux S. [Fractures and fracture-dislocations of the upper extremity of the humerus]. Rev Chir Orthop Reparatrice Appar Mot. 1969;55(5):387–496.
6. Neer CS, Brown TH, McLauglin HL. Fracture of the neck of the humerus with dislocation of the head fragment. Am J Surg. 1953;85(3):252–8.
7. Neer CS. Indications for replacement of the proximal humeral articulation. Am J Surg. 1955;89(4):901–7.
8. Neer CS. Displaced proximal humeral fractures. I. Classification and evaluation. J Bone Joint Surg Am. 1970;52(6):1077–89.
9. Neer CS. Four-segment classification of proximal humeral fractures: purpose and reliable use. J Shoulder Elb Surg. 2002;11(4):389–400.
10. Neer CS. The four-segment classification of displaced proximal humeral fractures. Instr Course Lect Am Acad Orthop Surg. 1975;24:160–8.
11. Siebenrock KA, Gerber C. The reproducibility of classification of fractures of the proximal end of the humerus. J Bone Joint Surg Am. 1993;75(12):1751–5.
12. Sidor ML, Zuckerman JD, Lyon T, Koval K, Cuomo F, Schoenberg N. The Neer classification system for proximal humeral fractures. An assessment of interobserver reliability and intraobserver reproducibility. J Bone Joint Surg Am. 1993;75(12):1745–50.
13. Burstein AH. Fracture classification systems: do they work and are they useful? J Bone Joint Surg Am. 1993;75(12):1743–4.
14. Bigliani LU, Flatow EL, Pollock R. Correspondence. J Bone Joint Surg Am. 1994;76-A(5):791–2.
15. Neer CS. Correspondence. J Bone Joint Surg Am. 1994;76-A(5):789.
16. Cowell HR. Patient care and scientific freedom. J Bone Joint Surg Am. 1994;76(5):640–1.
17. Jakob RP, Miniaci A, Anson PS, Jaberg H, Osterwalder A, Ganz R. Four-part valgus impacted fractures of the proximal humerus. J Bone Joint Surg Br. 1991;73(2):295–8.
18. Müller ME, Nazarian SKP. Classification AO des fractures: les os longs. Berlin: Springer; 1987.

References

19. Müller ME, Koch P, Nazarian S, Schatzker J. Principles of the classification of fractures. In: The comprehensive classification of fractures of long bones. Berlin, Heidelberg: Springer; 1990. p. 4–7. Available from: http://link.springer.com/10.1007/978-3-642-61261-9_2.
20. Marsh JL, Slongo TF, Agel J, Broderick JS, Creevey W, DeCoster TA, et al. Fracture and dislocation classification compendium – 2007: Orthopaedic Trauma Association classification, database and outcomes committee. J Orthop Trauma. 2007;21(10 Suppl):S1–S133. Available from: https://journals.lww.com/jorthotrauma/abstract/2007/11101/fracture_and_dislocation_classification_compendium.1.aspx.
21. Meinberg EG, Agel J, Roberts CS, Karam MD, Kellam JF. Fracture and dislocation classification compendium – 2018. J Orthop Trauma. 2018;32(Suppl 1):S1–S170. Available from: https://journals.lww.com/jorthotrauma/fulltext/2018/01001/fracture_and_dislocation_classification.1.aspx.
22. AO Foundation. Müller AO classification of fractures – long bones. 2010. Available from: https://www.akot.com.ar/especialidad/files/mueller_ao_class.pdf.
23. AO Trauma. AO/OTA fracture and dislocation classification compendium. 2018 Revisions. Available from: https://www.aofoundation.org/trauma/clinical-library-and-tools/journals-and-publications/classification.

Open Access This chapter is licensed under the terms of the Creative Commons Attribution 4.0 International License (http://creativecommons.org/licenses/by/4.0/), which permits use, sharing, adaptation, distribution and reproduction in any medium or format, as long as you give appropriate credit to the original author(s) and the source, provide a link to the Creative Commons license and indicate if changes were made.

The images or other third party material in this chapter are included in the chapter's Creative Commons license, unless indicated otherwise in a credit line to the material. If material is not included in the chapter's Creative Commons license and your intended use is not permitted by statutory regulation or exceeds the permitted use, you will need to obtain permission directly from the copyright holder.

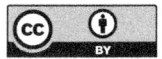

Why Do We Disagree When Classifying Shoulder Fractures?

10.1 Introduction

Poor observer agreement on radiology-based classifications of shoulder fractures has been known and discussed for nearly a century. In this quote from JAMA in 1932, the American surgeon Sumner M. Roberts highlighted the challenge of consistently interpreting shoulder radiographs:

> Doubtless, many who reviewed our series of roentgenograms would shift some of the cases from one group to another. Many of these fractures are comminuted in type, and even with the best of roentgenograms, it is a matter of personal opinion just where the fracture lines run and which are the primary ones. [1]

Without a gold standard to determine the accuracy of fracture classification, *observer agreement* may serve as an indirect measure. If two observers classify the same fracture differently, they cannot both be right. Two observers can, however, very well agree on something wrong. Numerous papers on the agreement between and within observers using the Neer and AO classifications have been published. Most reports have shown disappointing results and questioned the value of classifications in clinical practice and research. In Chap. 9, I focused on obstacles to using fracture classification systems. In this chapter, I will review the landscape of observer studies, comment on some of the cognitive processes involved in determining a classification category, and suggest which stages of the processes are prone to errors. Although observer studies of fracture classification systems have grown in number, the impact of poor observer agreement on clinical decisions and patient outcome remains little studied.

10.2 Classification in Everyday Clinic

Before focusing on the agreement on fracture classification systems, I will briefly consider their role in everyday clinical decision-making. While the organization may vary by institution, there are common traits. Imagine attending the morning rounds in a large orthopedic department. The team on duty presents the patients admitted, and treatment plans are determined. The radiographs are reviewed, and the senior surgeon summarizes: "This fracture is a comminuted fracture of the proximal humerus. It requires a prosthesis. Let's prepare the OR for replacement surgery and check if the 12-millimeter fracture stems are in stock. We have a surgeon who can fix it tomorrow."

In this case, the clinical decision does not involve considerations of classification categories.

The following case has a different radiographic fracture pattern. Again, the senior consultant surgeon's treatment plan is stated after a review of the radiographs: "This fracture fits perfectly to a locking plate. Without surgery, the fracture will never heal. This is a standard case for the trauma guys. Let's schedule the case for osteosynthesis."

Do we need a classification to arrive at surgical decisions? Many decisions and surgeries on shoulder fractures are performed without formal classification, even in preoperative planning.

Imagine two surgeons in conversation in the coffee room before the operation: "This is a comminuted fracture in a young person. Let's go for an osteosynthesis. The clinically most important part of the fracture complex is the greater tuberosity. It appears that the greater tuberosity is displaced posteriorly. To get optimal access, we can approach the tuberosity through a deltoid split."

In these examples, the decision-making process is not dependent on classification. Often, the description of the fracture pathoanatomy is not provided until the postoperative note. We do not entirely understand the direction of our clinical reasoning, but the examples demonstrate that important decisions are made from radiology-based pattern recognition rather than classification categories.

As clinicians (and as human beings), we rely heavily on pattern recognition to make decisions. The clinical experience and training, personal preferences, and the preferences of the surgical community inform clinical decisions. Evidence is not always considered when making initial decisions unless the decision-maker has up-to-date knowledge in the relevant field. Few shoulder fractures require immediate action, however allowing time to reflect and incorporate updated evidence.

Observer agreement depends on the observers' ability to master the assessments required to differentiate between categories. The process of reading and classifying fractures can be divided into two phases. First, the radiographs are interpreted to form a three-dimensional mental image of the fracture. Second, the three-dimensional image is translated into a category. It is unclear at which point the agreement is lost. Charles Neer underlined that a mental image of the fracture pattern should be created before arriving at a category:

The 4-segment classification is not meant to be a numerical classification that is oversimplified or patterned for easy roentgen classification, but rather is a "concept" or mental picture of the actual pathomechanics and pathoanatomy of displaced humeral fractures and the terminology to identify each category. [2]

The Neer and AO classifications involve transforming continuous data into binary data during the classification process. In the Neer classification, displacement is first transformed into *minimally displaced* or *displaced.* There will inevitably be measurement errors and borderline cases. Minor differences in the placement of the cursor or goniometer or a slight rotation of the patient's arm could lead to a change in classification. It is unlikely that new classifications involving displacement will solve this problem. Furthermore, conducting several assessments increases the risk of magnifying errors.

Studies on the stepwise classification process have been conducted for lower extremity fractures. An observer study on tibial plafond fractures revealed that the agreement on the adequacy of radiographs was lower than the agreement on fracture classification. Having observers mark articular fragments did not affect interobserver agreement. However, pre-marking the articular fragments improved agreement on the classification [3].

Recently, printed, handheld three-dimensional models have been accessible to clinicians for surgical planning and teaching. It has been suggested that models of proximal humerus fractures could improve agreement among residents and attending surgeons [4, 5]. Theoretically, these models could help the cognitive process of translating two-dimensional images into a three-dimensional fracture pattern. However, there are conflicting reports on whether this is effective [6].

10.3 Measures of Agreement

Most studies of the Neer and AO classifications use *Cohen's kappa*, *Cohen's weighted kappa*, or *intraclass correlation coefficient* to report the level of agreement [7]. The intraclass correlation coefficient is used in continuous data: displacement measured in millimeters, for example. Kappa is a measure of agreement between paired observations of categorical data, such as two observers classifying the same fracture or the same fracture classified by the same observer on two occasions. Kappa statistics (κ) adjust the observed agreement (p_0) for the expected agreement by chance (p_e):

$$\kappa = \frac{p_0 - p_e}{1 - p_e}$$

Kappa ranges from 1 (perfect agreement) to −1 (perfect disagreement) via 0 (agreement by chance). In binary categories, such as minimally displaced versus displaced, a kappa value of 0 indicates the agreement expected by chance (tossing a coin). A kappa value of 0.5 means the agreement is halfway between tossing a coin and perfect agreement. When dealing with ordinal data, where the level of severity increases with higher categories, assigning weights to kappa can help account for the differences between the categories. For instance, the distance between a two-part surgical neck fracture and a three-part greater tuberosity fracture is smaller than between a minimally displaced fracture and a four-part fracture-dislocation. The interpretation of weighted kappa presupposes reporting the assigned weights. Kappa statistics can handle most classification categories. Exceptions are very rare categories where a lesser kappa can be expected.

Numerous qualitative interpretations of kappa have been used, leading to potential inconsistency in reporting measures of agreement. Therefore, comparisons of interpretations should be approached cautiously [8]. Below, I refer to the interpretation of kappa for observer agreement by Landis and Koch: ≥ 0.81, almost perfect; 0.61–0.80, substantial; 0.41–0.60, moderate; 0.21–0.40, fair; ≤ 0.2, slight agreement [9].

10.4 An Introduction to Observer Studies

Observer studies provide information about the inherent error in a classification system. The degree of agreement between different ratings determines the validity of the results obtained using the classification system. This agreement is a measure of the quality of the measurement and depends on various factors, such as the cases (typically imaging material) and the observers (usually doctors or other decision-makers).

Interobserver agreement refers to the level of agreement between different observers assessing the same case; conversely, *intraobserver agreement* refers to the level of agreement within an observer evaluating the same case at different times. The agreement is not a fixed property of a classification system but, rather, of an interaction between the case, the observer, and the classification system [7]. The agreement depends on the context, which includes the quality and quantity of images, the sampling of cases, the distribution of fractures, the experience of the observers, the number of categories and cases, and the modifications made to the classification system. While numerous observer studies have been conducted on the Neer and the AO classifications, comparisons across studies should be made with caution due to the potential confounding of the estimates [10].

Studies of fracture classification systems differ from studies of diagnostic tests in that they lack a *gold standard* against which to measure. In classification-based intervention studies, a proxy for a gold standard, such as more advanced imaging, senior surgeon classification, radiologist assessment, consensus classification, or intraoperative classification, is often used. However, even intraoperative classification may change during the handling of the patient and tissue. Due to the lack of a gold standard, the *specificity* and *sensitivity* of the categorizations do not apply. The *true* fracture pattern remains unknown to the observer.

10.5 The Landscape of Observer Studies

Studies on the classification of shoulder fractures first emerged in the late 1980s [11, 12]. The studies can be categorized into four groups: those focused on proposing and testing new classifications, those examining modifications of existing classifications, those investigating the impact of imaging material, and those investigating interventions on observers to improve agreement.

Several new classification systems for shoulder fractures have been proposed. Some of these systems have been validated in observer studies, including Duparc [13, 14], AST [15], Edelson [16], Carrera [17], Codman/Hertel/HGLS [18, 19], Resch [20, 21], and Mayo-FJD [22]. In general, these new classifications show good performance in the hands of those who created them, possibly due to their familiarity with the classification principles or to bias. Other studies have modified existing classification systems and tested the agreement. However, reducing the number of Neer categories into 13 [23], 6 [24], 5 [12, 25], 4 [26], or 2 categories [27, 28] has not resulted in a markedly improved agreement between observers. Various subgroup analyses have been conducted, including the binary distinction of minimally displaced versus displaced fractures [29] and for two-part fractures [28] or four-part fractures [30] against all other categories. An observer study compared the agreement on the revised AO classification from 2018 (13 categories) with the AO classification from 2007 (27 categories) and reported an increased agreement in the latest version. The agreement on the *universal modifiers* and *qualifications* was not tested, and the challenging assessment of displacement was not addressed [31].

A considerable number of observer studies have been conducted in the hope of improving agreement through the addition of high-quality radiographs [32], two-dimensional CT scans [33], three-dimensional CT scans [34–40], and digital measurement tools [41]. Conflicting results have been reported, most with fair, slight, or moderate agreement. One study reported an increased rate of surgery when three-dimensional CT scans were used [42]. It is worth noting that although adding three-dimensional CT scans does not improve the agreement among observers, they may still be helpful for preoperative planning. However, the routine use of advanced imaging modalities in geriatric shoulder fractures should be revisited, except for the few patients considered for surgery. The amount of data rapidly increases—but we have no reason to believe that this leads to better clinical decisions regarding improved patient outcomes. No imaging modality, no matter how advanced, can replace the consideration of patient-related factors or, most importantly, patient involvement in the clinical decision-making process.

Several studies have examined the effect of training on improving observer agreement when classifying shoulder fractures. In a randomized trial, 185 observers were assigned to an online or no training module [27]. The observers were trained to distinguish between fractures involving the anatomical neck and those involving the surgical neck. However, the agreement among observers was only fair to poor in both groups, with no statistically significant improvement after training. As a result, the authors concluded that simplifying classifications and training observers did not lead to an improvement in the interobserver reliability for the diagnosis of proximal humerus fractures.

A study aimed to identify the reasons for disagreement in the classification of shoulder fractures. Three observers were asked to examine plain radiographs and CT scans to identify fracture lines and displacement and recommend treatments. Following a discussion, ten learning points were defined and implemented, slightly improving agreement [43].

In a randomized trial, my colleagues and I randomized 14 orthopedic doctors to either two training sessions in the Neer classification or no training [44]. The training used text and images from Neer's original papers [45, 46], and the observers classified plain radiographs in two sessions, 2 weeks apart. We reported a statistically and clinically significant improvement in interobserver agreement, particularly in the specialist group, where mean kappa improved from 0.30 to

0.79. While this study suggested that training can improve agreement, it also raised questions about the value of a classification system that requires repeated training of specialists to achieve an acceptable level of agreement.

Interestingly, there seems to be a tendency to overestimate the severity of fractures in observers without training. In a secondary analysis of our randomized training study [30], the *prevalence* of four-part fractures in the study sample decreased from 10% to 2% after training. In most cases, the original diagnosis of a four-part fracture was changed to a two-part fracture, indicating that assessing fracture displacement in the tuberosities was challenging without experience. We also found an increase in the detection of minimally displaced fractures after training.

Charles Neer remained convinced that observer variation was due to a lack of experience. In a comment on our training study [44], he wrote: "I consider your work to be very important because while other reliability studies have shown that interpretation without knowledge confuses the results and introduces inconsistency, your work has gone on to show that training of the interpreters markedly improves the above" (C.S. Neer, Personal correspondence with Stig Brorson, 8 May 2003).

10.6 Limitations of Observer Studies

Considering the population of observers and cases before comparing kappa values is important. As a measure of agreement, kappa is tied to a certain population of observers and cases. To compare kappa values, the marginal distribution of the categories must be comparable. This means that kappa values from populations with a high prevalence of displaced fractures cannot be compared to those from populations with a low prevalence of displaced fractures. Suppose the prevalence of a category is very high or very low. In these cases, the kappa value will decrease, making interpreting values for categories such as anatomical neck fractures or posterior fracture-dislocations challenging. In addition, kappa does not account for the *prognostic distance* between categories. While weighted kappa can help with this, the weights used are not always specified, and assigning different weights to categories could make comparisons between studies difficult. The number of observers also influences kappa. As the number of observers increases, standard error decreases, and kappa stabilizes on a mean value [47], making the comparison of studies with markedly different numbers of observers difficult.

In experimental settings, images are often selected to optimize the data provided for the observers. Observer agreement may be overestimated if the image material does not mimic the clinical setting. Observer studies commonly involve observers with a particular interest in shoulder fractures. This can result in overestimating agreement, and the findings cannot be generalized to a standard situation.

The agreement on classification can differ at various classification levels, such as Neer parts or AO types, groups, or subgroups. A more straightforward classification is generally used for patient management. In the emergency room, the decision-making is often binary. In cases of minimally displaced fractures, the patient is discharged, while a more experienced doctor will reassess displaced fractures. In such cases, the final decision is not in the young doctor's hands.

10.7 What Are the Clinical Implications of Disagreement on Classification?

Answering this question requires empirical investigation through prospective studies that test individual factors involved in clinical decision-making and their consequences for patient outcome. While there are currently few such studies, we do have some indications of which factors can influence clinical decision-making beyond the classification category. Disagreement on classification does not necessarily mean disagreement on treatment. Different classification categories may require identical treatments, while different treatments can be relevant within the same category.

Clinical decision-making involves more data than radiographic images. It includes age, gender, bone quality, fall history, comorbidities, concomitant injuries, trauma mechanism, patient preferences, local guidelines, usual care, surgeon-related factors, and numerous other known and unknown factors. Observer studies that rely solely on images may underestimate agreement. A study on tibial plafond fractures found that while additional CT scans did not increase agreement on classification, they did help determine the treatment plan [48]. In an observer study on hip fracture classification using the Garden classification, age was the defining factor for treatment planning rather than the classification category [49].

To examine the possible inconsistency in agreement between classification and recommended treatment, my colleagues and I invited five shoulder surgeons to categorize 193 radiographs using the 16-category Neer classification on two occasions [50]. We also asked the observers to suggest one of three treatment options: non-surgical treatment, locking plate osteosynthesis, or hemiarthroplasty. Information on the patient's age was added in the second round. In 36% of the ratings, the observer changed the category between the first and second rounds. Agreement on treatment recommendations was higher to a statistically significant degree compared to the agreement on fracture classification. The kappa values did not, however, exceed moderate levels.

10.8 Translation of Categories Between Classification Systems

Roughly half of the scientific literature on shoulder fractures is based on the Neer classification, while the other half is based on the AO classification. This raises the question of whether the two classification systems are interchangeable or if we need to become equally competent in each to interpret the literature. Many authors translate Neer two-part to unifocal fractures (AO Type A), Neer three-part to bifocal fractures (AO Type B), and Neer four-part to intraarticular fractures (AO Type C). As discussed below, such translations have limited clinical or scientific value.

From a clinical perspective, the crucial difference between the classification systems is the absence of a definition of displacement in the AO classification and the absence of a *varus/valgus* distinction in the Neer classification. In the 2018 version of the AO classification, displacement has been added as a *universal modifier* but has not been defined [51]. The Neer classification has also adopted elements from the AO classification. In his 2002 revision [2], Neer acknowledged that the *valgus-impacted four-part* fracture (AO C2.1) could not be classified, and he added this category as a *precursor* to the *classical* Neer four-part fracture with lateral displacement of the articular surface (Fig. 9.5).

A rigorous approach to classification facilitates the conduct, reporting, and interpretation of clinical trials. Two partly incommensurable fracture classification systems represent a challenge. In the AO classification, valgus-impacted fractures can appear as subgroups A2.3, B1.1, C1.1, and C2.1, which could be translated to one-part, two-part, three-part, and four-part patterns within the Neer classification. The varus-impacted fracture patterns can appear as the subgroups A2.2, B1.2, C1.2, C2.2, and C2.3, covering one-part, two-part, three-part, and four-part patterns within the Neer classification.

To analyze the actual use of the two classification systems, my colleagues and I reviewed studies classifying shoulder fractures according to both classification systems [50]. After contacting the authors, we obtained primary classification data on 2530 cases. We then organized the classification data in a cross-table with the 432 combinations between the 16 Neer categories and the 27 AO subgroups and assessed each combination as *plausible* (39%), *problematic* (34%), or *not plausible* (35%). Assessment of the plausibility of translations between Neer categories and AO subgroups for Type A fractures is shown in Fig. 10.1.

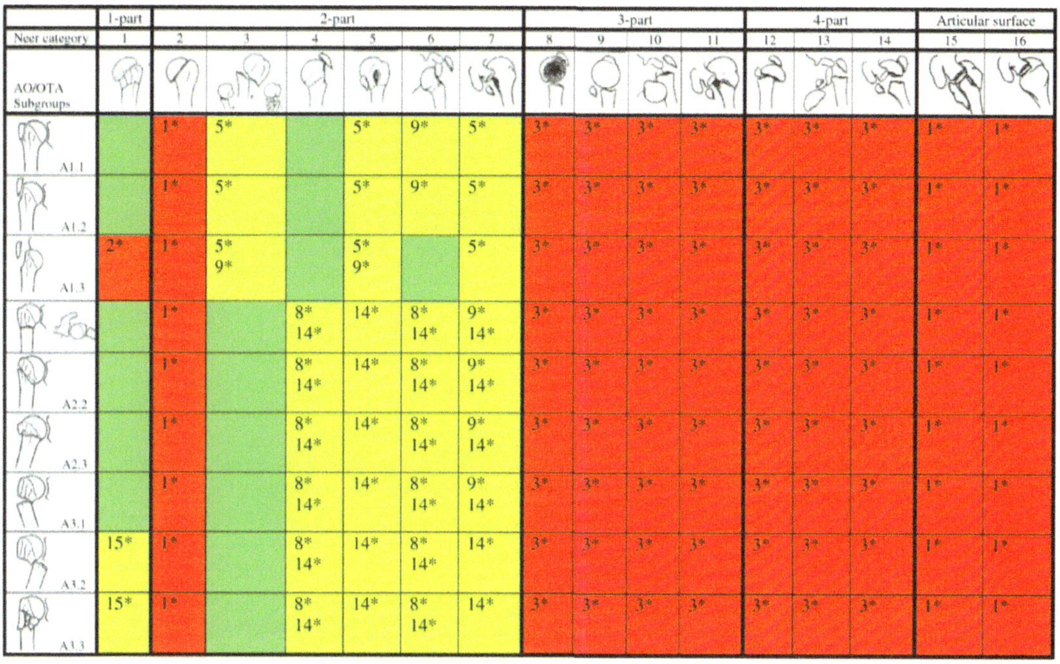

Fig. 10.1 Assessment of the plausibility of translations between Neer categories and AO subgroups. Green indicates plausible; yellow indicates problematic, and red indicates not plausible. Only Type A fractures are shown [50]

Interpretation examples: Type A fractures (AO) are unifocal and cannot appear as three- or four-part fractures (Neer). Anatomical neck fractures (Neer) are intraarticular and cannot be Type A (AO extraarticular). A fracture-dislocation (AO A1.3) cannot be minimally displaced (Neer). Through the retrieval of classification data, we found that Neer minimally displaced/one-part fractures could correspond to 15 different AO subgroups. In contrast, AO Type C fractures could appear as one-part, two-part, three-part, or four-part fractures within the Neer classification. Clinically important information is lost in translation. Consequently, my colleagues and I found it necessary to perform two separate systematic reviews on locking plate osteosynthesis covering AO Type C and Neer four-part fractures, respectively [52, 53].

10.9 Perspectives

The pursuit of an ideal classification for shoulder fractures has resulted in many observer studies reporting lower levels of agreement than expected. Not surprisingly, the observer studies arrive at different kappa values. Differences in observers, cases, imaging material, modified classifications, and bias toward classification and treatment preferences can explain some discrepancies. Instead of conducting more studies with doctors classifying images according to a classification sheet and calculating whether they perform better than the toss of a coin, more attention should be paid to the role of classification in clinical decision-making and patient outcomes after classification-based interventions. It is more urgent to understand agreement in clinical decisions than to understand agreement on a classification sheet in an experimental setting. The extent to which agreement on classification categories is essential for high-quality clinical decision-making and patient outcome is still unclear. Prospective studies are needed to determine the role of the various elements in the clinical decision-making process and their clinical importance.

References

1. Roberts SM. Fractures of the upper end of the humerus: an end-result study which shows the advantage of early active motion. JAMA J Am Med Assoc. 1932;98(5):367–73.
2. Neer CS. Four-segment classification of proximal humeral fractures: purpose and reliable use. J Shoulder Elb Surg. 2002;11(4):389–400.
3. Dirschl DR, Adams GL. A critical assessment of factors influencing reliability in the classification of fractures, using fractures of the tibial plafond as a model. J Orthop Trauma. 1997;11(7):471–6. Available from: https://journals.lww.com/jorthotrauma/fulltext/1997/10000/a_critical_assessment_of_factors_influencing.3.aspx.
4. Cocco LF, Yazzigi JAJ, Kawakami EFKI, Alvachian HJF, Dos Reis FB, Luzo MVM. Inter-observer reliability of alternative diagnostic methods for proximal humerus fractures: a comparison between attending surgeons and orthopedic residents in training. Patient Saf Surg. 2019;13:12. Available from: https://pssjournal.biomedcentral.com/articles/10.1186/s13037-019-0195-3.
5. Bougher H, Buttner P, Smith J, Banks J, Na HS, Forrestal D, et al. Interobserver and intraobserver agreement of three-dimensionally printed models for the classification of proximal humeral fractures. JSES Int. 2021;5(2):198–204.
6. Spek RW, Schoolmeesters BJ, Oosterhoff JH, Doornberg JN, van den Bekerom MP, Jaarsma RL, et al. 3D-printed handheld models do not improve recognition of specific characteristics and patterns of three-part and four-part proximal humerus fractures. Clin Orthop Relat Res. 2022;480(1):150–9. Available from: https://journals.lww.com/clinorthop/fulltext/2022/01000/3d_printed_handheld_models_do_not_improve.24.aspx.
7. Kottner J, Audige L, Brorson S, Donner A, Gajewski BJ, Hróbjartsson A, Roberts C, Shoukri M, Streiner D. Guidelines for reporting reliability and agreement studies (GRRAS) were proposed. J Clin Epidemiol. 2011;64(1):96–106. https://www.sciencedirect.com/science/article/abs/pii/S0895435610000971?via%3Dihub.
8. Audigé L, Bhandari M, Kellam J. How reliable are reliability studies of fracture classifications? A systematic review of their methodologies. Acta Orthop Scand. 2004;75(2):184–94. Available from: https://actaorthop.org/actao/article/view/19514.
9. Landis JR, Koch GG. The measurement of observer agreement for categorical data. Biometrics. 1977;33(1):159–74.
10. Brorson S, Hróbjartsson A. Training improves agreement among doctors using the Neer system for proximal humeral fractures in a systematic review. J Clin Epidemiol. 2008;61:7.
11. Ackermann C, Lam Q, Linder P, Kull C, Regazzoni. [Problems in classification of fractures of the proximal humerus]. Z Unfallchir Versicherungsmed Berufskr. 1986;79(4):209–15.
12. Kristiansen B, Andersen UL, Olsen CA, Varmarken JE. The Neer classification of fractures of the proximal humerus. An assessment of interobserver variation. Skeletal Radiol. 1988;17(6):420–2.
13. Schwartz C, Cuny C. Fractures of the proximal humerus. A prospective review of 188 cases. Eur J Orthop Surg Traumatol. 2003;13:1–12.
14. Nerot C, Thoreaux D, Hannouche D. Classification et étude inter-observateurs. Rev Chir Orthop Reparatrice Appar Mot. 1998;84(Suppl 1):129–35.
15. Cuny C, Baumann C, Mayer J, Guignand D, Irrazi M, Berrichi A, et al. AST classification of proximal humeral fractures: introduction and interobserver reliability assessment. Eur J Orthop Surg Traumatol. 2013;23(1):35–40.
16. Edelson G, Safuri H, Salami J, Vigder F, Militianu D. Natural history of complex fractures of the proximal humerus using a three-dimensional classification system. J Shoulder Elb Surg. 2008;17(3):399–409.
17. Carrerra EDF, Wajnsztejn A, Lenza M, Netto NA. Reproducibility of three classifications of proximal humeral fractures. Einstein (Sao Paulo). 2012;10(4):473–9.
18. Sukthankar AV, Leonello DT, Hertel RW, Ding GS, Sandow MJ. A comprehensive classification of proximal humeral fractures: HGLS system. J Shoulder Elb Surg. 2013;22(7):e1–6.
19. Iordens GIT, Mahabier KC, Buisman FE, Schep NWL, Muradin GSR, Beenen LFM, et al. The reliability and reproducibility of the Hertel classification for comminuted proximal humeral fractures compared with the Neer classification. J Orthop Sci. 2016;21(5):596–602.
20. Resch H, Tauber M, Neviaser RJ, Neviaser AS, Majed A, Halsey T, et al. Classification of proximal humeral fractures based on a pathomorphologic analysis. J Shoulder Elb Surg. 2016;25(3):455–62.
21. Majed A, Macleod I, Bull AM, Zyto K, Resch H, Hertel R, et al. Proximal humeral fracture classification systems revisited. J Shoulder Elb Surg. 2011;20(7):1125–32.
22. Foruria AM, Martinez-Catalan N, Pardos B, Larson D, Barlow J, Sanchez-Sotelo J. Classification of proximal humerus fractures according to pattern recognition is associated with high intraobserver and interobserver agreement. JSES Int. 2022;6(4):563–8. Available from: https://www.ncbi.nlm.nih.gov/pmc/articles/PMC9264021/.
23. Brien H, Noftall F, MacMaster S, Cummings T, Landells C, Rockwood P. Neer's classification system: a critical appraisal. J Trauma. 1995;38(2):257–60.
24. Sallay PI, Pedowitz RA, Mallon WJ, Vandemark RM, Dalton JD, Speer KP. Reliability and reproducibility of radiographic interpretation of proximal humeral fracture pathoanatomy. J Shoulder Elb Surg. 1997;6(1):60–9.

References

25. Siebenrock KA, Gerber C. The reproducibility of classification of fractures of the proximal end of the humerus. J Bone Joint Surg Am. 1993;75(12):1751–5.
26. Papakonstantinou MK, Hart MJ, Farrugia R, Gabbe BJ, Kamali Moaveni A, van Bavel D, et al. Interobserver agreement of Neer and AO classifications for proximal humeral fractures. ANZ J Surg. 2016;86(4):280–4. Available from: https://onlinelibrary.wiley.com/doi/10.1111/ans.13451.
27. Mellema JJ, Kuntz MT, Guitton TG, Ring D. The effect of two factors on interobserver reliability for proximal humeral fractures. J Am Acad Orthop Surg. 2017;25(1):69–76.
28. Sumrein BO, Mattila VM, Lepola V, Laitinen MK, Launonen AP. Intraobserver and interobserver reliability of recategorized Neer classification in differentiating 2-part surgical neck fractures from multi-fragmented proximal humeral fractures in 116 patients. J Shoulder Elb Surg. 2018;27(10):1756–61.
29. Brorson S, Bagger J, Sylvest A, Hrobjartsson A. Low agreement among 24 doctors using the Neer-classification; only moderate agreement on displacement, even between specialists. Int Orthop. 2002;26(5):271–3. Available from: https://www.ncbi.nlm.nih.gov/pmc/articles/PMC3620992/.
30. Brorson S, Bagger J, Sylvest A, Hrobjartsson A. Diagnosing displaced four-part fractures of the proximal humerus: a review of observer studies. Int Orthop. 2009;33(2):323–7. Available from: https://www.ncbi.nlm.nih.gov/pmc/articles/PMC2899076/.
31. Marongiu G, Leinardi L, Congia S, Frigau L, Mola F, Capone A. Reliability and reproducibility of the new AO/OTA 2018 classification system for proximal humeral fractures: a comparison of three different classification systems. J Orthop Traumatol. 2020;21(1):4. Available from: https://www.ncbi.nlm.nih.gov/pmc/articles/PMC7067934/.
32. Sidor ML, Zuckerman JD, Lyon T, Koval K, Cuomo F, Schoenberg N. The Neer classification system for proximal humeral fractures. An assessment of interobserver reliability and intraobserver reproducibility. J Bone Joint Surg Am. 1993;75(12):1745–50.
33. Bernstein J, Adler LM, Blank JE, Dalsey RM, Williams GR, Iannotti JP. Evaluation of the Neer system of classification of proximal humeral fractures with computerized tomographic scans and plain radiographs. J Bone Joint Surg Am. 1996;78(9):1371–5.
34. Sjödén GO, Movin T, Aspelin P, Güntner P, Shalabi A. 3D-radiographic analysis does not improve the Neer and AO classifications of proximal humeral fractures. Acta Orthop Scand. 1999;70(4):325–8. Available from: https://actaorthop.org/actao/article/view/20406.
35. Sjödén GO, Movin T, Güntner P, Aspelin P, Ahrengart L, Ersmark H, et al. Poor reproducibility of classification of proximal humeral fractures. Additional CT of minor value. Acta Orthop Scand. 1997;68(3):239–42. Available from: https://actaorthop.org/actao/article/view/20753.
36. Brunner A, Honigmann P, Treumann T, Babst R. The impact of stereo-visualisation of three-dimensional CT datasets on the inter- and intraobserver reliability of the AO/OTA and Neer classifications in the assessment of fractures of the proximal humerus. J Bone Joint Surg Br. 2009;91(6):766–71.
37. Foroohar A, Tosti R, Richmond JM, Gaughan JP, Ilyas AM. Classification and treatment of proximal humerus fractures: inter-observer reliability and agreement across imaging modalities and experience. J Orthop Surg Res. 2011;6:38. Available from: https://josr-online.biomedcentral.com/articles/10.1186/1749-799X-6-38.
38. Berkes MB, Dines JS, Little MT, Garner MR, Shifflett GD, Lazaro LE, et al. The impact of three-dimensional CT imaging on intraobserver and interobserver reliability of proximal humeral fracture classifications and treatment recommendations. J Bone Joint Surg Am. 2014;96(15):1281–6.
39. Martínez R, Santana F, Pardo A, Torrens C. One versus 3-week immobilization period for nonoperatively treated proximal humeral fractures: a prospective randomized trial. J Bone Joint Surg Am. 2021;103(16):1491–8.
40. Bruinsma WE, Guitton TG, Warner JP, Ring D. Interobserver reliability of classification and characterization of proximal humeral fractures: a comparison of two and three-dimensional CT. J Bone Joint Surg Am. 2013;95(17):1600–4.
41. Mahadeva D, Dias RG, Deshpande SV, Datta A, Dhillon SS, Simons AW. The reliability and reproducibility of the Neer classification system – digital radiography (PACS) improves agreement. Injury. 2011;42(4):339–42.
42. Torrens C, Marí R, Cuenca M, Ferrer T, Langohr K, Santana F. 3D reconstruction does not improve agreement and results in an increase in surgical indications in proximal humeral fractures. J Orthop. 2018;15(4):967–70. Available from: https://www.ncbi.nlm.nih.gov/pmc/articles/PMC6134158/.
43. Shrader MW, Sanchez-Sotelo J, Sperling JW, Rowland CM, Cofield RH. Understanding proximal humerus fractures: image analysis, classification, and treatment. J Shoulder Elb Surg. 2005;14(5):497–505.
44. Brorson S, Bagger J, Sylvest A, Hrobjartsson A. Improved interobserver variation after training of doctors in the Neer system. A randomised trial. J Bone Joint Surg Br. 2002;84(7):950–4.
45. Neer CS. Displaced proximal humeral fractures. I. Classification and evaluation. J Bone Joint Surg Am. 1970;52(6):1077–89.
46. Neer CS. Displaced proximal humeral fractures. II. Treatment of three-part and four-part displacement. J Bone Joint Surg Am. 1970;52(6):1090–103.
47. Thomsen NOB, Olsen LH, Nielsen ST. Kappa statistics in the assessment of observer variation: the significance of multiple observers classifying ankle fractures. J Orthop Sci. 2002;7(2):163–6.
48. Chan P, Klimkiewicz J, Luchetti W, Esterhai J, Kneeland J, Dalinka M, et al. Impact of CT scan on treatment plan and fracture classification of tibial plateau fractures. J Orthop Trauma. 1997;11(7):484–9.

Available from: https://journals.lww.com/jorthotrauma/abstract/1997/10000/impact_of_ct_scan_on_treatment_plan_and_fracture.5.aspx.

49. Oakes DA, Jackson KR, Davies MR, Ehrhart KM, Zohman GL, Koval KJ, et al. The impact of the garden classification on proposed operative treatment. Clin Orthop Relat Res. 2003;409:232–40. Available from: https://journals.lww.com/clinorthop/fulltext/2003/04000/the_impact_of_the_garden_classification_on.30.aspx.

50. Brorson S, Eckardt H, Audigé L, Rolauffs B, Bahrs C. Translation between the Neer- and the AO/OTA-classification for proximal humeral fractures: do we need to be bilingual to interpret the scientific literature? BMC Res Notes. 2013;6(1):69. Available from: https://www.ncbi.nlm.nih.gov/pmc/articles/PMC3610277/.

51. Meinberg EG, Agel J, Roberts CS, Karam MD, Kellam JF. Fracture and dislocation classification compendium – 2018. J Orthop Trauma. 2018;32(Suppl 1):S1–S170. Available from: https://journals.lww.com/jorthotrauma/fulltext/2018/01001/fracture_and_dislocation_classification.1.aspx.

52. Brorson S, Rasmussen JV, Frich LH, Olsen BS, Hróbjartsson A. Benefits and harms of locking plate osteosynthesis in intraarticular (OTA Type C) fractures of the proximal humerus: a systematic review. Injury. 2012;43(7):999–1005. https://www.clinicalkey.com/#!/content/journal/1-s2.0-S0020138311004025.

53. Brorson S, Frich LH, Winther A, Hróbjartsson A. Locking plate osteosynthesis in displaced 4-part fractures of the proximal humerus. Acta Orthop. 2011;82(4):475–81. Available from: https://actaorthop.org/actao/article/view/10945.

Open Access This chapter is licensed under the terms of the Creative Commons Attribution 4.0 International License (http://creativecommons.org/licenses/by/4.0/), which permits use, sharing, adaptation, distribution and reproduction in any medium or format, as long as you give appropriate credit to the original author(s) and the source, provide a link to the Creative Commons license and indicate if changes were made.

The images or other third party material in this chapter are included in the chapter's Creative Commons license, unless indicated otherwise in a credit line to the material. If material is not included in the chapter's Creative Commons license and your intended use is not permitted by statutory regulation or exceeds the permitted use, you will need to obtain permission directly from the copyright holder.

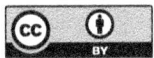

Part IV

Management: Eminence Meets Evidence

Interventions for Shoulder Fractures: The Evidence Base

11.1 Introduction

Many orthopedic surgeons take the benefits of surgery for granted. If they conduct clinical research, they mainly study surgical procedures in uncontrolled case series or compare them with other surgical interventions. A bibliometric review retrieved 1051 publications on shoulder fractures from multiple databases [1]. Forty-eight percent of the identified studies were uncontrolled case series. The majority were retrospective. Only 3% of the sample were randomized trials. Other studies included basic science, prognostic studies, and non-randomized comparative studies. By mapping the themes, 67% studied surgical treatments, 4% studied non-surgical treatments, and less than 2% studied rehabilitation. Thus, the typical study of shoulder fractures is an uncontrolled, retrospective case series of surgical interventions. A strong belief in a particular surgical implant or procedure may lead to bias in studies. Industry involvement may further encourage certain positive conclusions. Commercial funding is notably absent in studies that include non-surgical comparators.

11.2 Randomized Trials

Since 2003, Cochrane reviews have included evidence from randomized trials on shoulder fractures, following the *Cochrane Handbook for Systematic Reviews of Interventions* [2]. The handbook outlines the methods and processes involved in conducting a review. It guides the reviewers through every step of the review process, from formulating the research question to interpreting the final results. This includes planning the review, conducting a thorough search and selecting appropriate studies, collecting and analyzing data, assessing the risk of bias, performing statistical analysis, and interpreting the results. In the two latest Cochrane reviews [3, 4], my colleagues and I used the Grading of Recommendations Assessment, Development, and Evaluation (GRADE) [5] to assess the quality of outcome data and the certainty of findings.

The Cochrane review has reported on five versions comparing surgical and non-surgical interventions. Table 11.1 provides details on these versions. The first randomized trial, involving a comparison of hemiarthroplasty using the Neer prosthesis and closed manipulation under anesthesia in 32 patients, was conducted in 1984 [6]. In 1988, another trial compared closed reduction and percutaneous pinning with closed reduction under anesthesia in 30 patients [7]. Although both treatments were common in the 1980s, they have been replaced by other procedures. In 1997, a trial compared internal fixation with tension band or cerclage wiring to non-surgical treatment in 40 patients [8]. Later, around the year 2000, the locking plate technology was introduced (Chap. 12), gaining popularity almost instantly. Subsequently, in 2010, locking plate osteosynthesis was compared to non-surgical treatment in

Table 11.1 Cochrane reviews 2003–2022 reporting surgical versus non-surgical interventions for shoulder fractures

Year	Studies and participants, overall	Studies and participants, non-surgical comparator	Interventions and comparisons (number of participants)	Conclusions
2003	12 (578)	3 (102)	Hemiarthroplasty versus closed reduction (32) Pinning versus closed reduction (30) Tension band versus non-surgical (40)	It is unclear whether operative intervention, even for specific fracture types, will produce consistently better long-term outcomes
2010	16 (801)	4 (155)	Hemiarthroplasty versus closed reduction (32) Pinning versus closed reduction (30) Tension band versus non-surgical (40) Locking plate and cerclage versus non-surgical (50)[a]	The very limited evidence available does not confirm that surgery is preferable to conservative treatment, and complications associated with surgery need to be considered
2012	23 (1238)	6 (270)	Hemiarthroplasty versus closed reduction (32) Pinning versus closed reduction (30) Tension band versus non-surgical (40) Locking plate and cerclage versus non-surgical (50)[a] Locking plate versus non-surgical (60) Hemiarthroplasty versus non-surgical (55)	It remains unclear whether surgery, even for specific fracture types, will produce consistently better long-term outcomes, but it is likely to be associated with a higher risk of surgery-related complications and requirement for further surgery
2015	31 (1941)	8 (567)	Hemiarthroplasty versus closed reduction (32) Pinning versus closed reduction (30) Tension band versus non-surgical (40) Locking plate and cerclage versus non-surgical (50)[a] Locking plate versus non-surgical (60) Hemiarthroplasty versus non-surgical (55) Hemiarthroplasty versus non-surgical (50) Surgeon's choice versus non-surgical (250)[b]	There is high- or moderate-quality evidence that, compared with non-surgical treatment, surgery does not result in a better outcome at 1 and 2 years after injury for people with displaced proximal humeral fractures involving the humeral neck and is likely to result in a greater need for subsequent surgery

(continued)

Table 11.1 (continued)

Year	Studies and participants, overall	Studies and participants, non-surgical comparator	Interventions and comparisons (number of participants)	Conclusions
2022	47 (3179)	10 (717)	Hemiarthroplasty versus closed reduction (32) Pinning versus closed reduction (30) Tension band versus non-surgical (40) Locking plate and cerclage versus non-surgical (50) Locking plate versus non-surgical (60) Hemiarthroplasty versus non-surgical (55) Hemiarthroplasty versus non-surgical (50)[a] Surgeon's choice versus non-surgical (250)[b] Reverse arthroplasty versus non-surgical (62) Locking plate versus non-surgical (88)	There is high- or moderate-certainty evidence that, compared with non-surgical treatment, surgery does not result in a better outcome at 1 and 2 years after injury for people with the large majority of displaced proximal humeral fractures. It may increase the need for subsequent surgery. The available evidence does not cover the treatment of two-part tuberosity fractures and is insufficient to draw conclusions on fractures in younger adults, on high-energy trauma, or for less common fractures, such as fracture-dislocations and articular surface fractures

[a]Three patients excluded from the analysis
[b]125 treated surgically, locking plates in 90 patients

a trial involving 50 patients [9]. In 2011, a trial compared locking plate osteosynthesis to non-surgical treatment in 60 patients [10]. In 2011, a comparison was made between hemiarthroplasty and non-surgical treatment in 55 patients [11]. The following year, a similar comparison was made in 50 patients [12]. The ProFHER trial published in 2015 [13] randomly assigned 250 patients to either surgery by *surgeon's choice* or non-surgical treatment. Of the 125 patients assigned to surgery, 109 underwent a procedure, with 90 receiving locking plates. The remaining 19 patients in the surgery group received either hemiarthroplasty ($n = 10$), intramedullary nails ($n = 4$), or other implants ($n = 5$). In 2018, reverse shoulder arthroplasty was compared to non-surgical treatment in 62 patients [14], and in 2019, locking plates were compared to non-surgical treatment in 88 patients [15].

The 2022 update of the Cochrane review included 47 randomized trials with 3279 participants and 26 pairwise comparisons [4]. Out of these, 10 trials compared surgical and non-surgical interventions; 12 trials compared nonoperative interventions; 23 trials compared 2 methods of surgery, and 2 trials compared the timing of immobilization after surgery. Two-thirds of the patients were female, with 66% suffering three- or four-part fractures. Most trials had a lower age limit of 60 years. The only trial comparing reverse arthroplasty to non-surgical treatment had a lower age limit of 80 years [14]. Substantial changes in the preferences for implants were observed within the study period. Some treatments, such as closed reduction, percutaneous pinning, monoblock hemiarthroplasty, cerclage, and tension band wiring, are no longer used. The popularity of reverse total shoulder arthroplasty has by far exceeded hemiarthroplasty. Implants are constantly being developed and modified. The extent of the Cochrane review has reached almost 400 pages. To make the current review more accessible to clinicians, my colleagues and I have published a short version with the key messages [16].

11.3 A Failed Trial

Several incomplete randomized trials can be found by searching protocol databases. In 2009, my colleagues and I published a protocol for a national three-arm multicenter study [17]. The study compared patient-reported outcomes after hemiarthroplasty, locking plate osteosynthesis, and non-surgical treatment in older people with four-part fractures. The recruitment of participants was planned from ten different centers. Twenty-two patients were recruited for a study, but eight out of ten centers withdrew due to ethical concerns. The allocation of patients with four-part fractures to nonoperative treatment was then considered unethical. If the trial were conducted today, many surgeons would have ethical concerns about allocating patients with four-part fractures to locking plates. In addition, total reverse arthroplasties would likely have replaced hemiarthroplasties in most centers. The example demonstrates that the success of randomized trials depends on the context in which they are conducted. As technology evolves, so does the confidence in new treatment methods. From an ethical perspective, trials should ideally be performed when there is *equipoise*—a balance in pre-trial beliefs in the compared treatments. However, pre-trial beliefs vary over time and between countries, orthopedic societies, centers, and individual surgeons.

11.4 The Evidence Base for Rehabilitation Interventions

High-quality clinical trials are as essential for the documentation of outcomes after rehabilitation interventions as they are for documenting outcomes after surgical interventions. Training is often assumed to be inherently beneficial, and there is a lack of evidence-based rehabilitation regimes for patients with displaced shoulder fractures treated without surgery. A few trials indicate that immobilization for 3 weeks is no better than immobilization for a single week [18, 19]. A randomized trial has further reported that supervised training is not superior to non-supervised home-based exercises [20]. We cannot provide patients with clear advice on whether training is better than no training. My colleagues and I conducted a randomized study to determine whether training is superior to no training. We randomized 60 patients aged 60 or above with displaced shoulder fractures treated non-surgically to a single instruction in early return to ordinary daily life or usual training in the municipalities [21].

A great number of rehabilitation regimens have been derived from experiences with other shoulder conditions treated surgically, such as rotator cuff surgery or joint replacement. Restrictions in range of motion may delay recovery in patients without surgical reconstruction or an implant needing specific protection. Surgeons familiar with secondary displacement after locking plate osteosynthesis tend to exaggerate the consequences of secondary displacement after early movement in non-surgically treated patients. Radiological changes can be expected during the consolidation and healing process. It is still yet to be demonstrated that radiological changes predict patient-reported outcomes in non-surgically treated patients. Despite being biomechanically justified, movement restrictions, braces, and bandages cannot neutralize the deforming forces acting on the fractured parts. Rehabilitation interventions should meet the same requirements for clinical documentation as surgical interventions.

11.5 Systematic Reviews and Meta-analyses

Systematic reviews aim to identify, assess, and summarize the existing evidence. Suppose the trials included in the review are qualitatively and statistically comparable (low heterogeneity). The performance of a meta-analysis can be feasible in this case, allowing for more statistically safe effect estimates. In the last decade, a number of meta-analyses on shoulder fractures have been published. Surprisingly, discordant conclusions can be found among studies based on the same primary studies. This highlights the need for a critical reappraisal of the meta-analyses. Historically, meta-analyses summarizing results from randomized controlled trials have been considered the highest level of evidence. However, following some basic methodological rules is essential if the reliability of the results is to be ensured.

While the results from the comparisons between surgical and non-surgical treatments have been consistent throughout all editions of the Cochrane review, the certainty of the findings (GRADE) has increased. The 2022 edition reports no significant difference in patient-reported shoulder function between the surgical and non-surgical groups after 1 or 2 years of treatment (high-certainty evidence). Additionally, there was no clinically important difference in quality of life after 1 year of treatment (high-certainty evidence). However, it was found that the surgery group had a higher risk that additional surgery would be required (low-certainty evidence). Figure 11.1 reports the patient-reported shoulder function at 12 months. The mean differences were normalized to account for differences in outcome assessment instruments.

Confidence intervals for all trials cross the line of no difference. Figure 11.2 presents the risk of additional surgery after the initial surgery. We compared the risk of undergoing a new surgery with the risk of undergoing a late surgery after receiving non-surgical treatment initially. The outcome was binary, and a risk ratio was calculated. A risk ratio of 2 in favor of non-surgical treatment means that patients who opt for surgery

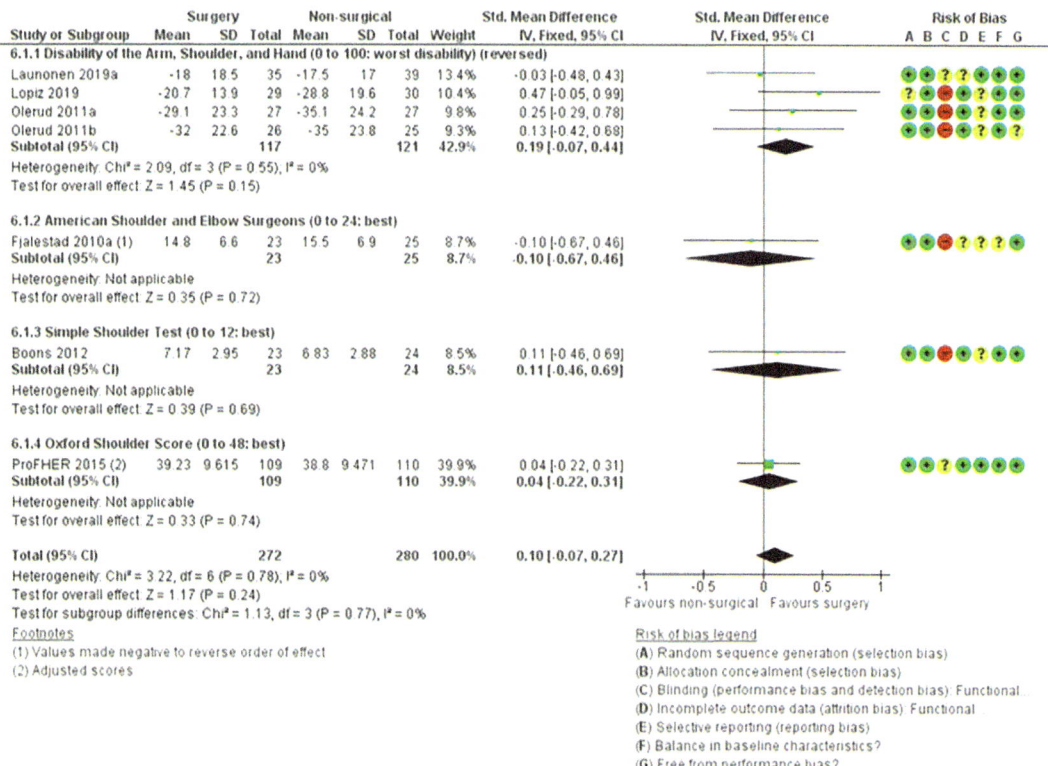

Fig. 11.1 Surgical versus non-surgical treatment. Patient-reported shoulder function after 12 months (With permission from John Wiley and Sons)

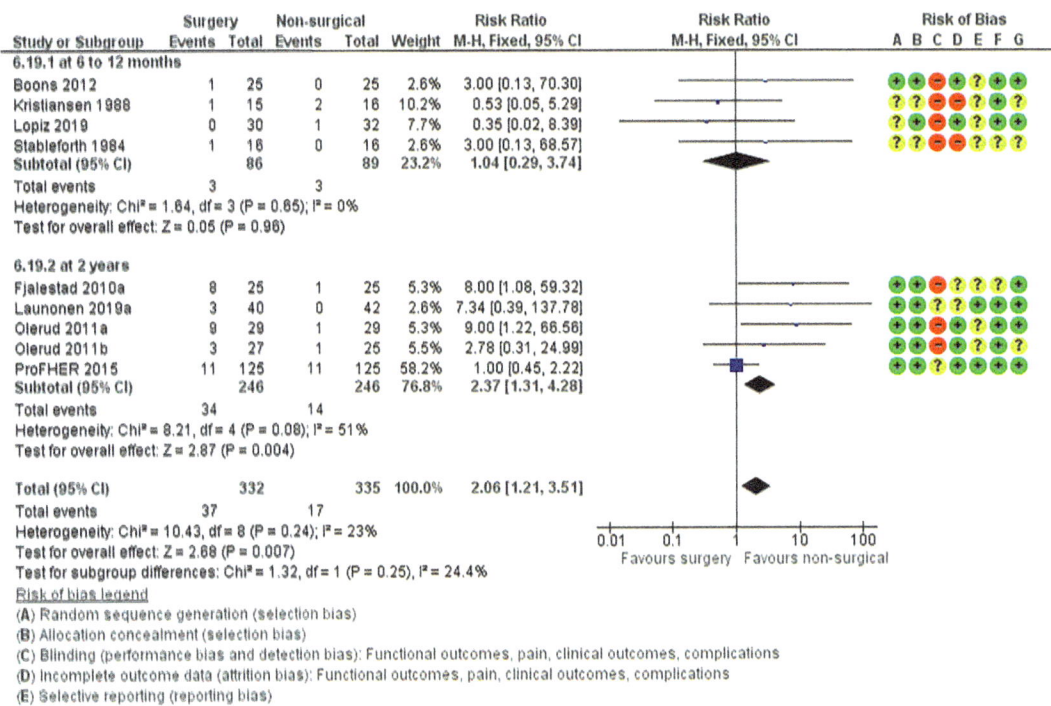

Fig. 11.2 Surgical versus non-surgical treatment. Risk of additional surgery within 2 years. (With permission from John Wiley and Sons)

have twice the risk of needing additional surgery compared to those who receive non-surgical treatment.

In summary, there was no high-certainty evidence for the superiority of surgical treatment compared to non-surgical treatment. The only difference is a higher risk of additional surgery. No surgical treatment modality differs from the general pattern. Based on the existing body of evidence comparing surgical and non-surgical treatments, it seems reasonable to conclude that we have now moved from *no evidence of a difference* to *evidence of no difference*.

11.6 Multiple Overlapping Meta-analyses

Summaries of data from studies on shoulder fractures tell us that low-quality meta-analyses have limitations. Numerous overlapping or partially overlapping systematic reviews and meta-analyses have compared outcomes after surgical and non-surgical treatments. Figure 11.3 compares the number of randomized controlled trials and the number of meta-analyses published between 1984 and 2018. The number of meta-analyses has by far exceeded the number of randomized trials. Multiple overlapping meta-analyses raise methodological concerns.

In a meta-epidemiological study [23], my colleagues and I identified 21 meta-analyses comparing surgical and non-surgical treatments of shoulder fractures, 19 pairwise meta-analyses, and two network meta-analyses. The 19 pairwise meta-analyses were based on up to eight randomized trials. Among the 19 meta-analyses, 18 were *critically low quality* as assessed by the AMSTAR 2 tool [24]. The critically low methodological quality was mainly due to a lack of protocol (18 out of 19), no reporting of excluded studies (16 out of 19), no reporting of the funding of the included studies (18 out of 19), and inappropriate sta-

11.7 Methodological Flexibility

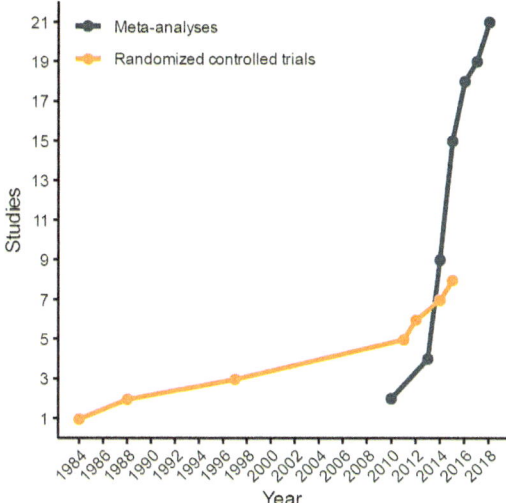

Fig. 11.3 The number of randomized controlled trials (brown) and meta-analyses (black) 1984–2018 [22]

tistical methods (16 out of 19). The conclusions reported in the 19 meta-analyses were extracted for shoulder function, quality of life, and harm.

The studies came to discordant conclusions for all domains. Although four meta-analyses shared their research question and were based on the same six primary studies, they nevertheless reached discordant conclusions for all three domains. This finding raises concerns about the use of low-quality meta-analyses in guiding clinical decision-making and further challenges the position of meta-analyses based on randomized trials as Level I evidence. Well-conducted meta-analyses serve important purposes by summarizing data and reducing statistical uncertainty. Multiple overlapping meta-analyses of critically low quality are, in the best case, redundant and, in the worst case, misleading. New meta-studies should await further primary studies, and editors should be more cautious in publishing meta-analyses without predefined and precise protocols.

The consequences of multiple overlapping meta-analyses of low quality can be approached empirically. *Methodological flexibility* refers to the methodological options used to conduct a meta-analysis. The *analytical scenarios* refer to the combination of the methodological choices taken. Without a protocol, the methodological flexibility is high, and different analytical scenarios can be obtained. The presence of a protocol specifying all steps of the meta-analysis markedly decreases methodological flexibility, thus limiting the risk of tilting the meta-analysis toward a certain conclusion. In another meta-epidemiological study, we studied the impact of methodological choices and possible conclusions [25]. We identified 23 meta-analyses based on 24 primary studies; some included non-randomized studies. Three protocols were identified by contacting the authors of the meta-analyses. After extracting data from the 23 meta-analyses, multiple meta-analyses were simulated using the same data pool but under differing analytical scenarios. Meta-analyses based on all possible combinations of the methodological choices were conducted. The distribution of effect estimates obtained with and without a protocol was mapped to demonstrate the impact of a protocol. Figure 11.4 illustrates the possibility of getting statistically significant effect estimates in shoulder function with or without following a protocol.

Conflicting effect estimates and discordant conclusions can be obtained without a protocol, even at the standard level of statistical significance ($p < 0.05$). Surgical or non-surgical treatment could be favored and supported by data. This is the case for shoulder function, quality of life, and harm. Figure 11.5 illustrates the distribution of effect estimates on harm outcomes with and without a protocol. Without a protocol, any

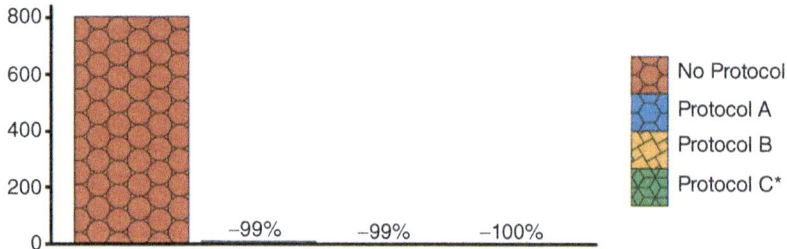

Fig. 11.4 The number of possible meta-analyses with statistically significant effect estimates for functional outcome without a protocol (brown) and with one of three protocols (A, B, C) [22]

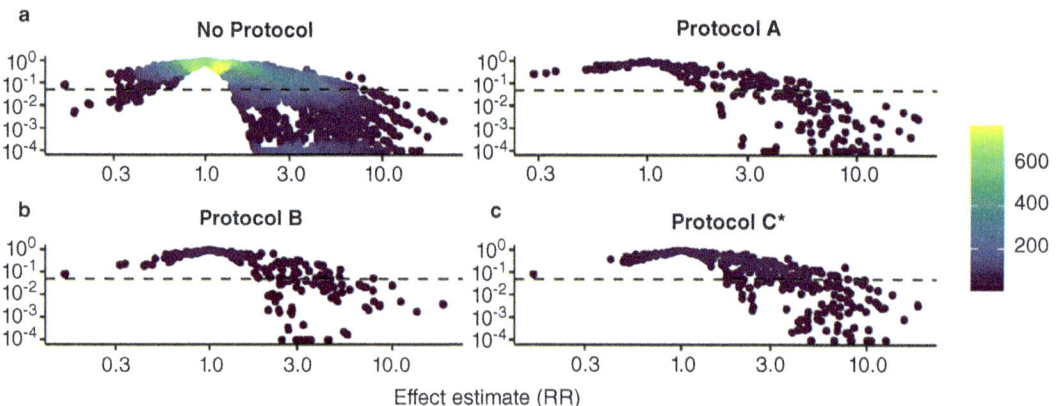

Fig. 11.5 Distributions of effect estimates for harm outcomes (risk ratio) without a protocol and with (A, B, C). Estimates below 1.0 favor surgical treatment. Values below the dotted line are significant at the 0.05 level [25]. (With permission from Elsevier)

conclusion can be supported; by following a protocol, surgical treatment is seen to be inferior regarding harm outcomes. The absence of a protocol raises serious concerns about bias toward preconceived assumptions regarding effects.

11.8 Network Meta-analyses

A substantial number of orthopedic interventions lack robust support from high-quality randomized trials. When the data pool is limited, meta-analyses can summarize the existing evidence and provide more statistically safe treatment estimates. Traditional meta-analyses are based on a pairwise comparison of effect estimates. Network meta-analyses can be used to estimate treatment effects when direct comparisons are absent or sparse. If two (or more) interventions share a common comparator, indirect comparison can be an option. This has raised hope for a stronger evidence base for interventions where direct comparisons are sparse or lacking altogether—for example, in comparing reverse shoulder arthroplasty to non-surgical treatment.

A network meta-analysis extends the traditional pairwise meta-analysis by comparing more than two interventions. Indirect comparisons rely on two critical assumptions: *transitivity* and *coherence*. Transitivity refers to the comparability of the studies included. Ideally, the included studies could all be part of the same imaginary multiarm randomized trial; this is only possible when potential effect modifiers such as age, gender, indications, or procedures are shared. Coherence is a statistical term referring to the estimates obtained through direct and indirect evidence. In the last few years, network meta-analyses on treatments of shoulder fractures have gained popularity; unfortunately, however, the methodological quality of current network meta-analyses is low. Substantial differences between the primary studies, including demographics, inclusion criteria, and differences between the interventions, make the conduct of network meta-analyses spurious. None of the network meta-analyses published so far had a predefined analysis plan, and they tend to favor surgical treatments.

The enthusiasm for the use of reverse shoulder arthroplasty in fracture cases has driven efforts to clarify the evidence base (Chap. 15). Until 2024, reverse shoulder arthroplasty in fractures was tested by only one randomized trial with 62 patients aged 80 years or above [14]. This study reported no superiority of surgery. Other studies have reported direct comparisons in favor of reverse arthroplasty compared to locking plates [26] and hemiarthroplasty [27, 28]. These two surgical treatments have previously been studied by direct comparison to non-surgical treatment [10–12, 15, 29, 30]. Interestingly, despite no difference found in any primary studies, network meta-analyses tend to indicate the superiority of surgical treatments over non-surgical treatments. Reverse arthroplasty was preferred in two studies: "RSA is the optimum treatment method for elderly patients" [31]; "RSA offers satisfactory improvements in clinical and functional outcomes when compared to other non-operative and operative treatment options" [32]. A third network meta-analysis was more reluctant to make conclusions [33].

All network meta-analyses were found to have considerable methodological flaws; none offered a publicly available protocol, and none reflected on transitivity. Given the differences in important effect modifiers, no network meta-analysis comparing the abovementioned treatment modalities can fulfill the transitivity assumption. Considerable age differences were found between patients receiving locking plates and patients receiving arthroplasty; similarly, the patients receiving surgical treatment differed markedly from patients receiving non-surgical treatment. Even the indications for surgery varied between the included studies. Incoherence was present due to the differences between direct and indirect comparisons. Network meta-analyses on shoulder fractures are likely to increase. Following guidance from network meta-analyses without a protocol or violating the assumptions of transitivity and coherence cannot be recommended.

11.9 Perspectives

How do we proceed toward safer estimates of treatment effects to better inform evidence-based decision-making? For reliable effect estimates, we need to ensure comparability at baseline, which is best obtained by randomization. It has become increasingly clear from randomized trials that two-, three-, and four-part fractures in older people should be treated without surgery. Evidence-based recommendations are still lacking for important patient subgroups. It is often assumed that when evidence is lacking, surgery is indicated. While this may be true for some patient subgroups, further empirical support is required to confirm it.

Collaboration in national or international multicenter trials is needed if studies of uncommon fracture patterns or subgroups of patients are to be sufficiently robust statistically. Most trials before the ProFHER trial have been *explanatory*, with a few selected surgeons performing the procedures under standardized conditions. The drawback is the lack of applicability and generalizability. Patients are rarely treated under ideal conditions. *Pragmatic* trials testing interventions under real-world conditions are, unfortunately, often considered unreliable and disregarded. The authors of the ProFHER trial [13], the first large pragmatic multicenter trial on shoulder fractures, reported no statistically significant or clinically important benefits of surgery for any outcome. The harsh criticism following the ProFHER trial was partly based on insufficient knowledge of the pragmatic design. One objection was that the study was unreliable because the surgeries had been performed by 66 surgeons from 32 hospitals—but these were surgeons performing the surgery in clinics every day. Interestingly, when a pragmatic trial reports no superiority of surgery in a real-world scenario, it is the study, not the treatment provided, that is criticized. The criticism the ProFHER trial received for the inclusion of only 20% of potentially eligible patients, raising concerns of selection bias [34, 35], stemmed from data from a screening protocol completed by the investigators. Only a few orthopedic trials account for pre-randomization behavior—something which should be considered an indicator of the study's quality. In the ProFHER trial, most patients were excluded due to predefined exclusion criteria. Most remaining patients refused to participate because they strongly preferred non-surgical treatment [36].

First, high-quality randomized trials should be conducted on patients younger than 60. The biology in younger patients with good bone stock may allow for osteosynthesis with lower failure rates. However, younger patients may have higher demands and shorter implant survival. Age as a selection criterion for treatment options is not ideal. Older people are fitter than they have been, and younger patients, resembling members of the older group, may be frail. Inclusion according to frailty assessment rather than age, for example, may offer a way of addressing the risk of combining data from these groups in future studies.

Second, we lack studies on the treatment of isolated greater tuberosity fractures. In younger patients, these fractures may resemble a total rotator cuff rupture with a bone avulsion, calling for a different clinical approach. Two-part anterior fracture-dislocations are relatively common, and it is unclear whether the bony fragment should be fixed if it falls in place after closed or open reduction. Even severe greater tuberosity displacement or retraction may be well tolerated in older people (Fig. 3.15).

Third, the popularity of reverse shoulder arthroplasty as a primary fracture treatment should be justified. The combination of primary non-surgical treatment, followed by the option of secondary reverse arthroplasty in clinical failures, should be examined. The massive use of reverse arthroplasty in primary fracture cases may lead to overtreatment and challenging revision surgery.

Fourth, the optimal treatment of fractures with involvement of the articular surface has not been defined. In many cases, including the greater tuberosity, a substantial part of the articular surface remains attached to the greater tuberosity. Seeing a part of the posterior surface visible on a CT scan, most surgeons are inclined to replace the articular surface—but strong data supporting the assumption of early posttraumatic osteoarthritis in these patients is, however, lacking. These patients often regain good function and pain relief despite a persistent step-off in the articular surface. If there is no pain, the insertion of an arthroplasty can be postponed until symptoms appear, preferably at an age where revision surgery is a lesser concern (Fig. 11.6).

Finally, limited patient flow at even the largest centers presents a challenge to conducting the abovementioned trials. Registry-based studies with high coverage and completeness may narrow the evidence gaps, especially when patient-reported outcomes are available. Reporting revision rates and implant survival

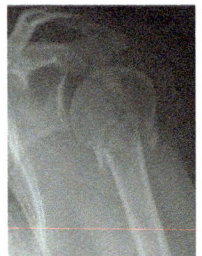
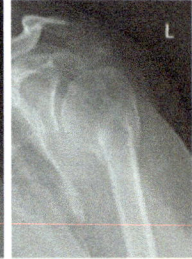
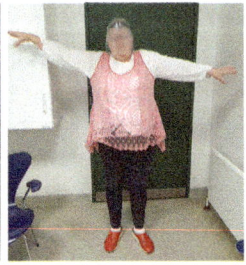
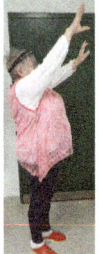
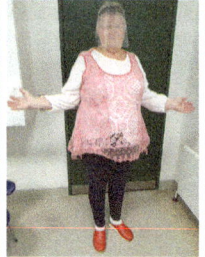
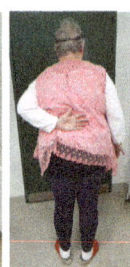

Fig. 11.6 Head-splitting fracture with a step-off in the articular surface in a 77-year-old female. The fracture healed in 12 weeks, and pain-free function was regained. The step-off remained. Radiographs at 2 and 24 weeks. Photos at 24 weeks

may provide helpful information for quality assessment [37], but it is an unreliable source of patient function, pain, and satisfaction [38]. Comparative studies of registry cohorts can be confounded by differences in diagnostics, population characteristics, surgical practice, patient preferences, and other variables not captured by the regression analysis.

References

1. Slobogean GP, Johal H, Lefaivre KA, MacIntyre NJ, Sprague S, Scott T, et al. A scoping review of the proximal humerus fracture literature. BMC Musculoskelet Disord. 2015;16(1):112. Available from: https://bmcmusculoskeletdisord.biomedcentral.com/articles/10.1186/s12891-015-0564-8.
2. Higgins JPT, Thomas J, Chandler J, Cumpston M, Li T, Page MJ, Welch V, editors. Cochrane handbook for systematic reviews of interventions, version 6.3. The Cochrane Collaboration; 2022. Available from: https://training.cochrane.org/handbook/archive/v6.3.
3. Handoll HH, Brorson S. Interventions for treating proximal humeral fractures in adults. Cochrane Database Syst Rev. 2015;(11):CD000434. Available from: http://doi.wiley.com/10.1002/14651858.CD000434.pub4.
4. Handoll HH, Elliott J, Thillemann TM, Aluko P, Brorson S. Interventions for treating proximal humeral fractures in adults. Cochrane Database Syst Rev. 2022;6(6):CD000434. Available from: https://www.cochranelibrary.com/cdsr/doi/10.1002/14651858.CD000434.pub5/abstract.
5. Schünemann H, Brożek J, Guyatt G, Oxman A. GRADE handbook. 2013 [cited 2023 Oct 4]. Available from: https://gdt.gradepro.org/app/handbook/handbook.html.
6. Stableforth PG. Four-part fractures of the neck of the humerus. J Bone Joint Surg Br. 1984;66(1):104–8.
7. Kristiansen B, Kofoed H. Transcutaneous reduction and external fixation of displaced fractures of the proximal humerus. A controlled clinical trial. J Bone Joint Surg Br. 1988;70(5):821–4.
8. Zyto K, Ahrengart L, Sperber A, Törnkvist H. Treatment of displaced proximal humeral fractures in elderly patients. J Bone Joint Surg Br. 1997;79(3):412–7.
9. Fjalestad T, Hole M, Jørgensen JJ, Strømsøe K, Kristiansen IS. Health and cost consequences of surgical versus conservative treatment for a comminuted proximal humeral fracture in elderly patients. Injury. 2010;41(6):599–605. https://www.sciencedirect.com/science/article/abs/pii/S0020138309005828.
10. Olerud P, Ahrengart L, Ponzer S, Saving J, Tidermark J. Internal fixation versus nonoperative treatment of displaced 3-part proximal humeral fractures in elderly patients: a randomized controlled trial. J Shoulder Elb Surg. 2011;20(5):747–55.
11. Olerud P, Ahrengart L, Ponzer S, Saving J, Tidermark J. Hemiarthroplasty versus nonoperative treatment of displaced 4-part proximal humeral fractures in elderly patients: a randomized controlled trial. J Shoulder Elb Surg. 2011;20(7):1025–33.
12. Boons HW, Goosen JH, Van Grinsven S, Van Susante JL, Van Loon CJ. Hemiarthroplasty for humeral four-part fractures for patients 65 years and older a randomized controlled trial. Clin Orthop Relat Res. 2012;470(12):3483–91. Available from: https://www.ncbi.nlm.nih.gov/pmc/articles/PMC3492647/.
13. Rangan A, Handoll H, Brealey S, Jefferson L, Keding A, Martin BC, et al. Surgical vs nonsurgical treatment of adults with displaced fractures of the proximal humerus: the PROFHER randomized clinical trial. JAMA. 2015;313(10):1037–47. Available from: https://jamanetwork.com/journals/jama/fullarticle/2190987.
14. Lopiz Y, Alcobía-Díaz B, Galán-Olleros M, García-Fernández C, Picado AL, Marco F. Reverse shoulder arthroplasty versus nonoperative treatment for 3- or 4-part proximal humeral fractures in elderly patients: a prospective randomized controlled trial. J Shoulder Elb Surg. 2019;28(12):2259–71.
15. Launonen AP, Sumrein BO, Reito A, Lepola V, Paloneva J, Jonsson KB, et al. Operative versus nonoperative treatment for 2-part proximal humerus fracture: a multicenter randomized controlled trial. PLoS Med. 2019;16(7):e1002855. Available from: https://www.ncbi.nlm.nih.gov/pmc/articles/PMC6638737/.
16. Brorson S, Elliott J, Thillemann T, Aluko P, Handoll H. Interventions for proximal humeral fractures: key messages from a Cochrane review. Acta Orthop. 2022;93:610–2. Available from: https://actaorthop.org/actao/article/view/3495/5768.
17. Brorson S, Olsen BS, Frich LH, Jensen SL, Johannsen HV, Sørensen AK, et al. Effect of osteosynthesis, primary hemiarthroplasty, and non-surgical management for displaced four-part fractures of the proximal humerus in elderly: a multi-centre, randomised clinical trial. Trials. 2009;10:51. https://trialsjournal.biomedcentral.com/articles/10.1186/1745-6215-10-51.
18. Martínez R, Santana F, Pardo A, Torrens C. One versus 3-week immobilization period for nonoperatively treated proximal humeral fractures: a prospective randomized trial. J Bone Joint Surg Am. 2021;103(16):1491–8.
19. Østergaard HK, Mechlenburg I, Launonen AP, Vestermark MT, Mattila VM, Ponkilainen VT. The benefits and harms of early mobilization and supervised exercise therapy after non-surgically treated proximal humerus or distal radius fracture: a systematic review and meta-analysis. Curr Rev Musculoskelet Med. 2021;14(2):107–29. Available from: https://www.ncbi.nlm.nih.gov/pmc/articles/PMC7990986/.
20. Østergaard HK, Launonen AP, Toft M, Fjalestad T, Sumrein BO, Døssing KV, et al. Physiotherapist-

20. supervised exercises versus non-supervised home-based exercises after non-surgically treated proximal humerus fracture: a multicentre randomised controlled trial. J Shoulder Elb Surg. 2024;33:994.
21. Liaghat B, Brorson S. Effect of structured rehabilitation versus non-structured rehabilitation following non-surgical management of displaced proximal humerus fractures: a protocol for a randomised clinical trial. BMJ Open. 2022;12(10):e064156. Available from: https://www.ncbi.nlm.nih.gov/pmc/articles/PMC9577899/pdf/bmjopen-2022-064156.pdf.
22. Sandau N. Why meta-analyses comparing proximal humerus fracture treatments report discordant conclusions. PhD thesis, University of Copenhagen. 2023.
23. Sandau N, Buxbom P, Hróbjartsson A, Harris IA, Brorson S. The methodological quality was low and conclusions discordant for meta-analyses comparing proximal humerus fracture treatments: a meta-epidemiological study. J Clin Epidemiol. 2022;142:100–9.
24. Shea BJ, Reeves BC, Wells G, Thuku M, Hamel C, Moran J, et al. AMSTAR 2: a critical appraisal tool for systematic reviews that include randomised or non-randomised studies of healthcare interventions, or both. BMJ. 2017;358:j4008. Available from: https://www.bmj.com/content/358/bmj.j4008.long.
25. Sandau N, Aagaard TV, Hróbjartsson A, Harris IA, Brorson S. A meta-epidemiological study found that meta-analyses of the same trials may obtain drastically conflicting results. J Clin Epidemiol. 2023;156:95–104.
26. Fraser AN, Bjørdal J, Wagle TM, Karlberg AC, Lien OA, Eilertsen L, et al. Reverse shoulder arthroplasty is superior to plate fixation at 2 years for displaced proximal humeral fractures in the elderly: a multicenter randomized controlled trial. J Bone Joint Surg Am. 2020;102(6):477–85.
27. Sebastiá-Forcada E, Cebrián-Gómez R, Lizaur-Utrilla A, Gil-Guillén V. Reverse shoulder arthroplasty versus hemiarthroplasty for acute proximal humeral fractures. A blinded, randomized, controlled, prospective study. J Shoulder Elb Surg. 2014;23(10):1419–26.
28. Jonsson EÖ, Ekholm C, Salomonsson B, Demir Y, Olerud P. Reverse total shoulder arthroplasty provides better shoulder function than hemiarthroplasty for displaced 3- and 4-part proximal humeral fractures in patients aged 70 years or older: a multicenter randomized controlled trial. J Shoulder Elb Surg. 2021;30(5):994–1006.
29. Fjalestad T, Hole MØ, Hovden IAH, Blücher J, Strømsøe K. Surgical treatment with an angular stable plate for complex displaced proximal humeral fractures in elderly patients: a randomized controlled trial. J Orthop Trauma. 2012;26(2):98–106. Available from: https://journals.lww.com/jorthotrauma/abstract/2012/02000/surgical_treatment_with_an_angular_stable_plate.6.aspx.
30. Fjalestad T, Hole MØ. Displaced proximal humeral fractures: operative versus non-operative treatment—a 2-year extension of a randomized controlled trial. Eur J Orthop Surg Traumatol. 2014;24(7):1067–73.
31. Du S, Ye J, Chen H, Li X, Lin Q. Interventions for Treating 3- or 4-part proximal humeral fractures in elderly patient: a network meta-analysis of randomized controlled trials. Int J Surg. 2017;48:240–6. Available from: https://www.sciencedirect.com/science/article/pii/S1743919117312499?via%3Dihub.
32. Davey MS, Hurley ET, Anil U, Condren S, Kearney J, O'Tuile C, et al. Management options for proximal humerus fractures – a systematic review and network meta-analysis of randomized control trials. Injury. 2022;53(2):244–9. https://www.sciencedirect.com/science/article/abs/pii/S0020138321010081.
33. Orman S, Mohamadi A, Serino J, Murphy J, Hanna P, Weaver MJ, et al. Comparison of surgical and non-surgical treatments for 3- and 4-part proximal humerus fractures: a network meta-analysis. Shoulder Elbow. 2020;12(2):99–108.
34. Theivendran K, Hassan S, Tambe A, Cresswell T, Clark DI. Not all patients with displaced proximal humerus fractures are suitable for sling treatment. BMJ. 2015;350:h1669.
35. von Keudell A, Vrahas MS, Weaver MJ. Surgical versus nonsurgical treatment of adults with displaced fractures of the proximal humerus: the PROFHER randomized clinical trial. J Orthop Trauma. 2016;30:e143. Available from: https://journals.lww.com/jorthotrauma/citation/2016/04000/surgical_versus_nonsurgical_treatment_of_adults.20.aspx.
36. Handoll H, Brealey S, Rangan A, Keding A, Corbacho B, Jefferson L, Chuang L-H, Goodchild L, Hewitt C, Torgerson D. The ProFHER (PROximal Fracture of the Humerus: Evaluation by Randomisation) trial – a pragmatic multicentre randomised controlled trial evaluating the clinical effectiveness and cost-effectiveness of surgical compared with non-surgical treatment for proximal fracture of the humerus in adults. Health Technol Assess (Rockv). 2015;19(24):1–280. Available from: https://www.ncbi.nlm.nih.gov/pmc/articles/PMC4781052/.
37. Brorson S, Salomonsson B, Jensen SL, Fenstad AM, Demir Y, Rasmussen JV. Revision after shoulder replacement for acute fracture of the proximal humerus. Acta Orthop. 2017;88(4):446–50. Available from: https://actaorthop.org/actao/article/view/9694.
38. Amundsen A, Rasmussen J, Olsen B, Brorson S. Low revision rate despite poor functional outcome after stemmed hemiarthroplasty for acute proximal humeral fractures: 2,750 cases reported to the Danish Shoulder Arthroplasty Registry. Acta Orthop. 2019;90(3):196. Available from: https://actaorthop.org/actao/article/view/529.

Open Access This chapter is licensed under the terms of the Creative Commons Attribution 4.0 International License (http://creativecommons.org/licenses/by/4.0/), which permits use, sharing, adaptation, distribution and reproduction in any medium or format, as long as you give appropriate credit to the original author(s) and the source, provide a link to the Creative Commons license and indicate if changes were made.

The images or other third party material in this chapter are included in the chapter's Creative Commons license, unless indicated otherwise in a credit line to the material. If material is not included in the chapter's Creative Commons license and your intended use is not permitted by statutory regulation or exceeds the permitted use, you will need to obtain permission directly from the copyright holder.

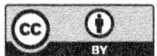

The Rise and Fall of an Implant: Locking Plates in Shoulder Fractures

12.1 Introduction

By the turn of the millennium, a new implant for fracture fixation in osteoporotic shoulder fractures had been developed and come to the market. The principle behind it was the provision of a more stable fixation of the humeral head after anatomical reduction of the fracture. By locking multiple convergent and divergent screws into an anatomically shaped lateral plate, a powerful and stiff construct was created (Fig. 12.1). In the following two decades, the locking plate technology became popular among traumatologists and shoulder surgeons. In 2019, one of the leading manufacturers announced that they had sold over 850,000 implants worldwide. It was estimated that every 7 min, a surgeon implanted the manufacturer's locking plate [1]. The implementation of the implant was supported by the principles of anatomical reduction and stable fixation, first stated by the AO group (Arbeitsgemeinschaft für Osteosynthesefragen) in 1958 [2]. The surgical technique guide from the manufacturer repeated these principles, thus linking marketing to research: "Instruments and implants approved by the AO Foundation" [3].

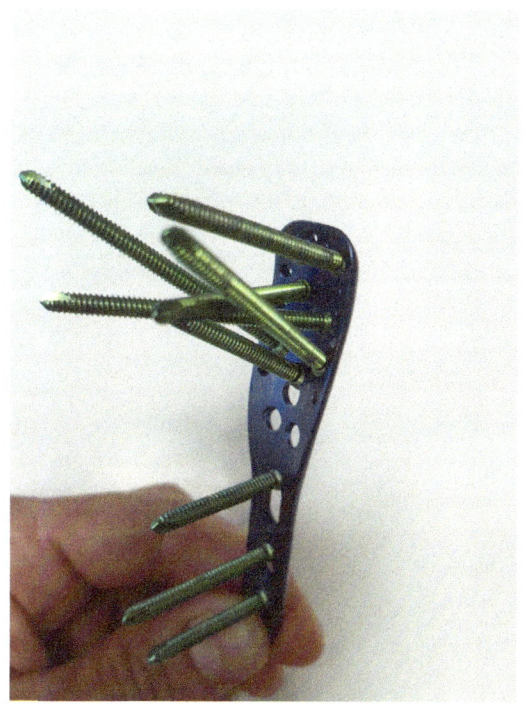

Fig. 12.1 Proximal humerus locking plate

12.2 The Biomechanical Properties of Locking Plates

Locking plate osteosynthesis aimed to provide an angle- and rotation-stable fracture fixation in osteoporotic bone. By transferring the biomechanical stress from the bone-plate interface to the locking mechanism of the screw into the plate, the traditional bi-cortical purchase of non-locking screws and the compression of the plate toward the bone were no longer needed (Fig. 12.2). The screws in the humeral head were locked into the plate and could not toggle or back out. The increased angular and axial stability, intended to reduce the risk of loss of reduction, gave hope for better fixation, especially in displaced fractures in osteoporotic bone.

The initial biomechanical testing of the locking plate technology yielded positive results. Cadaveric studies of the new implant showed superior biomechanical properties, including greater stiffness and higher varus bending load before failure (Fig. 12.3). However, while the axial load is of importance in lower limb reconstruction and quadrupeds, the most important deforming forces in shoulder fractures are horizontal and act on the tuberosities and the humeral shaft. The promising results from the laboratory gave support to a rapid clinical introduction of the implant: "We extrapolate that these improved biomechanical properties may prove advantageous in future clinical investigation" [5].

The promising preliminary results did not lead to systematic clinical testing of the implant in randomized trials. With effective manufacturer marketing, and justified by superior biomechanical properties, the use of locking plates sharply

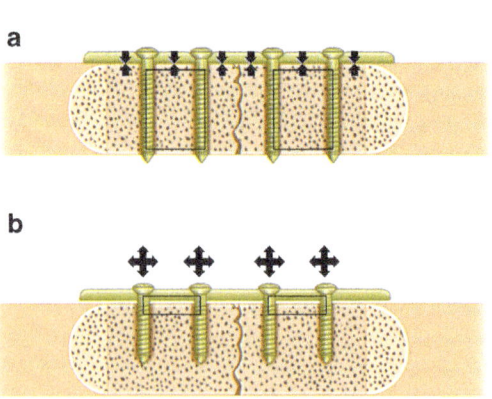

Fig. 12.2 In non-locking osteosynthesis (**a**), stability is obtained by compression of the plate against the bone by bi-cortical screws. In locking osteosynthesis (**b**), the screws are locked into the plate [4]. (With permission from Elsevier)

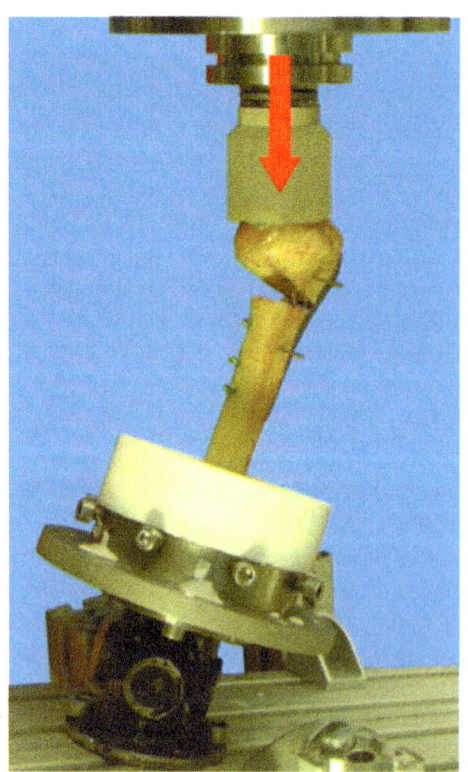

Fig. 12.3 Test of varus bending. The arrow indicates the load application [6]. (With permission from Elsevier)

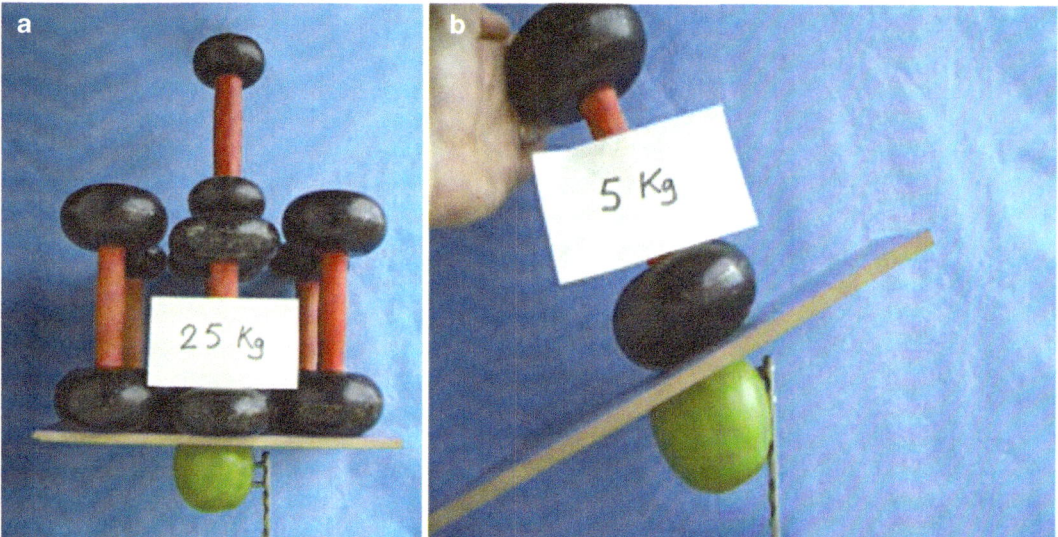

Fig. 12.4 Loading test demonstrating superior loading strength of a locking plate (**a**) compared with a non-locking plate (**b**) [7]. (With permission from Elsevier)

increased. Apart from small, uncontrolled clinical series, however, the clinical evidence remained sparse. The biomechanical evidence was incorporated into the curriculum for orthopedic residents taking internal fixation courses at all levels. Figure 12.4 demonstrates the limited purchase of non-locking screws in plate fixation of a fresh apple. A much better purchase is obtained when the fixation is performed with a locking plate. Unfortunately, we do not operate on fresh apples.

Regardless of the lack of supporting clinical evidence, biomechanical arguments were continuously used as supporting evidence. A leading implant manufacturer promoted their product under the slogan "Continued Trust in Stable Fixation." They advertised that their screw pattern covered 155% more volume of the humeral head than a similar plate from a competing company [1], assuming that more screws contributed to the implant's superiority. However, the implant's stiffness, a key biomechanical property, proved a clinical drawback.

12.3 How Does a Rigid Implant Work in an Osteoporotic Humeral Head?

In a surgical neck fracture in osteoporotic bone, some degree of humeral head collapse can be expected (Fig. 12.5). The progression typically ends with the bone healing in malunion. This process helps relieve the patient's pain and

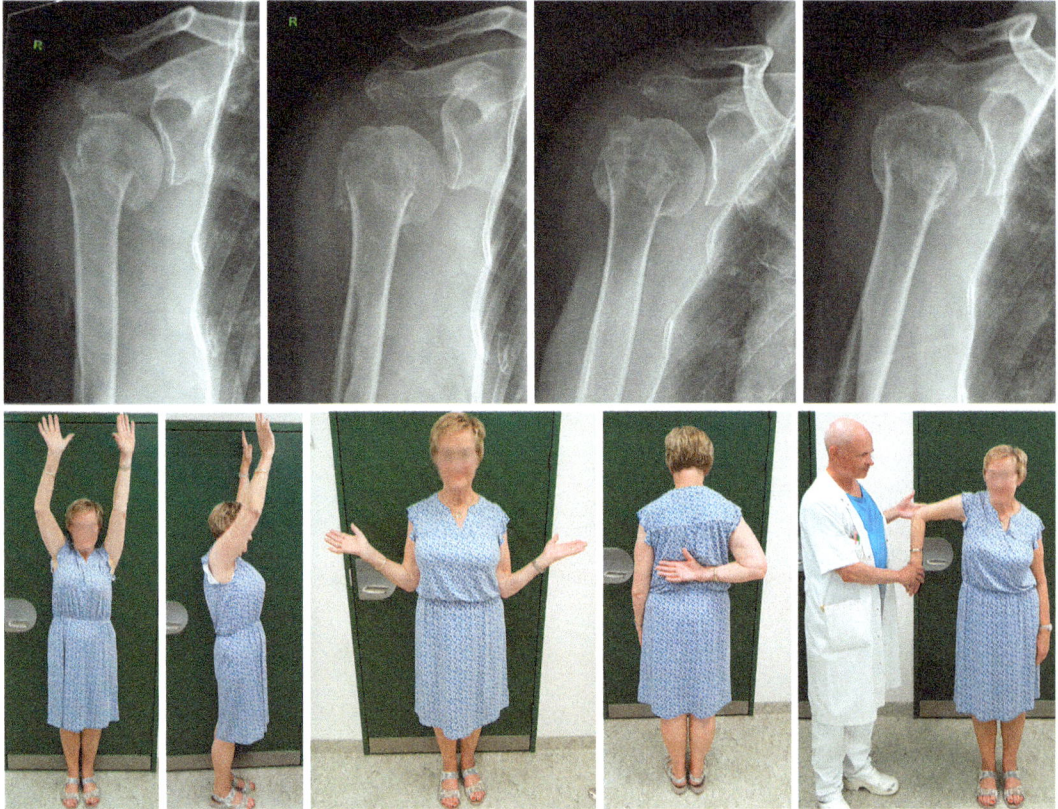

Fig. 12.5 The natural healing in an osteoporotic two-part surgical neck fracture treated non-surgically. Further impaction and partial humeral head collapse followed the initial varus displacement. Despite a fracture healing in malunion and shortening, the patient had excellent shoulder function and was pain-free. Radiographs were taken at 0, 3, 6, and 24 weeks. Photos at 24 weeks

enables rehabilitation. Regardless of anatomical reduction and satisfactory postoperative radiographs, changes in the humeral head will often proceed, leading to a cutout of the locking screws into the shoulder joint (Fig. 12.6). The osteoporotic humeral head is not strong enough to resist the stiff implant. Reverse shoulder arthroplasty is still an option as a salvage procedure, but the outcome is inferior to primary arthroplasty [8].

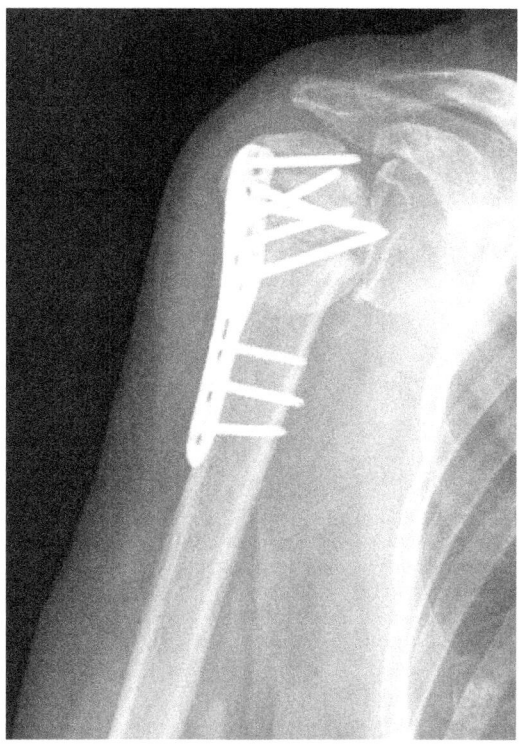

Fig. 12.6 Failure of a locking plate osteosynthesis. The humeral head has collapsed, and the screws protrude into the joint. The result is pain and damage to the cartilage and the glenoid bone

12.4 Indications for Locking Plate Osteosynthesis

When an orthopedic resident on call faces a challenging clinical case, digital platforms are available and commonly consulted. One of the most popular platforms worldwide is the AO Surgery Reference [9]. If shoulder fractures are searched, the platform recommends locking plates in "selected 2-part, 3-part, and 4-part fracture patterns."

In two-part fractures, osteoporotic bone is mentioned as a *supporting indication*. Another popular platform, *Orthobullets*, recommends locking plates in displaced two-part fractures [10]. If no colleague with up-to-date knowledge is available, the patient will be prepared for surgery with a locking plate. Few residents will have the time to search for high-quality clinical evidence or have the stamina to choose a non-surgical option for a patient with a displaced fracture. When preparing the patient for surgery, the resident will look for the surgical technique guide from the implant provider to check if implants and instruments are in stock. Again, the indication for surgery with a locking plate is confirmed. One of the leading implant providers states that the indications for locking plates are "dislocated two-, three-, and four-fragment fractures of the proximal humerus, including fractures involving osteopenic bone" [3].

This message raises a new challenge. What is a *dislocated fracture*? In orthopedic lingo, a dislocated fracture is used synonymously with any fracture not in anatomical position. In shoulder fractures, however, a *fracture-dislocation* has a distinct meaning. A fracture is *dislocated* if there is a complete separation of the humeral head and the glenoid accompanied by a fracture. This is an uncommon injury calling for immediate action. The confusion is more than semantic. If any shoulder fracture not in anatomical position is termed *dislocate*d, it provides grounds for surgical treatment of all displaced shoulder fractures. Recently, the implant provider changed the indication found in the surgical technique guide to "fractures and fracture dislocations ... particularly for patients with osteopenic bone" [11]. This statement authorizes the use of locking plates in any shoulder fracture.

Another popular indication is *fractures unsuitable for non-surgical treatment*, indicating that non-surgical treatment is the treatment of choice. Still, the phrasing authorizes operative treatment of any fracture. Fracture *instability* is another common indication for surgical intervention and intuitively appeals to orthopedic surgeons: "Whereas stable fractures are generally and successfully treated by closed means, the majority of unstable and displaced fractures require surgical treatment" [12].

An unstable fracture should be operated on. If you want to operate on a fracture, you term it *unstable*, which means it needs surgery: an unstable fracture is a surgical problem, and *surgical problems have surgical solutions*. This rhetoric puts evidence-based arguments and patient preferences under pressure. Justifying surgery by referral to fracture stability is a cornerstone in orthopedic reasoning—but when is a shoulder fracture *unstable*? This is rarely defined; if it is specified, it may refer to the stability of the fracture when tested by manipulation under fluoroscopy, meaning the patient needs to be anesthetized and prepared for open surgery to determine the stability. This is not a very useful criterion for determining indications for surgery. In clinical practice, a fracture is termed *unstable* if the position of the fragments has changed between two radiographic assessments. In osteoporotic bone, however, displaced shoulder fractures settle to some degree before they heal. It is still possible to achieve solid healing and pain-free shoulder function without needing to fix the fracture.

12.5 The Evidence Base for Locking Plates in Shoulder Fractures in Elderly

The first randomized trial comparing locking plate osteosynthesis to non-surgical treatment appeared in 2011 [13]. A Swedish group randomized 60 patients with three-part fractures and a mean age of 74. Follow-up was at 2 years and included range of motion, shoulder function (DASH and Constant Score), and health-related quality of life (EQ-5D). They reported 13% major reoperations and 17% minor reoperations. Screw penetration into the shoulder joint was reported in 17%. Re-displacement into varus was seen in 23% of the patients. Interestingly, the authors conclude:

> The results of the study indicate an advantage in functional outcome and quality of life in favor of the locking plate as compared to nonoperative treatment in elderly patients with a displaced 3-part fracture of the proximal humerus. [13]

A closer look at the data reveals that the predefined level of statistical significance was not reached for any outcome. At the moment the study was conducted, belief in the superiority of locking plates was at its highest. The implant was unlikely to be no better (or even worse) than non-surgical treatment. This led the authors to report non-significant results indicating an implant advantage. They assumed that if the study had been better powered, it would have shown the benefits of surgery.

In 2012, a Norwegian group randomized 50 patients aged 60 or above with three- and four-part fractures to locking plate or non-surgical treatment. Shoulder function was assessed after 1 year using Constant Score and ASES Score. As expected, the radiographic pattern was better in the surgical group, but no differences were found in shoulder function. They concluded:

> … there is no evidence that ORIF with an angular stable device of severely displaced B2 and C2 proximal humeral fractures in elderly patients using angular stable device [results] in better functional outcome compared with conservative closed treatment. [14]

In a pragmatic British multicenter trial from 2015, 250 patients (mean age 66) with mainly two- and three-part fractures were randomized to *surgeons' choice* or non-surgical treatment [15]. Surgeons chose a locking plate in 83% of all operative cases. No between-group differences in shoulder function (Oxford Shoulder Score) or health-related quality of life (Short Form-12) were reported at 6 or 12 months or subsequently after 2 and 5 years [16].

A Nordic group randomized 88 patients aged 60 or above with two-part fractures to locking plate osteosynthesis or non-surgical treatment. At 2-year follow-up, no differences were found in function (DASH, Constant Score, Oxford Shoulder Score) or health-related quality of life (EQ-5D). The authors concluded: "These results suggest that the current practice of performing surgery on the majority of displaced proximal 2-part fractures of the humerus in older adults may not be beneficial" [17].

In summary, the four randomized trials conducted thus far have not shown locking plate osteosynthesis to be superior to non-surgical treatment (Fig. 12.7). As discussed in the following section, it has become increasingly evident that complications specific to implants following locking plate osteosynthesis present a substantial challenge.

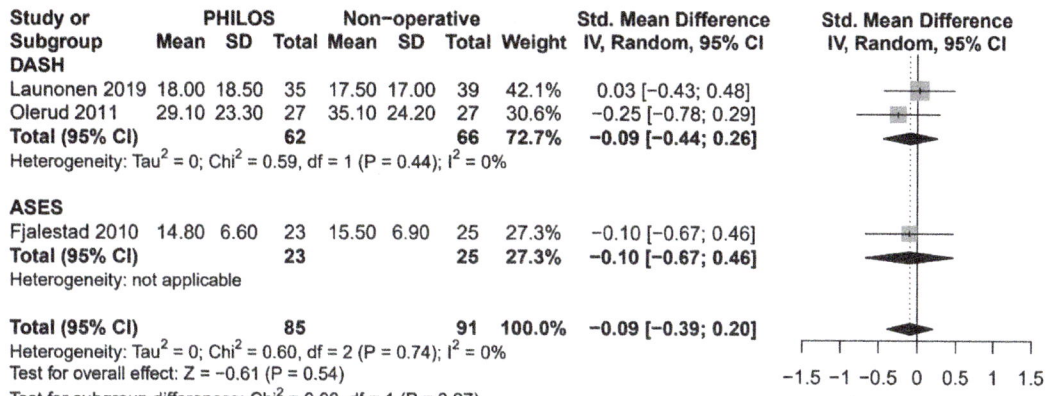

Fig. 12.7 Forest plot summarizing the functional outcome after 12 months in three randomized trials comparing locking plates with non-surgical treatment. All estimates cross the vertical line of no difference. Data from the ProFHER trial are not included because the patients were randomized to *surgeons' choice*, and baseline differences could not be controlled. However, adding the data does not change the pattern of this figure and Fig. 12.8

12.6 Failure of Locking Plate Osteosynthesis

Locking plates have been used in most shoulder fracture patterns. They have even been recommended in Neer four-part fractures and AO Type C fractures. No results from randomized trials were available until 2011, but my colleagues and I reviewed the available clinical series and reported complication rates of 16–64% and reoperation rates of 11–27% in four-part fractures [18]. In Type C fractures, avascular necrosis was reported in 4–33%, screw perforations in 5–20%, loss of fixation in 3–16%, impingement in 7–11%, and infections in 4–19% [19]. A review of 13 locking plate studies, including patients above 55 years, reported a complication rate of 29.5% and a reintervention rate of 19% [20]. The most common complication reported was screw cutout linked to poor bone quality (Fig. 12.6) [21]. A review including 374 four-part fractures reported an overall complication rate of 49% [22]. More recently, a respected shoulder clinic reported a series of 173 shoulder fractures in older people treated with locking plates [23].

Table 12.1 Risk factors for failure of locking plate osteosynthesis [24–29]

Lack of medial support
Low head-shaft angle
Varus collapse
Metaphyseal comminution
Osteoporosis
High age
Lack of anatomic reduction
Reduced humeral head height

The overall complication rate was 44%. The failure rate was 34%, defined as radiographic failure or need for reoperation.

Risk factors for clinical failure after locking plate osteosynthesis have been intensively studied to limit clinical failures. Table 12.1 summarizes risk factors for failure. Ironically, the risk factors create a picture of a patient very similar to the average older person with a displaced shoulder fracture. Thus, this implant is probably not the optimal solution for displaced shoulder fractures in older people.

The convincing biomechanical evidence and the concordance with the AO principles of anatomical reduction and stable fixation have led to a remarkable neglect of clinical failures. Faced with the failure of the trusted implant, orthopedic surgeons will often respond: "If the procedure fails, we need to improve the implant or perform the procedure differently." The orthopedic community has had a hard time accommodating that this implant is simply not working well in this fracture in this population. Consequently, numerous modifications have been proposed to decrease the clinical failure rate (Table 12.2).

In Chap. 11, I highlighted that the likelihood of undergoing additional surgery was twice as high after the initial surgery as opposed to non-surgical treatment. Specifically, for locking plates, the risk of additional surgery is more than eight times higher for the locking plate group, as depicted in Fig. 12.8.

Table 12.2 Examples of modifications to the procedure and implant for proximal humerus locking plates proposed or implemented to reduce the failure rate

Minimally invasive techniques
Cement augmentation
Additional screws
Dynamic locking screws
Thinner plates
Carbon fiber plates
Supplemental medial blade
Supplemental anterior plate
Double plating
Combined nail and plate osteosynthesis
Fibular strut augmentation
Autologous iliac crest bone graft
Endosteal strut plate
Titanium cage in the medullary channel
Arthroscopically examination for screw penetration

12.7 The Locking Plate Epidemic

This section will analyze geographical trends in the use of locking plates during the first two decades of the millennium. Several companies adopted the new technology and introduced a number of almost identical implants to the market. Before public tendering, communication between surgeons and manufacturers was crucial for the promotion of new implants. However, this may lead to a focus on biomechanical properties at the expense of documenting patient outcome. The rapidly growing use of locking plates may have been influenced by factors beyond clinical evidence, such as effective marketing, lack of awareness about the scientific literature, and a strong belief in surgical skills and the advantages of surgery [30].

Access to reliable data on treatment outcome is scarce beyond the four randomized trials. While several national databases have been established to cover joint replacement surgery, data quality on joint-preserving techniques remains poor. Insurance companies have some data available, but implant companies are hesitant to share it due to competition concerns. The most reliable data often comes from national administrative or reimbursement databases based on diagnoses and procedure codes.

In the Swedish Hospital Discharge Register, a 12-fold increase in the overall rate of plate osteosynthesis was reported between 2001 and 2012 [31]. The Finnish National Hospital Discharge Register reported a more than fourfold increase in locking plate osteosynthesis between 1998 and 2009. The steepest increase was seen between 2002 and 2009 [32]. The Danish National Patient

Study	PHILOS		Non-operative		Weight	Risk Ratio MH, Random, 95% CI	Risk Ratio MH, Random, 95% CI
	Events	Total	Events	Total			
Fjalestad 2010	8	25	1	25	40.5%	8.00 [1.08; 59.32]	
Launonen 2019	3	40	0	42	18.9%	7.35 [0.39; 137.81]	
Olerud 2011	9	29	1	29	40.6%	9.00 [1.22; 66.56]	
Total (95% CI)		94		96	100.0%	8.26 [2.31; 29.55]	
Heterogeneity: Tau^2 = 0; Chi^2 = 0.01, df = 2 (P = 0.99); I^2 = 0%							
Test for overall effect: Z = 3.25 (P < 0.01)							

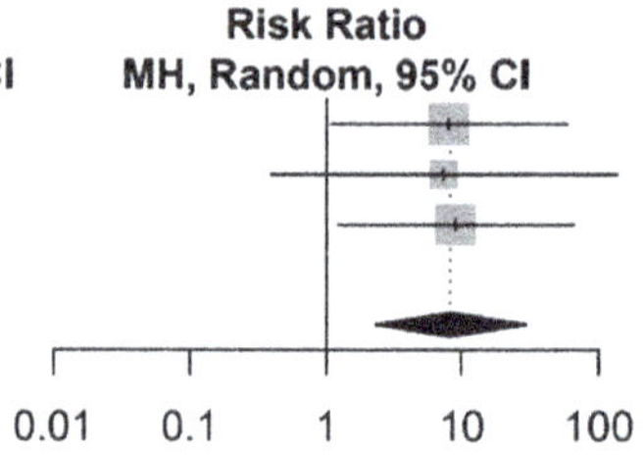

Fig. 12.8 Risk of additional surgery after locking plate osteosynthesis

Register reported a 13-fold increase in plate osteosyntheses between 2001 and 2011 [33]. A study based on the data from the Federal Statistical Office of Germany reported an increase in surgery of 39% between 2007 and 2016, with locking plates used in 48% of the surgeries [34]. In Portugal, the use of locking plate osteosynthesis in hospitalized patients increased from below 30% to above 45% between 2000 and 2016, according to the data from a national admission database [35].

While high-quality epidemiological data on implants are sparse outside Europe, similar trends have been reported. According to the Statewide Planning and Research Cooperative System database in New York State, the use of locking plates increased from 47% to 59% of surgeries between 2001 and 2010 [36]. Additionally, a sample from Medicare data reported a 29% increase in osteosynthesis between 2000 and 2005. A 20- to 30-fold difference in surgery rates between hospitals in the United States has been reported [37]. There have been limited studies on the epidemiology of shoulder fractures in Asia, although the use of locking plates is extensive. According to the Korean Health Insurance Review and Assessment Service database, the surgery rate increased from 25% in 2008 to 37% in 2016. In 2008, osteosynthesis accounted for 72% of surgical procedures, while in 2016, it accounted for 86% [38]. According to two Australian national healthcare databases, there has been a reverse trend in the number of surgeries performed. Although the trend immediately after the introduction of locking plates in 2002 is not covered, a decrease in surgeries overall has been reported. Moreover, 2008 surgeries accounted for 33%, while in 2017, the percentage decreased to 23%. Osteosynthesis accounted for 77% and 73%, respectively. The most significant decrease in surgery was observed between 2015 and 2017 [39].

In the Nordic countries, there has been a steady decline in the use of locking plates for osteosynthesis from the mid-2010s. While the registry-based studies cannot establish causal relationships, it is interesting to note that this trend coincides with the emergence of randomized trials [14–17] and meta-analyses [40, 41]. These studies have consistently reported that locking plate osteosynthesis is not superior to non-surgical treatment, which may, to some extent, explain the decline in the use of locking plates. A Swedish single center covering the period from 2011 to 2017 reported an overall surgery rate of 23%. Additionally, locking plates in surgeries decreased from 47% to 25% [42]. Meanwhile, a Finnish study based on two national registries reported a 50% decrease in the use of locking plates between 2013 and 2019. The reduction was primarily observed in patients aged 60 years or older. In 2019, the overall surgery rate was 13% [43]. In Denmark, my colleagues and I reported the percentage of surgeries for fractures decreased from 17% in 2013 to 11% in 2018 [33]. The rate of surgeries using locking plates remained steady at around 55%. In 2015, the Danish Orthopaedic Association published a national guideline recommending non-surgical treatment for two-, three-, and four-part fractures in older people.

In contrast to the Nordic trend, German practice seems unaffected by the clinical evidence. Locking plate osteosynthesis has remained the most popular procedure, with more than 35,000 surgeries in 2016 [34]. The difference in practice, even between geographically and culturally close countries, is remarkable. German-speaking orthopedic communities, having a strong biomechanical tradition, may have placed less emphasis on conducting high-quality clinical trials to validate the biomechanical findings in relevant populations.

12.8 Perspectives

Orthopedic surgeons have a strong inclination to bring broken bones together. This general approach does not, however, consider differences in upper and lower limb fractures, bone quality, the potential for spontaneous healing, functional demands, or the patient's preferences and values. It is unclear why prominent orthopedic surgeons continue to carry out low-value procedures despite the availability of high-quality clinical evidence. While surgical traditions and a culture of acting could be contributing factors, commercial interests, concerns over patient flow in private clinics, ignorance of scientific literature, or unquestioning confidence in one's abilities may also be at play [30]. It is reasonable to assume that insurance companies, coming to an increasing recognition of the lack of clinical evidence for the benefits of surgical treatment of shoulder fractures, will request less operative activity on older people. Healthcare administrators, politicians, and patient associations are likely to come to the same conclusion.

Many surgical procedures currently being practiced do not align with evidence-based practice. Evidence-based practice involves the integration of the best clinical evidence with clinical expertise and the patient's values and preferences [44]. For older people with shoulder fractures, locking plates are not the best option, despite the presence of clinical expertise in the operative procedure. This conclusion may be uncomfortable for some stakeholders. However, the de-implementation of surgical treatment for the majority of shoulder fracture patients must not lead to indifference toward this large population of fracture patients. High-quality care for non-surgically treated fracture patients is a core orthopedic responsibility.

References

1. DePuy Synthes. 3.5 mm LCP® Proximal Humerus Plate: value summary. 2019. p. 1–2. Available from: https://www.jnjmedtech.com/sites/default/files/user_uploaded_assets/pdf_assets/2019-03/108141-190224DSUS_ProxHum_SS_US_150.pdf.
2. Müller ME, Allgöwer M, Willenegger H. Technik der Operativen Frakturenbehandlung. Berlin, Heidelberg: Springer; 1963.
3. DePuy Synthes. PHILOS and PHILOS Long. Surgical technique. Synth GmbH. 2016. p. 1–36. Available from: https://www.kalteq.com/wp-content/uploads/2024/07/PHILOS-PHILOS-LONG.pdf.
4. Frigg R, Appenzeller A, Christensen R, Frenk A, Gilbert S, Schavan R. The development of the distal femur Less Invasive Stabilization System (LISS). Injury. 2001;32:24–31.
5. Chudik SC, Weinhold P, Dahners LE. Fixed-angle plate fixation in simulated fractures of the proximal humerus: a biomechanical study of a new device. J Shoulder Elb Surg. 2003;12(6):578–88.
6. Röderer G, Brianza S, Schiuma D, Schwyn R, Scola A, Gueorguiev B, et al. Mechanical assessment of local bone quality to predict failure of locked plating in a proximal humerus fracture model. Orthopedics. 2013;36(9):e1134–40. Available from: https://journals.healio.com/doi/10.3928/01477447-20130821-14?url_ver=Z39.88-2003&rfr_id=ori:rid:crossref.org&rfr_dat=cr_pub0pubmed.
7. Cronier P, Pietu G, Dujardin C, Bigorre N, Ducellier F, Gerard R. The concept of locking plates. Orthop Traumatol Surg Res. 2010;96(4):S17–36. Available from: https://www.sciencedirect.com/science/article/pii/S1877056810000587?via%3Dihub.
8. Kristensen MR, Rasmussen JV, Elmengaard B, Jensen SL, Olsen BS, Brorson S. High risk for revision after shoulder arthroplasty for failed osteosynthesis of proximal humeral fractures. Acta Orthop. 2018;89(3):345–50. Available from: https://actaorthop.org/actao/article/view/7206.
9. Jaeger M. Proximal humerus. AO Surgical Reference; 2018. Available from: https://surgeryreference.aofoundation.org/orthopedic-trauma/adult-trauma/proximal-humerus.
10. Orthobullets. Proximal humerus fractures. 2022. Available from: https://www.orthobullets.com/trauma/1015/proximal-humerus-fractures.
11. DePuy Synthes. 3.5 mm LCP® Proximal Humerus Plates: surgical technique. 2021. p. 1–60. Available from: https://p1.aprimocdn.net/jjamp/en/depuy-synthes/surgical-technique-guide/3.5-mm-lcp-proximal-humerus-platesdsustrm10161133.pdf.
12. Plecko M, Kraus A. Internal fixation of proximal humerus fractures using the locking proximal humerus plate. Oper Orthop Traumatol. 2005;17(1):25–50.
13. Olerud P, Ahrengart L, Ponzer S, Saving J, Tidermark J. Internal fixation versus nonoperative treatment of displaced 3-part proximal humeral fractures in elderly patients: a randomized controlled trial. J Shoulder Elb Surg. 2011;20(5):747–55.
14. Fjalestad T, Hole MØ, Hovden IAH, Blücher J, Strømsøe K. Surgical treatment with an angular stable plate for complex displaced proximal humeral fractures in elderly patients: a randomized controlled trial. J Orthop Trauma. 2012;26(2):98–106. Available from: https://journals.lww.com/jorthotrauma/abstract/2012/02000/surgical_treatment_with_an_angular_stable_plate.6.aspx.
15. Rangan A, Handoll H, Brealey S, Jefferson L, Keding A, Martin BC, et al. Surgical vs nonsurgical treatment of adults with displaced fractures of the proximal humerus: the PROFHER randomized clinical trial. JAMA. 2015;313(10):1037–47. Available from: https://jamanetwork.com/journals/jama/fullarticle/2190987.
16. Handoll HH, Keding A, Corbacho B, Brealey SD, Hewitt C, Rangan A. Five-year follow-up results of the PROFHER trial comparing operative and non-operative treatment of adults with a displaced fracture of the proximal humerus. Bone Joint J. 2017;99-B(3):383–92. Available from: https://boneandjoint.org.uk/article/10.1302/0301-620X.99B3.BJJ-2016-1028.

References

17. Launonen AP, Sumrein BO, Reito A, Lepola V, Paloneva J, Jonsson KB, et al. Operative versus non-operative treatment for 2-part proximal humerus fracture: a multicenter randomized controlled trial. PLoS Med. 2019;16(7):e1002855. Available from: https://www.ncbi.nlm.nih.gov/pmc/articles/PMC6638737/.
18. Brorson S, Rasmussen JV, Frich LH, Olsen BS, Hróbjartsson A. Benefits and harms of locking plate osteosynthesis in intraarticular (OTA Type C) fractures of the proximal humerus: a systematic review. Injury. 2012;43(7):999–1005. Available from: https://www.sciencedirect.com/science/article/abs/pii/S0020138311004025.
19. Brorson S, Frich LH, Winther A, Hróbjartsson A. Locking plate osteosynthesis in displaced 4-part fractures of the proximal humerus. Acta Orthop. 2011;82(4):475–81. Available from: https://actaorthop.org/actao/article/view/10945.
20. Oldrini LM, Feltri P, Albanese J, Marbach F, Filardo G, Candrian C. PHILOS synthesis for proximal humerus fractures has high complications and reintervention rates: a systematic review and meta-analysis. Life. 2022;12(2):311. Available from: https://www.mdpi.com/2075-1729/12/2/311.
21. Panagiotopoulou VC, Varga P, Richards RG, Gueorguiev B, Giannoudis PV. Late screw-related complications in locking plating of proximal humerus fractures: a systematic review. Injury. 2019;50(12):2176–95. Available from: https://www.sciencedirect.com/science/article/abs/pii/S0020138319306989?via%3Dihub.
22. Sproul RC, Iyengar JJ, Devcic Z, Feeley BT. A systematic review of locking plate fixation of proximal humerus fractures. Injury. 2011;42(4):408–13. Available from: https://www.sciencedirect.com/science/article/abs/pii/S002013831000793X?via%3Dihub.
23. Barlow JD, Logli AL, Steinmann SP, Sems SA, Cross WW, Yuan BJ, et al. Locking plate fixation of proximal humerus fractures in patients older than 60 years continues to be associated with a high complication rate. J Shoulder Elb Surg. 2020;29(8):1689–94.
24. Laflamme G-Y, Moisan P, Chapleau J, Goulet J, Leduc S, Benoit B, et al. Novel technical factors affecting proximal humerus fixation stability. J Orthop Trauma. 2021;35(5):259–64. Available from: https://journals.lww.com/jorthotrauma/abstract/2021/05000/novel_technical_factors_affecting_proximal_humerus.7.aspx.
25. Wang Q, Sheng N, Rui B, Chen Y. The neck-shaft angle is the key factor for the positioning of calcar screw when treating proximal humeral fractures with a locking plate. Bone Joint J. 2020;102-B(12):1629–35. Available from: https://boneandjoint.org.uk/article/10.1302/0301-620X.102B12.BJJ-2020-0070.R1.
26. Krappinger D, Bizzotto N, Riedmann S, Kammerlander C, Hengg C, Kralinger FS. Predicting failure after surgical fixation of proximal humerus fractures. Injury. 2011;42(11):1283–8. Available from: https://www.sciencedirect.com/science/article/abs/pii/S002013831100026X.
27. Jung S-W, Shim S-B, Kim H-M, Lee J-H, Lim H-S. Factors that influence reduction loss in proximal humerus fracture surgery. J Orthop Trauma. 2015;29(6):276–82. Available from: https://journals.lww.com/jorthotrauma/abstract/2015/06000/factors_that_influence_reduction_loss_in_proximal.4.aspx.
28. Newton AW, Selvaratnam V, Pydah SK, Nixon MF. Simple radiographic assessment of bone quality is associated with loss of surgical fixation in patients with proximal humeral fractures. Injury. 2016;47(4):904–8. Available from: https://www.sciencedirect.com/science/article/abs/pii/S0020138315008505.
29. Haws BE, Samborski SA, Karnyski S, Soles G, Gorczyca JT, Nicandri GT, et al. Risk factors for loss of reduction following locked plate fixation of proximal humerus fractures in older adults. Injury. 2023;54(2):567–72. Available from: https://www.sciencedirect.com/science/article/abs/pii/S0020138322008713.
30. Brorson S. Locking plate osteosynthesis in geriatric shoulder fractures: why do we continue to perform a low-value procedure? Acta Orthop. 2022;93:355–7. Available from: https://actaorthop.org/actao/article/view/2208.
31. Sumrein BO, Huttunen TT, Launonen AP, Berg HE, Felländer-Tsai L, Mattila VM. Proximal humeral fractures in Sweden—a registry-based study. Osteoporos Int. 2017;28(3):901–7.
32. Huttunen TT, Launonen AP, Pihlajamäki H, Kannus P, Mattila VM. Trends in the surgical treatment of proximal humeral fractures – a nationwide 23-year study in Finland. BMC Musculoskelet Disord. 2012;13(1):261. Available from: https://bmcmusculoskeletdisord.biomedcentral.com/articles/10.1186/1471-2474-13-261.
33. Brorson S, Viberg B, Gundtoft P, Jalal B, Ohrt-Nissen S. Epidemiology and trends in management of acute proximal humeral fractures in adults: an observational study of 137,436 cases from the Danish National Patient Register, 1996-2018. Acta Orthop. 2022;93:750–5. Available from: https://actaorthop.org/actao/article/view/4578.
34. Klug A, Gramlich Y, Wincheringer D, Schmidt-Horlohé K, Hoffmann R. Trends in surgical management of proximal humeral fractures in adults: a nationwide study of records in Germany from 2007 to 2016. Arch Orthop Trauma Surg. 2019;139(12):1713–21.
35. Relvas Silva M, Linhares D, Leite MJ, Nunes B, Torres J, Neves N, et al. Proximal humerus fractures: epidemiology and trends in surgical management of hospital-admitted patients in Portugal. JSES Int. 2022;6(3):380–4.

36. Khatib O, Onyekwelu I, Zuckerman JD. The incidence of proximal humeral fractures in New York State from 1990 through 2010 with an emphasis on operative management in patients aged 65 years or older. J Shoulder Elb Surg. 2014;23(9):1356–62.
37. Bell J-E, Leung BC, Spratt KF, Koval KJ, Weinstein JD, Goodman DC, et al. Trends and variation in incidence, surgical treatment, and repeat surgery of proximal humeral fractures in the elderly. J Bone Joint Surg Am. 2011;93(2):121–31.
38. Jo Y-H, Lee K-H, Lee B-G. Surgical trends in elderly patients with proximal humeral fractures in South Korea: a population-based study. BMC Musculoskelet Disord. 2019;20(1):136. Available from: https://bmcmusculoskeletdisord.biomedcentral.com/articles/10.1186/s12891-019-2515-2.
39. McLean AS, Price N, Graves S, Hatton A, Taylor FJ. Nationwide trends in management of proximal humeral fractures: an analysis of 77,966 cases from 2008 to 2017. J Shoulder Elb Surg. 2019;28(11):2072–8.
40. Handoll HH, Brorson S. Interventions for treating proximal humeral fractures in adults. Cochrane Database Syst Rev. 2015;(11):CD000434. Available from: http://doi.wiley.com/10.1002/14651858.CD000434.pub4.
41. Handoll HH, Elliott J, Thillemann TM, Aluko P, Brorson S. Interventions for treating proximal humeral fractures in adults. Cochrane Database Syst Rev. 2022;6(6):CD000434. Available from: https://www.cochranelibrary.com/cdsr/doi/10.1002/14651858.CD000434.pub5/abstract.
42. Bergdahl C, Wennergren D, Swensson-Backelin E, Ekelund J, Möller M. No change in reoperation rates despite shifting treatment trends: a population-based study of 4,070 proximal humeral fractures. Acta Orthop. 2021;92(6):651–7. Available from: https://actaorthop.org/actao/article/view/1445.
43. Leino OK, Lehtimäki KK, Mäkelä K, Äärimaa V, Ekman E. Proximal humeral fractures in Finland: trends in the incidence and methods of treatment between 1997 and 2019. Bone Joint J. 2022;104-B(1):150–6.
44. Sackett DL. Evidence-based medicine and treatment choices. Lancet. 1997;349:570.

Open Access This chapter is licensed under the terms of the Creative Commons Attribution 4.0 International License (http://creativecommons.org/licenses/by/4.0/), which permits use, sharing, adaptation, distribution and reproduction in any medium or format, as long as you give appropriate credit to the original author(s) and the source, provide a link to the Creative Commons license and indicate if changes were made.

The images or other third party material in this chapter are included in the chapter's Creative Commons license, unless indicated otherwise in a credit line to the material. If material is not included in the chapter's Creative Commons license and your intended use is not permitted by statutory regulation or exceeds the permitted use, you will need to obtain permission directly from the copyright holder.

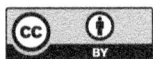

The Use of Reverse Shoulder Arthroplasty in Shoulder Fractures

13.1 Reverse Shoulder Arthroplasty in Fracture Management

Paul Grammont (1940–2012) developed the reverse shoulder prosthesis in 1985 for the treatment of advanced rotator cuff arthropathy. At that time, no treatment could be offered to these patients suffering severe pain and disability. The design appeared in the literature in 1993 [1]. Grammont also used his new prosthesis in an unpublished series of 22 patients with acute fractures and fracture-dislocations between 1989 and 1993 [2]. Grammont observed that the deltoid's function could be improved by medially and inferiorly shifting the center of rotation (Fig. 13.1). This adjustment created a new biomechanical environment for the deltoid muscle, allowing it to compensate for the lack of or weakness in the rotator cuff muscles by increasing tension and improving the lever arm for the deltoid abduction. Function is provided by recruiting anterior and posterior deltoid fibers to serve as abductors [3].

The device depends on the deltoid muscle for function, making it useful for patients with severe

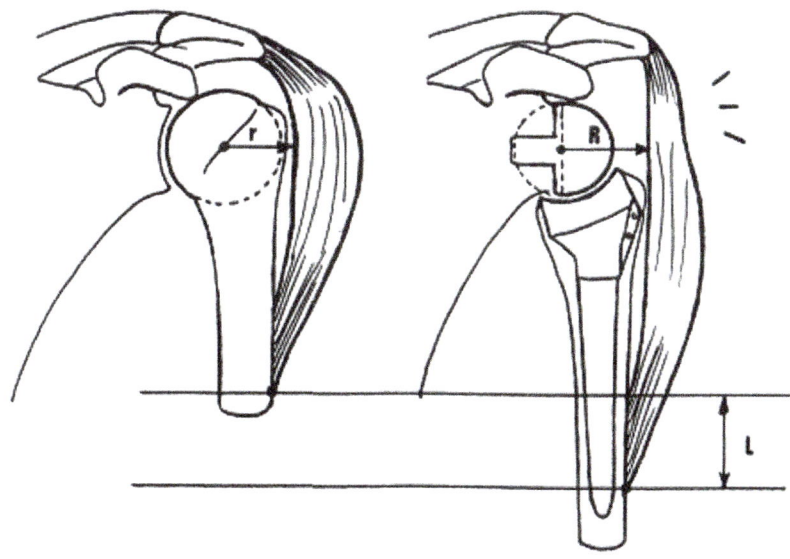

Fig. 13.1 The principle of medialization and distalization in the Grammont type of reverse arthroplasty. The design involves using a large glenoid hemisphere without a neck to articulate with a small humeral cup [4]. (With permission from Elsevier)

rotator cuff deficiency. While it was initially designed for patients with rotator cuff arthropathy, older people with displaced shoulder fractures face similar challenges. In three- and four-part fractures, the rotator cuff insertions are detached from the humeral head and need reattachment to regain rotational movement. This can be obtained with or without surgical fixation. However, tuberosity healing often fails, whether to native bone or implants. Furthermore, many older people have preexisting rotator cuff insufficiency, rotator cuff tears during the trauma, or *acute in chronic* tears. This is the rationale for using reverse shoulder arthroplasty as the first-line treatment in elderly with three- and four-part fractures and fracture-dislocations (Fig. 13.2). The procedure's popularity or familiarity, however, is no guarantee of clinical benefit.

The popularity of reverse arthroplasty in fracture management is remarkable, as it provides a nonanatomical solution. While osteosynthesis or anatomical prostheses aim to provide anatomical reconstructions, Grammont introduced a nonanatomical solution. Subsequent developments of reverse arthroplasty have focused on facilitating tuberosity fixation and ingrowth. The basic design, although biomechanically meaningful, is nonanatomical.

Some insights into the use of reverse shoulder arthroplasty can be obtained from the annual reports of national joint replacement registries. In the 2023 report from the British National Joint Registry, more than 600 reverse arthroplasties were implanted for fractures in 2022. The cumulative number of reverse arthroplasties inserted since 2014 was 4380 [5]. The cumulative number of reverse arthroplasty for fractures in Australia since 2008 was 7648 [6]. Based on the data from the American National Inpatient Sample, an increase in reverse arthroplasty for fractures from

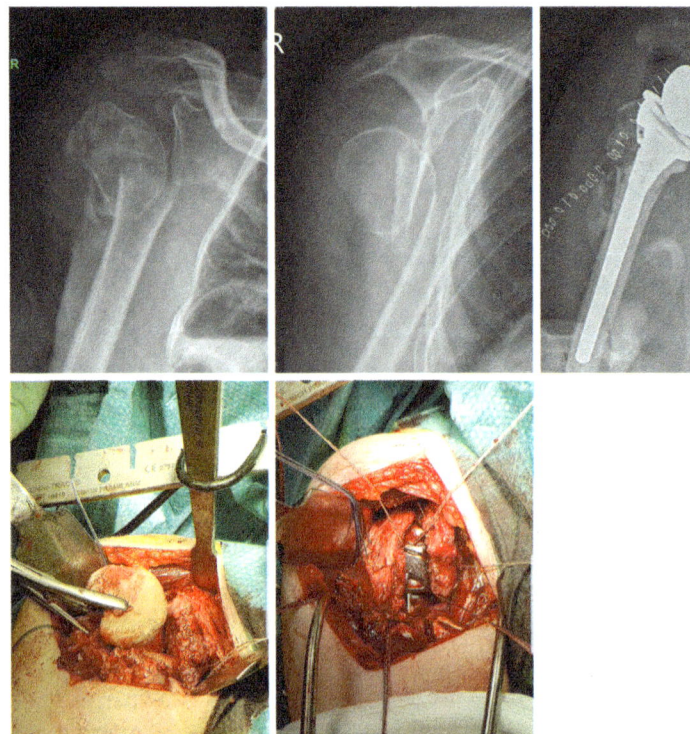

Fig. 13.2 A 74-year-old self-reliant female suffering a painful two-part surgical neck fracture without bony contact. A reverse arthroplasty was inserted, preceded by an osteotomy of the tuberosities. Subsequently, the tuberosities were fixed to the stem, and the rotator cuff was reconstructed. Pre- and postoperatively radiographs. Peroperative photos of the humeral head removal and closure of the rotator interval

2558 surgeries in 2012 to 8904 in 2017 has been reported [7].

Published reports on the outcome after reverse arthroplasty for shoulder fractures appeared in the mid-2000s [8]. In 2003, the American Food and Drug Administration approved reverse arthroplasty for "grossly rotator cuff deficient joint with severe arthropathy or a previous failed joint replacement with a grossly rotator cuff deficient joint" [9]. Many series and reviews have been published. Reapplying the search string my colleagues and I used for a systematic review on reverse arthroplasty in fractures in 2013 [8] reveals an increase in PubMed references from 190 in 2013 to 1578 in 2024. The procedure is now well-established globally as the preferred surgical treatment for displaced shoulder fractures in older people. The abundance of research reports may add to the misconception that the clinical effect is firmly documented.

13.2 The Evidence Base for Reverse Shoulder Arthroplasty in Fracture Management

Although many authors report treatment effects, only five randomized trials (<1%) have been conducted and can provide reliable estimates of treatment effects [10–14]. This section focuses on the two randomized trials comparing reverse shoulder arthroplasty to non-surgical treatment [10, 11].

The first trial was published in 2019 [10]. In total, 62 patients aged 80 years or older with three- or four-part fractures were randomized to reverse arthroplasty or non-surgical treatment. The primary outcomes were the non-adjusted and adjusted Constant-Murley scores at 1 year. The predefined minimal clinically important difference was set at 8 points. A statistically and clinically non-significant difference of 6 points in favor of surgery was found. The authors concluded that reverse arthroplasty offers minimal benefits over non-operative treatment.

The second randomized trial appeared in 2024 with the title *Reverse Shoulder Arthroplasty or Nothing for Patients with Displaced Proximal Humeral Fractures* [11]. As the title suggests, the options were reverse arthroplasty or nothing. Even their rehabilitation protocol seems included in "nothing." The study is one of the few randomized trials in the field, which means a more difficult and time-consuming design than most observational studies. The protocol was registered in ClinicalTrials in 2018, while the publication was done in 2024. The conclusion in the abstract reads:

> Treatment with reverse shoulder arthroplasty provides superior functional outcomes compared with conservative treatment for patients presenting with an acute proximal humeral fracture. The difference in CMS is close to the clinically significant thresholds, and some harms are associated with the operative treatment.

Let us take a closer look at the data behind this puzzling conclusion. The study was a two-group multicenter, superiority, randomized trial that allocated patients aged 70 to 90 with a three- or four-part fracture to reverse shoulder arthroplasty or non-surgical treatment. The primary outcome measure was the unadjusted Constant-Murley score at a 1-year follow-up. The primary analysis was the between-group difference in the overall Constant-Murley score. The sample size calculation relied on a predefined minimal clinically important difference of 10 points in the Constant-Murley score. A mean difference of 8.84 points was reported.

Although the primary outcome was below the predefined threshold for clinical importance, several outcomes turned out to be statistically significant. In their discussion, the authors sought to justify a positive interpretation by considering the adjusted Constant-Murley score and breaking down the score for sub-analyses. They also referred to authors who had suggested a lower minimal clinically important difference for the Constant-Murley score. Their conclusion was that the clinical relevance of their findings was unclear:

> Patients presenting a displaced proximal humeral fracture allocated to the RSA group obtained better outcomes than those assigned to nonoperative treatment. However, the benefit was unlikely to be perceived by participants. The risk of presenting a poor outcome based on the adjusted Constant-Murley score was higher in the nonoperative group [11].

The strength of a randomized trial depends on a rigorous methodology and a clear interpretation. A treatment cannot be claimed to be superior if the average difference between the groups is less than the predefined minimal clinically important difference for the primary outcome. Drawing conclusions based on a misinterpretation of data is an example of *spin*: reporting practices that distort the interpretation of results and so mislead readers into viewing results in a more favorable light [15].

13.3 The Limited Impact of a Negative Finding

Why was the enthusiasm for reverse arthroplasty for fractures not affected by the first trial, and why was the second trial's data so challenging to interpret? Some answers can be found by examining the research activity in the 5 years between the two trials.

During this period, more than 200 observational studies and reviews were published; the majority of these were retrospective series or cohort studies with historical controls. The question of whether reverse arthroplasty was better than non-surgical treatment was neglected to a remarkable degree. All studies shared the assumption that reverse arthroplasty was superior in treating shoulder fractures. Observational studies with historical controls can be heavily confounded as patient selection and indications are rarely recorded and reported. Selection bias may occur if patients with specific pathologies and other patient-related factors are selected for surgery.

The numerous studies published on reverse shoulder arthroplasty during this period reported data on, among others, surgical approaches [16], the effect of tuberosity fixation [17, 18], the use of fracture stems versus conventional stems [19, 20], the use of cemented versus uncemented stems [21, 22], suture techniques for tuberosity fixation [23], tension band technique [24], the impact of humeral inclination on tuberosity healing [25, 26], an offset modular system with bone graft [27], medialized or lateralized center of rotation [28], the effect of humeral inclination and lateral offset of the glenosphere [29], excision of the supraspinatus tendon [30], and rehabilitation after reverse arthroplasty [31, 32].

The perceived superiority of reverse arthroplasty for fractures was justified by comparison with cohorts of other indications for reverse arthroplasty, including elective indications [33, 34], degenerative conditions [35], and rotator cuff deficiency [25]. A series of publications compared acute and delayed procedures [36, 37] and reported outcomes after reverse arthroplasty for failed osteosynthesis [38, 39].

To demonstrate the superiority of reverse arthroplasty, several network meta-analyses were conducted [40–42]. In Chap. 12, I discussed some of the problems of conducting network meta-analyses for surgical interventions. Most importantly, the indirect comparison of more than two interventions relies on the assumption of *transitivity*. The study populations included should be comparable at baseline, like in an imaginary randomized multiarm trial. The studies included in the three network meta-analyses varied substantially regarding indications, procedures, age, and gender. Moreover, none of the network meta-analyses seemed to follow a predefined protocol or analysis plan, which allowed for various *analytical scenarios* and conclusions. We need direct comparisons of reverse arthroplasty and non-surgical treatment in randomized trials to obtain reliable effect estimates. Network meta-analyses are not applicable to heterogeneous surgical populations and interventions.

At least three ongoing trials compare reverse arthroplasty with non-surgical treatment. The ReShAPE trial is a combined randomized and observational cohort study, including patients aged 70 or older with three- or four-part fractures [43]. It aims to recruit 72 patients. The primary outcome is the American Shoulder and Elbow Society score at 1 year. The Nordic DeltaCon trial aims to include 154 patients aged 65–85 with three- or four-part fractures [44]. The primary outcome is QuickDASH score at 2 years. The ProFHER-2 trial is a three-arm trial aiming to include 380 patients aged 65 or above with three- or four-part fractures or fracture-dislocations from 40 NHS hospitals in the United Kingdom [45]. The patients with three- and four-part fractures are allocated in a 2:2:1 fashion to reverse arthroplasty, hemiarthroplasty, or non-surgical treatment. Patients with fracture-dislocations are allocated 1:1 to reverse arthroplasty or hemiarthroplasty. The primary outcome is the Oxford Shoulder Score at 2 years. The challenge of recruitment to orthopedic randomized trials is illustrated in protocol registrations of the three ongoing trials in 2016, 2018, and 2018. Designing a trial to determine the optimal time for surgery is challenging and requires a multicenter setup and a common core outcome set. If only about 5–10% of fractures in older people require surgery, the pool of eligible participants becomes restricted. A randomization process would need to take place at baseline. Some in the delayed surgery group may cross over to non-surgical treatment. Future trials are required for evidence-based decision-making in the most challenging cases.

13.4 The "Red Wine Effect" of Fracture Prostheses

National arthroplasty registries with high completeness can provide reliable data on implant survival. By merging data from Nordic arthroplasty registries, my colleagues and I reported a satisfactory cumulative implant survival rate of 96% for 6756 hemiarthroplasties and reverse arthroplasties in acute fractures [46]. However, we also found that implant survival did not mirror patient outcomes in hemiarthroplasty procedures for fractures. In 2719 patients from the Danish Shoulder Arthroplasty Register, the 10-year cumulative implant survival rate was 95%. Still, we found that 25% of the patients had less than 50% of their patient-reported shoulder function left, and 11% had less than 30% left [47]. Revision of failed reverse arthroplasty can be challenging, and an unknown number of patients with failed reverse arthroplasties may not be offered revision or are not fit for surgery.

Surprisingly, following patient-reported outcomes over time from registry data may seem like the patients' outcomes are improving, akin to a red wine that improves with age. This may cause some enthusiasm among implant providers and wishful surgeons. However, the apparent improvement is not a property of the implant or procedure but a consequence of patients with a poor outcome, leaving the cohort in a population with high mortality [48].

13.5 "The Surgeon's Fallacy"

In this section, I will discuss a commonly used strategy for justifying the use of reverse arthroplasty in fracture patients. This reasoning is typically used at scientific meetings when presenting observational data on the benefits of reverse arthroplasty. Although there may be variations of this argument, it essentially goes as follows:

> "Reverse arthroplasty is better than hemiarthroplasty."
> "Reverse arthroplasty is better than locking plates."
> "Let's use reverse arthroplasty!"

The first premise is an empirical claim that reverse arthroplasty is superior to hemiarthroplasty. Two randomized trials have investigated this question. A Swedish group randomized 99 patients aged 70 or above with three- and four-part fractures to hemiarthroplasty or reverse arthroplasty [13]. The primary outcome was the unadjusted Constant-Murley score at the final follow-up (minimum 2 years). The minimal clinically important difference was predefined at 10 points. A statistically and clinically significant mean difference of 11.1 points was reported. The authors concluded that reverse arthroplasty provided better shoulder function than hemiarthroplasty.

Similarly, a Spanish group randomized 62 patients aged 70 or above with three- and four-part fractures, fracture-dislocations, and head-splitting fractures to hemiarthroplasty or reverse arthroplasty [12]. The primary outcome was the unadjusted Constant-Murley score at 2 years of follow-up. The predefined minimal clinically important difference was set at 15 points. A statistically and clinically significant mean difference of 16.1 points was reported. It was concluded that reverse arthroplasty resulted in less pain, better function, and a lower revision rate.

In a combined analysis of the two trials, 19 complications were reported. These occurred more frequently in the hemiarthroplasty group (14 out of 81) compared to the reverse arthroplasty group (5 out of 79). Most reoperations (8 out of 10) were performed on patients from the hemiarthroplasty group, with conversion to reverse arthroplasty. Therefore, data from these two randomized trials support the premise that reverse arthroplasty is superior to hemiarthroplasty.

The second premise is another empirical claim that reverse shoulder arthroplasty is superior to locking plate osteosynthesis. This question was addressed in the multicenter DelPhi trial, which randomized 124 patients aged 65–85 with AO B2 or C2 fractures to locking plate or reverse shoulder arthroplasty [14]. The primary outcome was the unadjusted Constant-Murley score at the 2-year follow-up. The minimal clinically important difference was predefined at 10 points. A statistically and clinically significant mean difference of 13.4 points in favor of reverse arthroplasty was found. The authors concluded their data suggested an advantage of reverse arthroplasty over locking plate osteosynthesis in treating displaced proximal humeral fractures in older people. There were fewer complications in the reverse group (7/64) than in the locking plate group (11/60). Four reoperations were performed in the reverse group compared to seven in the locking plate group. Thus, the second premise of the superiority of reverse arthroplasty over locking plate osteosynthesis is supported by data from a randomized trial.

Now let us consider the conclusion that reverse arthroplasty should be used in shoulder fractures. While we found high-quality evidence to support its superiority compared to hemiarthroplasty and locking plate osteosynthesis, our findings are still compatible with the conclusion that reverse arthroplasty is less harmful than the other surgical options. In other words, we need to anchor our trials and demonstrate that any of these procedures are superior to no procedure. So far, ten randomized trials have reported no superiority of surgical procedures compared to non-surgical treatment. The studies have included hemiarthroplasty [49, 50], locking plate [51–53], hemiarthroplasty or locking plate [54], surgeon's choice [55], or reverse arthroplasty [10, 11]. Therefore, the conclusion is not valid. It might well be the case that reverse arthroplasty is superior to hemiarthroplasty and locking plate—but we still have to demonstrate that any of these implants is better than no implant.

13.6 Perspectives

The question of acute versus delayed surgery can only be answered through randomization. Retrospective or prospective cohort studies cannot answer the question as residual confounding at baseline cannot be controlled. It is unclear if the acutely operated share the same characteristics as the delayed group. Patients who are not suitable for surgery or are hesitant to undergo surgery are not primarily operated on. However, if patients return with unbearable pain, they are more likely to undergo surgery. One might argue that if observational studies suggest acute surgery to be better than delayed surgery, why not perform acute surgery on all patients? Even if late surgery has a worse outcome than primary RSA, this does not justify that all patients should undergo acute surgery. This may lead to unnecessary surgeries and a substantial burden of revision surgeries. The trend toward operating on younger patients and less severe fractures and the steadily increasing number of implantations is concerning. Complications include dislocation, infection, hematoma, instability, nerve injury, reflex sympathetic dystrophy, acromion or scapular spine fractures, scapular notching, periprosthetic fractures, and baseplate failure. Revision surgery can be challenging, and excessive bone loss can be expected over time. Using a salvage procedure as the first-line treatment can have consequences for the patient. Current practice will be judged by the next generation of patients and surgeons.

References

1. Grammont PM, Baulot E. Delta shoulder prosthesis for rotator cuff rupture. Orthopedics. 1993;16(1):65–8.
2. Sirveaux F, Navez G, Roche O MD. Reverse Prosthesis for Proximal Humerus Fracture, Technique and Results. Tech Should Surg. 2008;9:15–22. Available from: https://web.archive.org/web/20170809120803id_/; http://www.kinex.cl/papers/Hombro/ReverseProsthesis for Proximal.pdf
3. Boileau P. Biographical sketch: Paul M. Grammont, MD (1940). Clin Orthop Relat Res. 2011;469(9):2422–3.
4. Boileau P, Watkinson DJ, Hatzidakis AM, Balg F. Grammont reverse prosthesis: design, rationale, and biomechanics. J Shoulder Elb Surg. 2005;14(1 Suppl S):147S–61S.
5. Healthcare Quality Improvement Partnership Ltd. (HQIP). National Joint Registry, 20th Annual Report. 2023; Available from: https://www.hqip.org.uk/resource/national-joint-registry-20th-annual-report-2023
6. The Australian Orthopaedic Association National Joint Replacement Registry. Annual report: hip, knee and shoulder arthroplasty. 2023.; Available from: https://aoanjrr.sahmri.com/annual-reports-2023
7. Best MJ, Aziz KT, Wilckens JH, McFarland EG, Srikumaran U. Increasing incidence of primary reverse and anatomic total shoulder arthroplasty in the United States. J Shoulder Elb Surg. 2021;30(5):1159–66.
8. Brorson S, Rasmussen J, Olsen B, Frich L, Jensen S, Hróbjartsson A. Reverse shoulder arthroplasty in acute fractures of the proximal humerus: a systematic review. Int J Shoulder Surg. 2013;7(2):70–8. Available from: https://www.ncbi.nlm.nih.gov/pmc/articles/PMC3743034/
9. Food and Drug Administration: Department of Health & human Services. Delta Total Shoulder Prosthesis 2003;(November 18). Available from: https://www.accessdata.fda.gov/cdrh_docs/pdf2/K021478.pdf
10. Lopiz Y, Alcobía-Díaz B, Galán-Olleros M, García-Fernández C, Picado AL, Marco F. Reverse shoulder arthroplasty versus nonoperative treatment for 3- or 4-part proximal humeral fractures in elderly patients: a prospective randomized controlled trial. J Shoulder Elb Surg. 2019;28(12):2259–71.
11. Miquel J, Cassart E, Santana F, Martínez R, Valls L, Salomó-Domènech M, et al. Reverse shoulder arthroplasty or nothing for patients with displaced proximal humeral fractures. A randomized controlled trial. J Shoulder Elb Surg. 2024;S1058-2746(24):00224-6.
12. Sebastiá-Forcada E, Cebrián-Gómez R, Lizaur-Utrilla A, Gil-Guillén V. Reverse shoulder arthroplasty versus hemiarthroplasty for acute proximal humeral fractures. A blinded, randomized, controlled, prospective study. J Shoulder Elb Surg. 2014;23(10):1419–26.
13. Jonsson EÖ, Ekholm C, Salomonsson B, Demir Y, Olerud P. Reverse total shoulder arthroplasty provides better shoulder function than hemiarthroplasty for displaced 3- and 4-part proximal humeral fractures in patients aged 70 years or older: a multicenter randomized controlled trial. J Shoulder Elb Surg. 2021;30(5):994–1006.
14. Fraser AN, Bjørdal J, Wagle TM, Karlberg AC, Lien OA, Eilertsen L, et al. Reverse shoulder arthroplasty is superior to plate fixation at 2 years for displaced proximal humeral fractures in the elderly: a multicenter randomized controlled trial. J Bone Joint Surg Am. 2020;102(6):477–85.
15. Chiu K, Grundy Q, Bero L. "Spin" in published biomedical literature: a methodological systematic review. PLoS Biol. 2017;15(9):e2002173. Available from: https://journals.plos.org/plosbiology/article?id=10.1371/journal.pbio.2002173
16. Schuette HB, Starcher NJ, Goubeaux CC, DeGenova DT, Triplet JJ, Mehta S, et al. Reverse shoulder arthroplasty for proximal humerus fractures: a comparison of the deltoid split and deltopectoral approaches. Arch Orthop Trauma Surg. 2023;143(8):4663–9.
17. Gunst S, Louboutin L, Swan J, Lustig S, Servien E, Nove-Josserand L. Does healing of both greater and lesser tuberosities improve functional outcome after reverse shoulder arthroplasty for fracture? A retrospective study of twenty-eight cases with a computed tomography scan at a minimum of one-year follow-up. Int Orthop. 2021;45(3):681–7. Available from: https://link.springer.com/article/10.1007/s00264-020-04928-9
18. Porcellini G, Montanari M, Giorgini A, Micheloni GM, Bonfatti R, Tarallo L. Great tuberosity fixation does not affect healing and clinical outcomes in RSA performed in proximal humeral fractures in elderly patients. Musculoskelet Surg. 2024;108(1):107–14.
19. Onggo JR, Nambiar M, Onggo JD, Hau R, Pennington R, Wang KK. Improved functional outcome and tuberosity healing in patients treated with fracture stems than nonfracture stems during shoulder arthroplasty for proximal humeral fracture: a meta-analysis and systematic review. J Shoulder Elb Surg. 2021;30(3):695–705.
20. Sasanuma H, Iijima Y, Saito T, Saitsu A, Saito T, Matsumura T, et al. Efficacy of fracture stem in reverse shoulder arthroplasty for 3- or 4-part proximal humerus fractures. J Orthop Sci. 2023;28(6):1266–73.
21. Rossi LA, Guillermina BM, Buljubasich M, Atala N, Tanoira I, Bongiovanni S, et al. Cemented versus uncemented reverse shoulder arthroplasty for acute proximal humeral fractures. J Shoulder Elb Surg. 2022;31(2):261–8.
22. Kramer M, Olach M, Zdravkovic V, Manser M, Jost B, Spross C. Cemented vs. uncemented reverse total shoulder arthroplasty for the primary treatment of proximal humerus fractures in the elderly-a retrospective case-control study. BMC Musculoskelet Disord. 2022;23(1):1043. Available from: https://bmcmusculoskeletdisord.biomedcentral.com/articles/10.1186/s12891-022-05994-3

23. Troiano E, Peri G, Calò I, Colasanti GB, Mondanelli N, Giannotti S. A novel "7 sutures and 8 knots" surgical technique in reverse shoulder arthroplasty for proximal humeral fractures: tuberosity healing improves short-term clinical results. J Orthop Traumatol. 2023;24(1):18. Available from: https://jorthoptraumatol.springeropen.com/articles/10.1186/s10195-023-00697-4
24. Takayama K, Yamada S, Kobori Y, Shiode H. The clinical outcomes and tuberosity healing after reverse total shoulder arthroplasty for acute proximal humeral fracture using the turned stem tension band technique. J Orthop Sci. 2022;27(2):372–9.
25. Schmalzl J, Piepenbrink M, Buchner J, Picht S, Gerhardt C, Lehmann L-J. Higher primary stability of tuberosity fixation in reverse fracture arthroplasty with 135° than with 155° humeral inclination. J Shoulder Elb Surg. 2021;30(6):1257–65.
26. O'Sullivan J, Lädermann A, Parsons BO, Werner B, Steinbeck J, Tokish JM, et al. A systematic review of tuberosity healing and outcomes following reverse shoulder arthroplasty for fracture according to humeral inclination of the prosthesis. J Shoulder Elb Surg. 2020;29(9):1938–49.
27. Fortané T, Beaudouin E, Lateur G, Giraudo P, Kerschbaumer G, Boudhissa M, et al. Tuberosity healing in reverse shoulder arthroplasty in traumatology: use of an offset modular system with bone graft. Orthop Traumatol Surg Res. 2020;106(6):1113–8. Available from: https://www.sciencedirect.com/science/article/pii/S1877056820302139?via%3Dihub
28. Carrazana-Suarez LF, Panico LC, Smolinski MP, Blake RJ, McCroskey MA, Sykes JB, et al. Humeral offset as a predictor of outcomes after reverse shoulder arthroplasty. J Shoulder Elb Surg. 2022;31(6S):S158–65.
29. Holschen M, Körting M, Khourdaji P, Bockmann B, Schulte TL, Witt K-A, et al. Treatment of proximal humerus fractures using reverse shoulder arthroplasty: do the inclination of the humeral component and the lateral offset of the glenosphere influence the clinical outcome and tuberosity healing? Arch Orthop Trauma Surg. 2022;142(12):3817–26.
30. Bonnevialle N, Ohl X, Clavert P, Favard L, Frégeac A, Obert L, et al. Should the supraspinatus tendon be excised in the case of reverse shoulder arthroplasty for fracture? Eur J Orthop Surg Traumatol. 2020;30(2):231–5.
31. Tuphe P, Caubriere M, Hubert L, Lancigu R, Sakek F, Loisel F, et al. Early rehabilitation after reverse total shoulder prosthesis on fracture of proximal humerus in elderly patients provides better functional outcome. Eur J Orthop Surg Traumatol. 2023;33(7):2951–7.
32. Tong CH, Fang CX. Rehabilitation progress following reverse total shoulder replacement and internal fixation for geriatric three and four-part proximal humerus fractures – a propensity score matched comparison. BMC Musculoskelet Disord. 2023 Jul;24(1):566. Available from: https://bmcmusculoskeletdisord.biomedcentral.com/articles/10.1186/s12891-023-06669-3
33. Crespo AM, Luthringer TA, Frost A, Khabie L, Roche C, Zuckerman JD, et al. Does reverse total shoulder arthroplasty for proximal humeral fracture portend poorer outcomes than for elective indications? J Shoulder Elb Surg. 2021;30(1):40–50.
34. Paras T, Raines B, Kohut K, Sabzevari S, Chang Y-F, Yeung M, et al. Clinical outcomes of reverse total shoulder arthroplasty for elective indications versus acute 3- and 4-part proximal humeral fractures: a systematic review and meta-analysis. J Shoulder Elb Surg. 2022;31(1):e14–21.
35. Spek RW, Spekenbrink-Spooren A, Vanhommerig JW, Jonkman N, Doornberg JN, Jaarsma RL, et al. Primary reverse total shoulder arthroplasty for fractures requires more revisions than for degenerative conditions 1 year after surgery: an analysis from the Dutch Arthroplasty Register. J Shoulder Elb Surg. 2023;32(12):2508–18.
36. Lu V, Jegatheesan V, Patel D, Domos P. Outcomes of acute vs. delayed reverse shoulder arthroplasty for proximal humerus fractures in the elderly: a systematic review and meta-analysis. J Shoulder Elb Surg. 2023;32(8):1728–39.
37. Barger J, Stenquist DS, Mohamadi A, Weaver MJ, Dyer GSM, von Keudell A. Acute versus delayed reverse total shoulder arthroplasty for the management of proximal Humerus fractures. Injury. 2021;52(8):2272–8. Available from: https://www.sciencedirect.com/science/article/abs/pii/S0020138321004903
38. Colasanti CA, Anil U, Adams J, Pennacchio C, Zuckerman JD, Egol KA. Primary versus conversion reverse total shoulder arthroplasty for complex proximal humeral fractures in elderly patients: a retrospective comparative study. J Shoulder Elb Surg. 2023;32(8):e396–407.
39. Sebastia-Forcada E, Lizaur-Utrilla A, Cebrian-Gomez R, Miralles-Muñoz FA, Lopez-Prats FA. Outcomes of reverse Total shoulder arthroplasty for proximal humeral fractures: primary arthroplasty versus secondary arthroplasty after failed proximal humeral locking plate fixation. J Orthop Trauma. 2017;31(8):e236–40. Available from: https://journals.lww.com/jorthotrauma/fulltext/2017/08000/outcomes_of_reverse_total_shoulder_arthroplasty.10.aspx
40. Zheng Y, Tang N, Zhang W-J, Shi W, Zhao W-W, Yang K. Comparative efficacy and safety of medical treatments for proximal humerus fractures: a systematic review and network meta-analysis. BMC Musculoskelet Disord. 2024;25(1):17. Available from: https://bmcmusculoskeletdisord.biomedcentral.com/articles/10.1186/s12891-023-07053-x
41. Huang Z, Dong H, Ye C, Zou Z, Wan W. A network meta-analysis of multiple modalities for the treatment of complex proximal humeral fractures in older adults. Injury. 2023;54(10):110958. Available from:

https://www.sciencedirect.com/science/article/pii/S0020138323006447

42. Davey MS, Hurley ET, Anil U, Condren S, Kearney J, O'Tuile C, et al. Management options for proximal humerus fractures – a systematic review and network meta-analysis of randomized control trials. Injury. 2022;53(2):244–9. Available from: https://www.sciencedirect.com/science/article/abs/pii/S0020138321010081

43. Smith GCS, Bateman E, Cass B, Damiani M, Harper W, Jones H, et al. Reverse Shoulder Arthroplasty for the treatment of Proximal humeral fractures in the Elderly (ReShAPE trial): study protocol for a multicentre combined randomised controlled and observational trial. Trials [Internet]. 2017;18(1):91. Available from: http://trialsjournal.biomedcentral.com/articles/10.1186/s13063-017-1826-6

44. Launonen AP, Fjalestad T, Laitinen MK, Lähdeoja T, Ekholm C, Wagle T, et al. Nordic Innovative Trials to Evaluate osteoPorotic Fractures (NITEP) collaboration: the Nordic DeltaCon trial protocol—non-operative treatment versus reversed total shoulder arthroplasty in patients 65 years of age and older with a displaced proximal humer. BMJ Open. 2019;9(1):e024916. Available from: http://bmjopen.bmj.com/lookup/doi/10.1136/bmjopen-2018-024916

45. Rangan A, Gwilym S, Keding A, Corbacho B, Kottam L, Arundel C, et al. Reverse shoulder arthroplasty versus hemiarthroplasty versus non-surgical treatment for older adults with acute 3- or 4-part fractures of the proximal humerus: study protocol for a randomised controlled trial (PROFHER-2: PROximal fracture of Humerus Eval). Trials. 2023;24(1):270. Available from: https://trialsjournal.biomedcentral.com/articles/10.1186/s13063-023-07259-3

46. Brorson S, Salomonsson B, Jensen SL, Fenstad AM, Demir Y, Rasmussen JV. Revision after shoulder replacement for acute fracture of the proximal humerus. Acta Orthop. 2017;88(4):446–50. Available from: https://actaorthop.org/actao/article/view/9694

47. Amundsen A, Rasmussen J, Olsen B, Brorson S. Low revision rate despite poor functional outcome after stemmed hemiarthroplasty for acute proximal humeral fractures: 2,750 cases reported to the Danish Shoulder Arthroplasty Registry. Acta Orthop. 2019;90(3) Available from: https://actaorthop.org/actao/article/view/529

48. Amundsen A, Brorson S, Olsen BS, Rasmussen JV. Ten-year follow-up of stemmed hemiarthroplasty for acute proximal humeral fractures. Bone Joint J. 2021;103-B(6):1063–9. Available from: https://boneandjoint.org.uk/article/10.1302/0301-620X.103B6.BJJ-2020-1753.R1

49. Boons HW, Goosen JH, Van Grinsven S, Van Susante JL, Van Loon CJ. Hemiarthroplasty for humeral four-part fractures for patients 65 years and older: a randomized controlled trial. Clin Orthop Relat Res. 2012;470(12):3483–91. Available from: https://www.ncbi.nlm.nih.gov/pmc/articles/PMC3492647/

50. Olerud P, Ahrengart L, Ponzer S, Saving J, Tidermark J. Hemiarthroplasty versus nonoperative treatment of displaced 4-part proximal humeral fractures in elderly patients: a randomized controlled trial. J Shoulder Elb Surg. 2011;20(7):1025–33.

51. Olerud P, Ahrengart L, Ponzer S, Saving J, Tidermark J. Internal fixation versus nonoperative treatment of displaced 3-part proximal humeral fractures in elderly patients: a randomized controlled trial. J Shoulder Elb Surg. 2011;20(5):747–55.

52. Fjalestad T, Hole MØ, Hovden IAH, Blücher J, Strømsøe K. Surgical treatment with an angular stable plate for complex displaced proximal humeral fractures in elderly patients: a randomized controlled trial. J Orthop Trauma. 2012;26(2):98–106. Available from: https://journals.lww.com/jorthotrauma/abstract/2012/02000/surgical_treatment_with_an_angular_stable_plate.6.aspx

53. Launonen AP, Sumrein BO, Reito A, Lepola V, Paloneva J, Jonsson KB, et al. Operative versus non-operative treatment for 2-part proximal humerus fracture: a multicenter randomized controlled trial. PLoS Med. 2019;16(7):e1002855. Available from: https://www.ncbi.nlm.nih.gov/pmc/articles/PMC6638737/

54. Launonen AP, Sumrein BO, Reito A, Lepola V, Paloneva J, Berg HE, et al. Surgery with locking plate or hemiarthroplasty versus nonoperative treatment of 3-4-part proximal humerus fractures in older patients (NITEP): An open-label randomized trial. PLoS Med [Internet]. 2023;20(11):e1004308. Available from: https://journals.plos.org/plosmedicine/article?id=10.1371/journal.pmed.1004308

55. Rangan A, Handoll H, Brealey S, Jefferson L, Keding A, Martin BC, et al. Surgical vs nonsurgical treatment of adults with displaced fractures of the proximal humerus: the PROFHER randomized clinical trial. JAMA. 2015;313(10):1037–47. Available from: https://jamanetwork.com/journals/jama/fullarticle/2190987

Open Access This chapter is licensed under the terms of the Creative Commons Attribution 4.0 International License (http://creativecommons.org/licenses/by/4.0/), which permits use, sharing, adaptation, distribution and reproduction in any medium or format, as long as you give appropriate credit to the original author(s) and the source, provide a link to the Creative Commons license and indicate if changes were made.

The images or other third party material in this chapter are included in the chapter's Creative Commons license, unless indicated otherwise in a credit line to the material. If material is not included in the chapter's Creative Commons license and your intended use is not permitted by statutory regulation or exceeds the permitted use, you will need to obtain permission directly from the copyright holder.

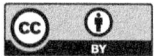

Part V

Benefits and Harms

Outcome After Shoulder Fractures

14.1 Introduction

Agreeing upon the relevant measuring instruments before collecting and comparing outcome data is essential. Should the instruments be objective, subjective, or a combination of both? Deciding who administers the instruments and determines the relevant domains and items is also essential. Over the years, surgeons have favored objective outcomes, which usually involve measuring factors such as range of motion, strength, and radiographic assessments. The line between objective and subjective outcomes is not clearly defined, but could impact the risk of bias in clinical trials [1]. Using *composite* outcomes like the Constant-Murley Score (CMS) may further challenge the assessment of the risk of bias in the measurement. Objective outcome measures influence how surgeons interpret the treatment results and can aid in assessing surgical quality. However, they may not necessarily align with patients' values and preferences. To practice evidence-based surgery, we need to consider the clinical expertise, the best available evidence, and the patient's values and preferences [2]. Patients must be consulted to know if our treatments are successful. If we rely only on the surgeon's assessment of patient outcome, there is a risk of missing important information from the treatment recipient. In this chapter, I will discuss the use of outcome instruments following shoulder fractures.

14.2 The Landscape of Outcome Assessment Instruments

There is no agreed-upon core outcome set for patients with shoulder fractures. Current outcome assessment measures have been adapted from other populations and contexts unrelated to fractures. Rheumatologists have attempted to identify all outcome measures used in randomized trials and prospective comparative studies for all shoulder conditions and have taken steps to establish a core outcome set for shoulder disorders [3]. They have identified 31 unique outcome measures from randomized trials, including ratings of complications, hardware problems, and CMS [4].

A systematic review identified 22 outcome measures in 74 research reports of outcome following shoulder fractures. A considerable variability in outcome choice was found [5]. The CMS was the most popular instrument (65%), followed by the Disabilities of the Arm, Shoulder and Hand (DASH) score (31%), pain visual analog scale (27%), and the American Shoulder and Elbow Surgeons (ASES) shoulder score (18%).

My colleagues and I included 47 randomized trials in the latest Cochrane review [6]. Most trials used a combination of instruments, commonly a shoulder-specific instrument and a generic health-related quality-of-life (HRQoL) instrument. The CMS was the most popular instrument used in 33 of 47 trials. Fourteen trials reported a DASH or QuickDASH score. Oxford Shoulder Score (OSS) was used in six trials, while five older trials used the Neer score. Three studies used the ASES score. Nine trials reported the generic HRQoL instrument EuroQol-five dimensions (EQ-5D). Four studies used Short-Form (SF-12 or SF-36).

14.3 Properties of Outcome Assessment Instruments

A few distinctions can be helpful before discussing the use of outcome instruments in shoulder fracture patients. Outcome assessment instruments can be divided into *physician-reported* and *patient-reported* instruments. In patient-reported outcomes (PROs), the assessment comes directly from the patient without any interpretation. Although several PROs are used to evaluate shoulder fracture patients, no PRO has been developed specifically for shoulder fracture patients. Measuring instruments can be divided into *patient-administered and observer-administered* instruments. The CMS is an example of an instrument that includes patient-reported data (pain and activities of daily living) but is administered by the observer, usually the treatment provider. Thus, the patient reports pain to the surgeon, who registers the pain and calculates the score. Outcome assessment instruments can further be *condition-specific* or *generic*. Although we have no shoulder fracture-specific instruments, several have been developed for other shoulder conditions (OSS and ASES) or upper extremity-specific instruments (DASH). Generic instruments include questionnaires to assess health-related quality of life like EQ-5D or SF-36.

Finally, outcome-measuring instruments can be *patient-derived* or *physician-derived*. Most PROs are physician-derived: the physician decides what is important for the patient to report to them. Although the patient reports the outcome, the extent to which the reported outcome captures areas of interest for the patient is less clear. In patient-derived PROs, the instrument is developed with the patient as an important collaborator. Typically, items are chosen and discussed in focus groups, and hierarchies of items are decided. A questionnaire is defined based on the selected items and subsequently validated in the relevant population. Patient-derived PROs have been developed in other medical specialties [7, 8] and can be expected to be introduced for orthopedic conditions.

14.4 The Constant-Murley Score and Its Limitations

CMS is the most popular outcome instrument for assessing outcome in patients with shoulder fractures. A PubMed search on ("Shoulder Fractures"[Mesh]) AND (constant score) revealed 844 studies referring to the Constant Score out of 4285 papers on shoulder fractures. The score was developed as a general tool for assessing shoulder function [9, 10]. CMS is an observer-administered, composite outcome, including patient- and physician-reported items. The score ranges from 0 to 100, with 100 being the best. The instrument consists of four parts: pain (0–15, no pain = 15 p), activities of daily living (0–20), range of motion (0–40), and strength (0–25). The questions cover the previous 24 hours. Objective outcomes (65/100) outweigh subjective outcomes (35/100). The measuring of strength relies on a dynamometer. The total score can be modified (or normalized) according to age and gender or be compared with the opposite shoulder function [11, 12].

When using CMS to assess older people with shoulder fractures, it is essential to consider certain limitations:

- Biases from both patients and observers may influence observer-administered outcomes.
- The use of a dynamometer requires standardization.
- Testing strength three times on each side is time-consuming and challenging for patients, observers, and trial logistics.
- Covering every shoulder pathology makes distinguishing impacts from different or overlapping conditions challenging.

- Pain measurement is poorly defined and often reported without reference to activity or time; assessing pain on a 0–15-point scale is unintuitive, and low observer agreement has been reported [13].
- The range of motion and the amount of weight lifted at 90° of abduction may not be very important for older people with shoulder fractures. For an elderly patient, having a pain-free shoulder with less than 90° of arm abduction may be acceptable; having less than 90° of arm movement automatically results in a deduction of 25 points; however, meaning a floor effect can be expected for strength assessment in older people. The instrument subtracts a disproportionate number of points for decreased range of motion and strength.

The patient in Fig. 14.1 illustrates a discrepancy between outcome assessment with CMS and patient perception. The treatment aim, expressed by the patient at the first visit, was to hold her grandchild again. This aim was obtained after 12 weeks. The patient was pain-free and had a good sleep at night. She remained self-reliant with a flexion at 120°. However, abduction remained at 80°. The total CMS was 47/100, indicating that less than half of the shoulder function was left. This did not reflect the patient's perception.

The relationship between objective and subjective outcome assessment instruments has not been thoroughly studied in shoulder fracture patients. The common assumption that the appearance of shoulder fractures on radiographs can predict the patient's condition must be revisited, especially for older people. More knowledge about the predictive value of radiographic findings in older people with shoulder fractures is needed. Pain may be a better predictor of fail-

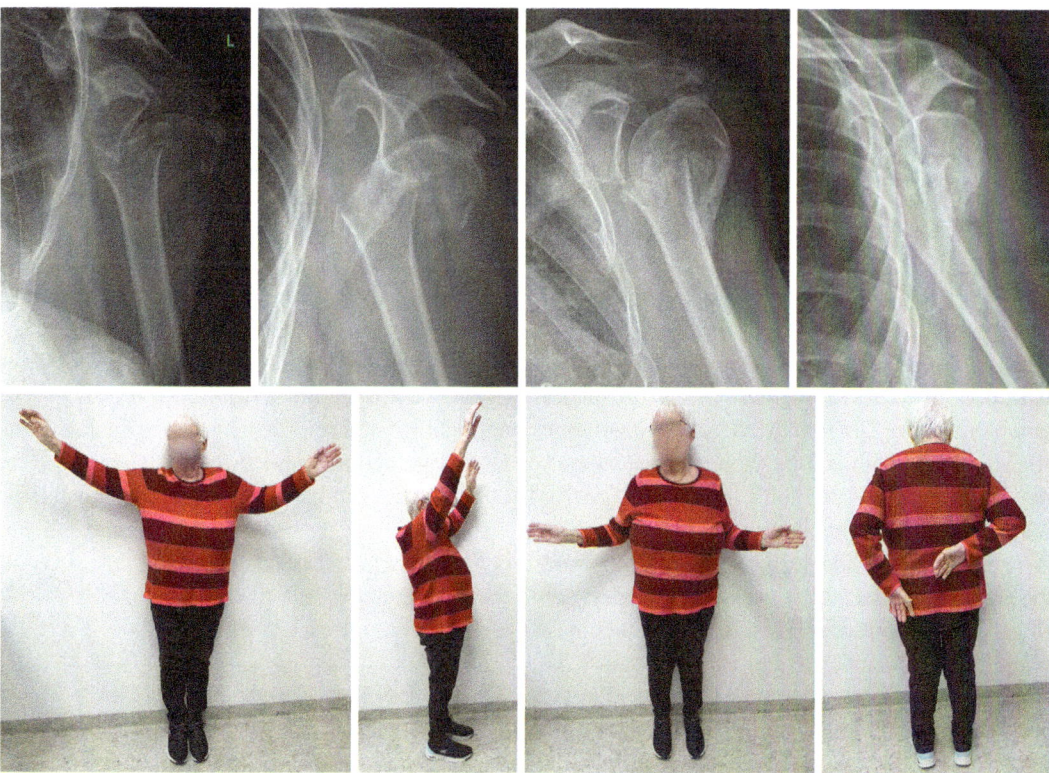

Fig. 14.1 A 77-year-old female with a medially and anteriorly translated two-part surgical neck fracture. The fracture healed in malunion, but a firm lateral callus bridge was formed. The patient was pain-free after 6 weeks. Radiographs at admission and 12 weeks. Clinical photos at 12 weeks

ure than radiographic appearance. Treatment decisions should not be exclusively based on radiographs, except in rare cases of fracture-dislocations and head-splitting fractures. Even severe malunion can be compatible with pain relief and patient satisfaction. We need the patients' expertise to arrive at qualified clinical decisions.

14.5 Patient-Reported Outcomes

Several patient-reported and patient-administrated outcome assessment instruments have been developed for shoulder and upper limb disability. Although these tools were not originally designed for patients with shoulder fractures, being developed for chronic shoulder conditions rather than traumatic conditions, they have been used to assess cases of fracture patients since the 1990s. The instruments aim to reflect relevant aspects in the restoration of activities of daily living among shoulder patients.

OSS is a patient-administrated shoulder-specific questionnaire. It was developed in 1996 to assess results after elective shoulder operations [14]. It consists of 12 questions or items, each answered on a 5-category Likert scale referring to the last 4 weeks. The total score is 0–48, with 48 being the best. Several other ways to report the total score have been used. Percentages of a full score can be calculated for comparison. Several studies have reported that OSS correlates well with CMS. Baker [15] reported 3- and 12-month outcomes using CMS and OSS in a population (mean age 61) with nonoperatively treated shoulder fractures. The Pearson's correlation coefficient between OSS and CMS was 0.84 (0.77–0.87). A regression equation for predicting CMS from OSS was proposed. Correlation studies may justify the pooling of data from different outcomes, but outcome instruments often do not measure the same. Although they may appear identical if the reported scores correlate well, pooling data from a patient-reported outcome instrument and a composite outcome like CMS is not recommended.

The DASH score from 1996 was designed for the assessment of disabilities of the upper extremity [16]. It is patient-administrated and contains 30 items. The instrument has demonstrated good psychometric properties but is lengthy for the patients. The QuickDASH has comparable psychometric properties and is shorter.

The ASES score from 1994 combines a patient self-assessment (pain) 50/100 with a cumulative assessment of activities of daily living 50/100 (10 items, including 2 items for sports). The instrument's psychometric properties have not been tested.

Several other patient-reported questionnaires have been proposed and used but have not been validated in patients with shoulder fractures.

The Shoulder Pain and Disability Index (SPADI) was developed in 1991 to assess disability and pain in patients with shoulder disorders, including rotator cuff tears, impingement syndrome, frozen shoulder, and instability [17]. The University of California-Los Angeles (UCLA) shoulder scale was developed in 1981 to assess the result after shoulder arthroplasty [18]. The Western Ontario Osteoarthritis of the Shoulder (WOOS) index is a questionnaire developed in 2001 to measure the shoulder-related quality of life in patients with shoulder osteoarthritis [19]. It is used by the Danish and Swedish shoulder arthroplasty registries to evaluate patients with shoulder replacement, including fracture arthroplasties. My colleagues and I have tested WOOS using classical test theory [20] and item response theory using a Rasch model [21]. Recently, WOOS has been validated in fracture patients treated with shoulder arthroplasty [22]. The national joint registries in New Zealand, the United Kingdom, and Norway are collecting OSS for patients treated with fracture prostheses. To my knowledge, no national fracture register collects patient-reported outcome after osteosynthesis or non-surgical management.

14.6 Perspectives

Various outcome instruments with different properties are available to assess recovery following shoulder fractures. While no instrument has been specifically developed for this patient group, some instruments designed to evaluate chronic shoulder conditions have been utilized. The absence of agreement on assessment instruments has several implications. Bias assessment relies on the outcome instruments when assessing and interpreting clinical research. Further, data from patient-reported outcomes and objective outcomes cannot be quantitatively analyzed together. This is a challenge for summarizing clinical evidence. The focus on range of motion, strength, and radiographic alignment may shift attention from the patient's preferences to the surgeon's preferences. But it is nevertheless essential to recognize that patients' preferences vary, and the average preference may not apply to the individual patient. There is a need to involve the patient more in the assessment process to ensure that the treatment creates value for the patient.

Ideally, what qualities should an instrument possess to assess outcomes in older people following shoulder fractures? The tool should be based on patient input, including relevant questions and capturing values and preferences. It should be sensitive to symptoms specific to the condition, and its validation should be performed on the appropriate patient population.

Qualitative research can help capture social and psychological factors. A qualitative study reported semi-structured interviews with 15 older people with shoulder fractures. The authors identified seven main themes: pain, lack of sleep, shoulder function, emotional state, social support network, relationships with healthcare professionals, and relationships with healthcare institutions [23]. They concluded that the ability to adapt is essential and suggested that adaptive behavior should be part of a future PRO.

For some time, I have been asking my shoulder fracture patients about their concerns at different stages of recovery. The responses included "Will I be able to hold my grandchild again?" "Can I take care of my husband, who has dementia?" "Can I keep the silverware for my neighbor's 25th wedding anniversary?" "Will I be able to drive again?" "Can I do the vacuuming?" "Can I attend choir practice while wearing the sling?" Older people seem concerned about specific daily activities, particularly those related to emotional and social aspects of life. These activities require a certain level of movement and strength—but it is crucial to remain receptive and prioritize according to the patient's concerns.

References

1. Moustgaard H, Bello S, Miller FG, Hróbjartsson A. Subjective and objective outcomes in randomized clinical trials: definitions differed in methods publications and were often absent from trial reports. J Clin Epidemiol. 2014;67(12):1327–34.
2. Sackett DL. Evidence-based medicine. How to Practise and Teach EBM. Edinburgh: Churchill Livingstone; 1997.
3. Ramiro S, Page MJ, Whittle SL, Huang H, Verhagen AP, Beaton DE, et al. The OMERACT Core domain set for clinical trials of shoulder disorders. J Rheumatol. 2019;46(8):969–75. Available from: https://www.jrheum.org/content/46/8/969.long
4. Buchbinder R, Page MJ, Huang H, Verhagen AP, Beaton D, Kopkow C, et al. A preliminary Core domain set for clinical trials of shoulder disorders: a report from the OMERACT 2016 shoulder Core outcome set special interest group. J Rheumatol. 2017;44(12):1880–3. Available from: https://www.jrheum.org/content/44/12/1880.long
5. Richard GJ, Denard PJ, Kaar SG, Bohsali KI, Horneff JG, Carpenter S, et al. Outcome measures reported for the management of proximal humeral fractures: a systematic review. J Shoulder Elb Surg. 2020;29(10):2175–84.
6. Handoll HH, Elliott J, Thillemann TM, Aluko P, Brorson S. Interventions for treating proximal humeral fractures in adults. Cochrane Database Syst Rev. 2022;6(6):CD000434. Available from: https://www.cochranelibrary.com/cdsr/doi/10.1002/14651858.CD000434.pub5/abstract
7. Jelin E, Wisløff T, Moe MC, Heiberg T. Development and testing of a patient-derived questionnaire for treatment of neovascular age-related macular degeneration: dimensions of importance in treatment of neovascular age-related macular degeneration. Acta Ophthalmol. 2018;96(8):804–11. Available from: https://onlinelibrary.wiley.com/doi/10.1111/aos.13847
8. Gossec L, de Wit M, Kiltz U, Braun J, Kalyoncu U, Scrivo R, et al. A patient-derived and patient-reported outcome measure for assessing psoriatic arthritis: elaboration and preliminary validation of the Psoriatic Arthritis Impact of Disease (PsAID) questionnaire, a 13-country EULAR initiative. Ann Rheum Dis. 2014;73(6):1012–9. Available from: https://www.sciencedirect.com/science/article/abs/pii/S0003496724149023?via%3Dihub
9. Constant CR. Age related recovery of shoulder function after injury. Cork: University College; 1986.

10. Constant CR, Murley AH. A clinical method of functional assessment of the shoulder. Clin Orthop Relat Res. 1987;214:160–4.
11. Katolik LI, Romeo AA, Cole BJ, Verma NN, Hayden JK, Bach BR. Normalization of the Constant score. J Shoulder Elb Surg. 2005;14(3):279–85.
12. Constant CR, Gerber C, Emery RJH, Søjbjerg JO, Gohlke F, Boileau P. A review of the Constant score: modifications and guidelines for its use. J Shoulder Elb Surg. 2008;17(2):355–61.
13. Rocourt MHH, Radlinger L, Kalberer F, Sanavi S, Schmid NS, Leunig M, et al. Evaluation of intra-tester and intertester reliability of the Constant-Murley shoulder assessment. J Shoulder Elb Surg. 2008;17(2):364–9.
14. Dawson J, Fitzpatrick R, Carr A. Questionnaire on the perceptions of patients about shoulder surgery. J Bone Joint Surg Br. 1996;78(4):593–600.
15. Baker P, Nanda R, Goodchild L, Finn P, Rangan A. A comparison of the Constant and Oxford shoulder scores in patients with conservatively treated proximal humeral fractures. J Shoulder Elb Surg. 2008;17(1):37–41.
16. Hudak PL, Amadio PC, Bombardier C. Development of an upper extremity outcome measure: the DASH (disabilities of the arm, shoulder and hand) [corrected]. The Upper Extremity Collaborative Group (UECG). Am J Ind Med. 1996;29(6):602–8.
17. Roach KE, Budiman-Mak E, Songsiridej N, Lertratanakul Y. Development of a shoulder pain and disability index. Arthritis Care Res. 1991;4(4):143–9.
18. Amstutz HC, Sew Hoy AL, Clarke IC. UCLA anatomic total shoulder arthroplasty. Clin Orthop Relat Res. 1981;155:7–20.
19. Lo IK, Griffin S, Kirkley A. The development of a disease-specific quality of life measurement tool for osteoarthritis of the shoulder: the Western Ontario Osteoarthritis of the Shoulder (WOOS) index. Osteoarthr Cartil. 2001;9(8):771–8. Available from: https://www.sciencedirect.com/science/article/pii/S1063458401904741?via%3Dihub
20. Rasmussen JV, Jakobsen J, Olsen BS, Brorson S. Translation and validation of the Western Ontario Osteoarthritis of the Shoulder (WOOS) index; the Danish version. Patient Relat Outcome Meas. 2013;4:49–54. Available from: https://www.dovepress.com/translation-and-validation-of-the-western-ontario-osteoarthritis-of-th-peer-reviewed-fulltext-article-PROM
21. Moeini S, Rasmussen JV, Wirenfelt Klausen T, Brorson S. Rasch analysis of the Western Ontario osteoarthritis of the shoulder index; the Danish version. Patient Relat Outcome Meas 2016.; Available from: https://www.dovepress.com/rasch-analysis-of-the-western-ontario-osteoarthritis-of-the-shoulder-i-peer-reviewed-fulltext-article-PROM
22. Demir Y, Sjöberg H, Stark A, Salomonsson B. Western Ontario osteoarthritis of the shoulder index (WOOS) – a validation for use in proximal humerus fractures treated with arthroplasty. BMC Musculoskelet Disord. 2023;24(1):450. Available from: https://bmcmusculoskeletdisord.biomedcentral.com/articles/10.1186/s12891-023-06578-5
23. Sabharwal S, Archer S, Cadoux-Hudson D, Griffiths D, Gupte CM, Reilly P. Exploring elderly patients' experiences of recovery following complex proximal humerus fracture: a qualitative study. J Health Psychol. 2021;26(6):880–91.

Open Access This chapter is licensed under the terms of the Creative Commons Attribution 4.0 International License (http://creativecommons.org/licenses/by/4.0/), which permits use, sharing, adaptation, distribution and reproduction in any medium or format, as long as you give appropriate credit to the original author(s) and the source, provide a link to the Creative Commons license and indicate if changes were made.

The images or other third party material in this chapter are included in the chapter's Creative Commons license, unless indicated otherwise in a credit line to the material. If material is not included in the chapter's Creative Commons license and your intended use is not permitted by statutory regulation or exceeds the permitted use, you will need to obtain permission directly from the copyright holder.

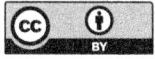

Complications After Shoulder Fractures

15.1 Introduction

Consistent reporting of benefits and harms is crucial for high-quality patient care and research, whether the interventions are surgical or non-surgical. Not enough attention has been given to defining and specifying the various harmful outcomes that may result from a given intervention. The fact that randomized trials comparing surgical and non-surgical interventions have been unable to identify the superiority of any treatment modality has increased the interest in possible differences in harms. Balanced clinical decision-making calls for valid harm data. This chapter introduces a consensus-based standardized terminology for complication terms and definitions.

15.2 Complications After Non-surgical Treatment of Shoulder Fractures

When recommending non-surgical treatment, concerns are raised about the potential complications that may arise without anatomical reduction, internal fixation, or joint replacement. There is a lack of validated definitions and terms for complications. Consistency in reporting is required to summarize harm outcomes across studies of interventions, whether surgical or non-surgical. Many of the complications described in the literature concern surgical procedures and implants. This reflects a bias toward surgical treatment in the scientific literature. A bibliometric study reported that around 70% of the papers on shoulder fractures focused on surgical interventions. Non-surgical treatments accounted for less than 5% of the papers [1].

To identify and describe terms and definitions for complications arising after treating shoulder fractures, my colleagues and I conducted two systematic reviews [2, 3]. We identified over 700 terms; some were synonymous, some were partly overlapping, and some were distinct. The terms and definitions reported after non-surgical treatment were extracted, and complication terms associated with non-surgical management were analyzed qualitatively [2]. After excluding redundant terms, we identified 67 distinct terms for unfavorable local events after non-surgical treatments. We found no general definition of a complication.

The terms could be classified into seven broad event groups. The largest group, *osteochondral*, covered 39 terms, including malunion, delayed union, nonunion, osteonecrosis, tuberosity migration or resorption, secondary displacement, and arthritis. All terms in this group were radiologically defined. Twenty-one terms were grouped as *soft tissue (deep)*, including impingement, rotator cuff problems, and joint stiffness. The remaining event groups included instability, shoulder pain, nerve injury, and superficial soft tissue problems. Only seven terms were accompanied by a definition; six were radiologically defined, and one regarded loss of strength.

15.3 Complications After Surgical Treatment of Shoulder Fractures

In the second systematic review, we reported 694 local event terms for complications after surgical treatment, with 345 related to locking plates [3]. Only 36 of the 694 identified event terms were defined. Some event terms were specific to an implant—acromion fracture, scapular notching, and screw penetration, for example; others overlapped across treatment modalities: for example, infection, nonunion, and implant failure. Events related to the injured shoulder were classified into nine major event groups: osteochondral, implant/device, infection, instability, pain, peripheral neurological, vascular, soft tissue (deep), and soft tissue (superficial). The events that occurred locally were categorized into 39 specific complications. Most of these terms were radiology-based, which included screw perforation/cutout, secondary fracture displacement, scapular notching, delayed union, and malunion. No overall definition of a complication was found, however. The most commonly reported complication terms were implant failure, infection, loss of reduction, impingement, pain, stiffness, dislocation, avascular necrosis, and malunion.

15.4 Toward a Core Event Set for Complication Reporting

To promote consistency in reporting complications after head-preserving treatments, we gathered an international panel of 231 clinicians experienced in treating patients with shoulder fractures [4]. Using a modified Delphi method, the participants reached a consensus (>90% agreement) on a core set of intraoperative, postoperative, and nonoperative local event terms. Two iterations were performed before the predefined level of consensus was reached. Three groups of intraoperative events and eight groups of postoperative and nonoperative events were defined (Table 15.1).

Table 15.1 Consensus-based event groups for reporting complications after head-preserving treatments for proximal humerus fractures

	Event group	Event terms (selected)	Period
Intraoperative	Device	Instrument problem (breakage, failure) Implant problem (breakage, screw penetration to joint) Cementation problem (augmentation)	Between skin incision and skin closure
–	Osteochondral	Articular cartilage damage Iatrogenic fracture	–
–	Soft tissue	Skin, muscle, tendon, joint, capsule, labrum Blood vessels (bleeding requiring intervention) Nerve damage	–
Postoperative/nonoperative	Implant/device (surgical)	Mispositioning Implant loosening (radiolucency) Screw or bolt back out Implant breakage Implant migration	12 months
–	Device (non-surgical)	Breakage of loosening of external device (bandage)	During the use of the device

(continued)

Table 15.1 (continued)

	Event group	Event terms (selected)	Period
–	Osteochondral (surgical)	New fracture around the implant Screw or bolt cutout	24 months
–		Loss of fracture reduction	
	(surgical and non-surgical)	Bone formation/resorption Tuberosity migration/resorption	
–		Head necrosis	
–		Delayed union/nonunion	
–	Shoulder instability	Subluxation Dislocation Dynamic instability	12 months
–	Peripheral neurological	Cervical or brachial plexus Branch neuropathy Autonomic (CRPS)	3 months
–	Vascular	Hematoma requiring evacuation Thrombosis at the involved extremity Ischemia requiring intervention	30 days
–	Infection	Fracture-related infection	24 months
–	Soft tissue (superficial)	Requiring additional treatment Early events: Edema, emphysema, burn, delayed wound healing, hypersensitivity, necrosis, bulla Late events: Hypertrophic scar and keloid	30 days to 6 months
–	Soft tissue (deep)	External muscular envelope (deltoid, pectoralis major) Subacromial/deltoid/coracoid bursa (space) Rotator cuff tendon/muscle and biceps tendon Capsule-synovium	12 months

Modified from [4]. A comparable core event set for complications after shoulder arthroplasty can be found in [5]

15.5 Radiographic Monitoring

Standardized monitoring is essential for ensuring reliable and reproducible outcome reporting. Most follow-up protocols for shoulder fractures include radiographic monitoring. There is an ongoing debate about routine radiographic monitoring, whether after surgical or non-surgical treatment. The terms and definitions of commonly used radiological findings are not clear. Consequently, we expanded the consensus-based study on complication terms to include the timing and type of diagnostic images. Through an iterative process, my colleagues and I proposed a consensus-based list of definitions for imaging parameters and a monitoring protocol for supporting the management of shoulder fractures (Table 15.2) [6]. The consensus terms and definitions still require clinical validation.

The preferred imaging views and modalities differed between and within countries. Sixty-five percent of the participants would add an axillary view to the plain perpendicular anterior-posterior and scapular Y-views. Forty-one percent of the participants would add CT and 3D reconstructions to the monitoring protocol. Only about half of the participants would stop monitoring the patients when the healing of the fracture was confirmed.

Table 15.2 Consensus-based definitions of radiological monitoring parameters [6]

Parameter	Definition and specifications
Fracture anatomical reduction (surgical)	Are greater tuberosity and head reduced anatomically? Are greater tuberosity and shaft reduced anatomically? Are greater and lesser tuberosities reduced anatomically? Are lesser tuberosity and head reduced anatomically? Are lesser tuberosity and shaft reduced anatomically?
Fracture healing	Healing: the presence of mineralized callus visible on at least two orthogonal radiographs or CT
Delayed healing: the absence of bridging callus on at least one of four cortices on two orthogonal radiographs taken at 3 months after fracture
Nonunion: absence of bridging callus on at least one of four cortices on two orthogonal radiographs taken at 6 months after fracture
Bone resorption	The progressive disappearance of bone from the proximal humerus (either medullary or cortical) in excess to that expected during normal fracture healing
Epiphyseal: humeral head avascular necrosis is one form of epiphyseal bone resorption
Metaphyseal: involvement of the calcar region and/or the tuberosities (greater or lesser)
Diaphyseal: involvement of endosteal or periosteal regions
Head necrosis	Epiphyseal bone resorption compared to immediate postoperative or initial nonoperative radiographs. Divided into four stages
Bone formation	The progressive apposition of bone on or within the humerus, more than that required for fracture healing
Orthotopic bone formation (ossification) is bone formation within the confines of the bone, including the periosteum (e.g., excessive callus formation)
Heterotopic bone formation (ossification) is excess bone formation within or between tissues that are not destined to be or become bone under normal healing or loading conditions
Varus/valgus of head	Slippage of the head in varus or valgus position leading to a secondary cutout of the screws through the head
Tuberosity migration	Any perceived migration, in comparison to initial radiographs

15.6 What Is a Radiological Complication?

The concept of *radiological complications* assumes a link between radiological appearance and patient outcome. After surgical procedures, radiological measures play a role in the postoperative assessment as a quality marker of the quality of reduction and the implant position. The role of radiological monitoring after non-surgical treatment has yet to be defined, however. Monitoring after surgical procedures cannot be transferred to non-surgically treated patients. Radiologically defined complications favor surgery as surgery aims to restore or replace the anatomy assessed by postoperative radiographs. Close to 100% of non-surgically treated displaced fractures result in radiological complications (malunion), whereas more than 30% of locking plates lead to radiological complications. Studying the link between radiological complications and patient outcome is crucial for informed decisions and patient-centered care. It is interesting to note that most complications following non-surgical treatment are identified through imaging.

While surgeons typically refer to images when they suspect a complication, it is not always clear if these radiological findings correlate with the patient's clinical condition, especially after non-

15.6 What Is a Radiological Complication?

surgical treatment in older people. A wide range of radiological abnormalities seem to be surprisingly well tolerated in older people. Radiologically defined complication terms reflect our interpretation of the underlying biology of the injury. For example, the greater tuberosity will point toward the acromion in displaced fractures with varus rotation of the humeral head. Consequently, the distance between the inferior surface of the acromion and the humeral head at an anterior-posterior view is decreased, often interpreted as *impingement*. There is a widely accepted belief in orthopedics that if a patient is experiencing pain in the subacromial area, it is because the bony parts are impinging on the subacromial bursa and the supraspinatus tendon. However, the pain experienced by the patient is poorly correlated with the distance between the bony parts, and subacromial pain remains to be satisfactorily explained. The subacromial space is a three-dimensional structure with several degrees of freedom, allowing the greater tuberosity to pass under the acromion without collision, which should be considered when assessing the acromiohumeral distance radiologically (Fig. 3.10). The clinical impact of several radiologically defined complication terms needs further consideration.

Avascular necrosis is an interpretation of pathology interpreted from radiological characteristics. The radiological appearance is interpreted as a loss of perfusion and gradual avascular necrosis of the humeral head. The radiological changes are poorly related to patient outcome. The diagnosis is rarely verified, except in humeral head removal with subsequent pathological examination, which is not performed routinely.

While the term *fracture union* is frequently used, its relationship with patient outcome is unclear. It is defined as mineralized callus visible on at least two orthogonal radiographs. The mineralized lateral and posterior callus bridges are visible on radiographs; the endosteal callus is challenging to define but is visible on CT scans. Both are illustrated in the illustrations by Robert William Smith from 1847 (Figs. 3.9 and 3.10) [7]. In cultures where open reduction and internal fixation are the treatment of choice in varus displaced fractures, much attention is paid to restoring medial (calcar) support. However, lateral bone bridging and endosteal callus formation seem to compensate for the lack of calcar support in older people. A CT scan without medial healing is expected at that point. If the radiological union is not obtained, different degrees of pathoanatomical changes are diagnosed, extending from *delayed union* to *prolonged delayed union* to *nonunion*. However, a lack of radiological healing can be found in patients after pain-free shoulder function has been regained (Fig. 15.1).

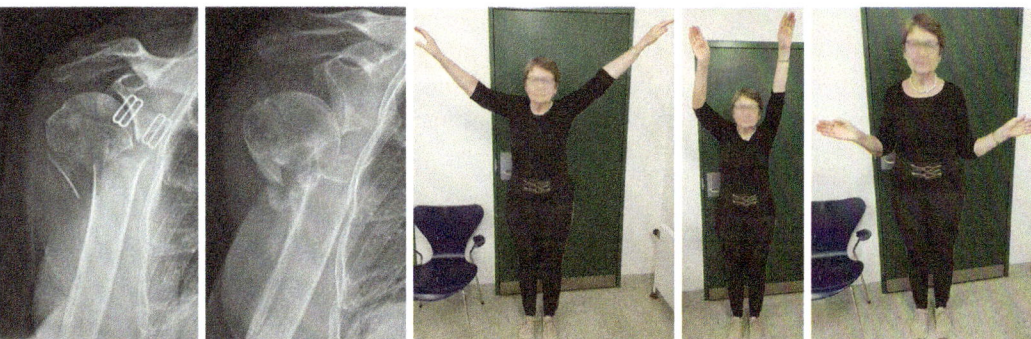

Fig. 15.1 An illustration of the discrepancy between the clinical and radiological outcomes in a 73-year-old woman with a medially translated surgical neck fracture. Radiographs were taken at admission and 6 months, along with photos at 6 months. Although the radiographs showed nonunion, the patient had a pain-free shoulder and normal shoulder function

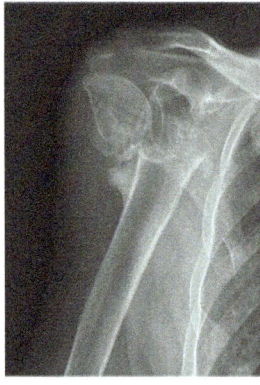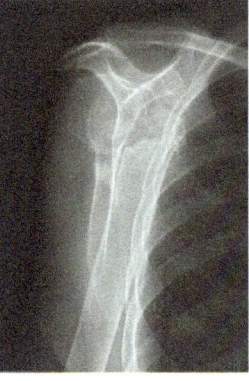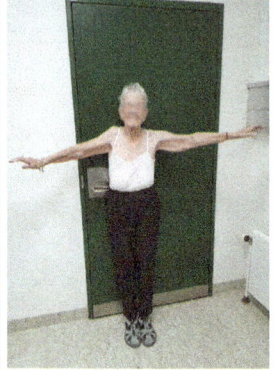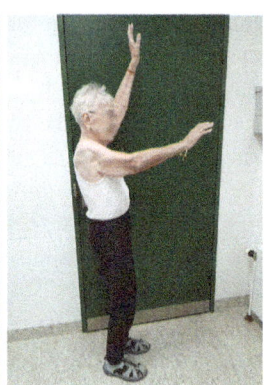

Fig. 15.2 Radiological and clinical nonunion in an 89-year-old female with a two-part surgical neck fracture. The patient had no pain and refused surgery. The case illustrates the shoulder's mobility without bony continuity in the proximal humerus. The strength was limited, but the patient was satisfied. Radiographs and clinical photos at 6 months

Some older individuals may prefer a reduction in strength to avoid surgery. Even when there is no bony contact between the humeral head and shaft, some level of shoulder function can be retained, as shown in Fig. 15.2.

Primary fracture displacement can be considered a continuum, with an arbitrary set cutoff value for defining the point at which displacement is held to occur. Most radiologically defined complications can be viewed as a continuum converted to a binary classification. Common complication terms like *varus* or *valgus* displacement, *humeral head collapse*, *tuberosity migration*, and *translation of the humeral shaft* are arbitrarily defined categories used for clinical communication and decision-making. The extent to which they have prognostic value has yet to be demonstrated. It was assumed in our radiological monitoring protocol that binary questions were less prone to observer variation [6]; this, however, also requires demonstration.

Previous studies on clinicians' ability to determine an arbitrary cutoff in a continuum have been disappointing. In an observer study among 24 orthopedic doctors classifying 42 pairs of plain radiographs, my colleagues and I reported a kappa value of 0.41 on the binary distinction between displaced and non-displaced [8]. We have no reason to believe that observer agreement would be higher for other radiologically defined categories.

Head collapse is another radiologically defined complication defined from a continuum. It can be found in most head-preserving treatments, whether surgical or non-surgical. The consequences for the patient are, however, very different. Penetration of locking screws into the glenohumeral joint is a devastating complication associated with pain, additional surgery, and poor functional outcome (Fig. 15.3).

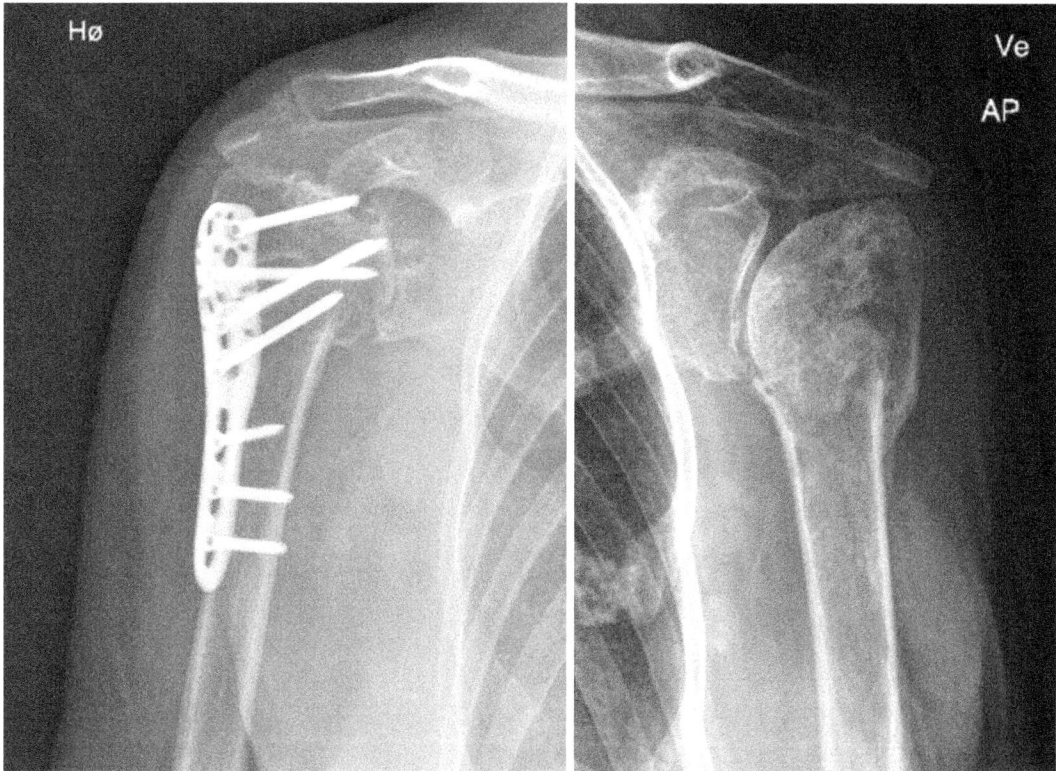

Fig. 15.3 Example of humeral head collapse with and without a head-preserving implant

15.7 Malunion: Friend or Foe?

It was not easy to obtain consensus on the definition of *malunion*. Malunion means healing in a nonanatomical position. Malunion can appear after surgical and non-surgical treatment, but has different meanings and clinical implications. Etymologically, malunion is associated with negative connotations, as the prefix *mal* means bad or wrong. In contrast, *osteosynthesis* has positive connotations, as *osteo* refers to bone and *synthesis* refers to putting things together. It appeals to the intrinsic human trait of mending broken things.

Osteosynthesis aims to restore the anatomy and to provide stable internal fixation in anatomical position. After head-preserving surgery, malunion can occur due to poor reduction, secondary loss of reduction, or failed tuberosity fixation. With rigid implants (locking plates and locking nails), the consequence of malunion will often be penetration of the locking screws into the glenohumeral joint. After joint replacement, malunion of the tuberosities can occur. After non-surgical treatment of displaced fractures in adults, some degree of malunion is expected. Malunion seems well tolerated, especially in older people, where callus bridging and progressive mineralization can be expected, even in severely displaced fractures (Fig. 15.4).

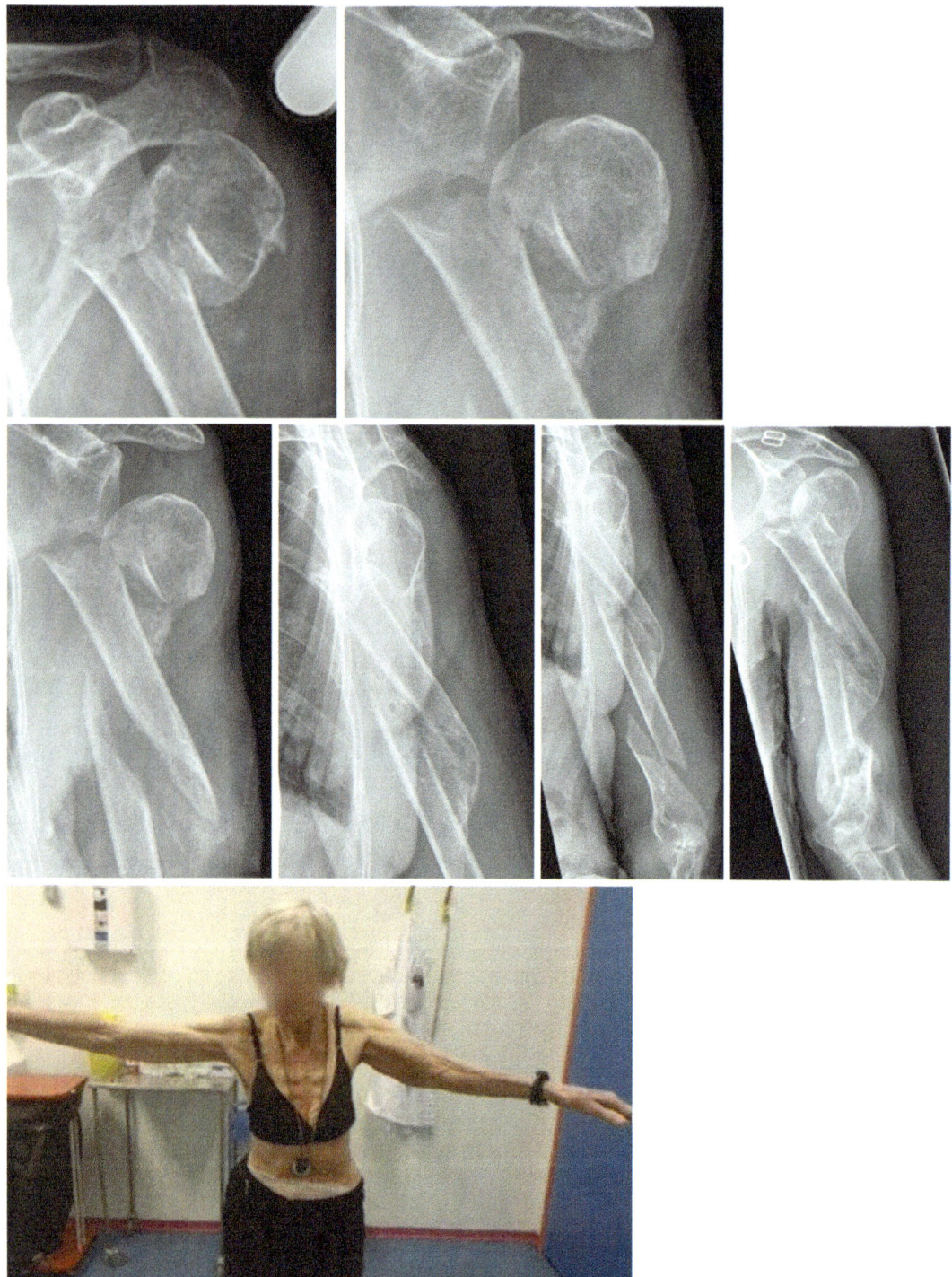

Fig. 15.4 The natural healing of three successive displaced humerus fractures involving the proximal humerus, the humeral shaft, and the distal humerus. The patient refused surgery but regained pain-free shoulder function below shoulder level. *Vis medicatrix naturae* (the healing power of nature) should not be underestimated in fracture management

15.8 Impairment of Rotational Mobility and Proprioception

Loss of mobility and strength can be expected in older people after shoulder fractures—but the literature does not discuss impairment of proprioception that may also ensue. Despite successful healing, for example, some patients cannot perform precise and targeted movements with their outstretched arm when pouring coffee. Malunion may be linked to proprioception compromised on account of alterations in the anatomy of the proximal humerus. Regaining internal and external rotation requires proper healing of the tuberosities in anatomical position. The greater tuberosity plays a vital role in balancing the shoulder joint. Posterior displacement of the greater tuberosity is often followed by impairment of external rotation regardless of the treatment modality. The tuberosity may remain displaced posteriorly despite satisfactory restoration on anterior-posterior radiographs. The use of locking plates in osteosynthesis may have unwanted consequences for patient mobility if greater tuberosity displacement is not addressed during the procedure, regardless of the focus on restoring the medial cortex and the head-shaft angle.

15.9 Perspectives

The surgical culture is decisive for determining when a complication occurs in a fracture patient. In a culture where treatment success is judged by radiographic alignment, bringing broken bones together and providing stable fixation is rational behavior. Treatments differing from usual care and resulting in fracture healing in a nonanatomical position are considered failures or neglected cases. However, without including the patient's assessment, radiology-based assessments and decisions are blind. The missing link is the association between radiographic parameters and patient outcome. Until such links are empirically established, imaging modalities should not be used as the sole basis for clinical decision-making and outcome assessment.

References

1. Slobogean GP, Johal H, Lefaivre KA, MacIntyre NJ, Sprague S, Scott T, et al. A scoping review of the proximal humerus fracture literature. BMC Musculoskelet Disord. 2015;16(1):112. Available from: https://bmcmusculoskeletdisord.biomedcentral.com/articles/10.1186/s12891-015-0564-8
2. Brorson S, Alispahic N, Bahrs C, Joeris A, Steinitz A, Audigé L, et al. Complications after non-surgical management of proximal humeral fractures: a systematic review of terms and definitions. BMC Musculoskelet Disord. 2019;20(1):91. Available from: https://bmcmusculoskeletdisord.biomedcentral.com/articles/10.1186/s12891-019-2459-6
3. Alispahic N, Brorson S, Bahrs C, Joeris A, Steinitz A, Audigé L. Complications after surgical management of proximal humeral fractures: a systematic review of event terms and definitions. BMC Musculoskelet Disord. 2020;21(1):327. Available from: https://bmcmusculoskeletdisord.biomedcentral.com/articles/10.1186/s12891-020-03353-8
4. Audigé L, Brorson S, Durchholz H, Lambert S, Moro F, Joeris A. Core set of unfavorable events of proximal humerus fracture treatment defined by an international Delphi consensus process. BMC Musculoskelet Disord. 2021;22(1):1002. Available from: https://bmcmusculoskeletdisord.biomedcentral.com/articles/10.1186/s12891-021-04887-1
5. Audige L, Schwyzer H-K, Durchholz H. Core set of unfavorable events of shoulder arthroplasty: an international Delphi consensus process. J Shoulder Elb Surg. 2019;28(11):2061–71.
6. Lambert S, Brorson S, Joeris A, Durchholz H, Moro F, Audigé L. International consensus for a core radiological monitoring protocol of proximal humerus fractures. Injury. 2022;53(10):3326–31. Available from: https://www.sciencedirect.com/science/article/pii/S0020138322005010
7. Smith RW. A treatise on fractures in the vicinity of joints and on certain forms of accidental and congenital dislocations. Dublin: Hodges and Smith; 1847. Available from: https://wellcomecollection.org/works/msz6zwcq
8. Brorson S, Bagger J, Sylvest A, Hrobjartsson A. Low agreement among 24 doctors using the Neer-classification; only moderate agreement on displacement, even between specialists. Int Orthop. 2002;26(5):271–3. Available from: https://www.ncbi.nlm.nih.gov/pmc/articles/PMC3620992/

Open Access This chapter is licensed under the terms of the Creative Commons Attribution 4.0 International License (http://creativecommons.org/licenses/by/4.0/), which permits use, sharing, adaptation, distribution and reproduction in any medium or format, as long as you give appropriate credit to the original author(s) and the source, provide a link to the Creative Commons license and indicate if changes were made.

The images or other third party material in this chapter are included in the chapter's Creative Commons license, unless indicated otherwise in a credit line to the material. If material is not included in the chapter's Creative Commons license and your intended use is not permitted by statutory regulation or exceeds the permitted use, you will need to obtain permission directly from the copyright holder.

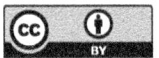

Bridging the Evidence-Practice Gap in Shoulder Fracture Management

16.1 Introduction

Many procedures and implants have been introduced based on biomechanical reasoning, a limited number of clinical cases, and effective marketing, rather than on results from well-conducted randomized trials. This presents a dilemma for the treating surgeons. On the one hand, new effective treatments should be available to patients without unnecessary delay; on the other hand, surgeons have a responsibility not to perform unnecessary or harmful treatments. The absence of results from randomized trials leaves patients and surgeons in an *evidence gap*. A new dilemma arises if randomized trials are subsequently conducted. If the new evidence does not align with established practice, an *evidence-practice gap* will emerge.

How do surgeons think and act when evidence from randomized trials does not conform with established practice? Surgeons familiar with certain implants and procedures are often reluctant to change their practice despite conflicting evidence. This reluctance can result in a delay in de-implementing unnecessary or harmful treatments.

In this chapter, I will first discuss obstacles to accommodating the increasing evidence of non-superiority of surgical treatment for shoulder fractures. Second, I will both discuss what happens if we do not operate on older people with displaced shoulder fractures and present preliminary data from a large prospective cohort study of patients treated non-surgically; I will also propose systematic data collection to support surgeons in clinical decision-making and narrow the evidence-practice gap.

16.2 Barriers to Accommodate Evidence

How have orthopedic surgeons responded to the message of the non-superiority of surgical interventions for proximal humerus fractures? The following four statements, each followed by a critical response, paraphrase reactions following our Cochrane review in 2015 [1].

Statement One: "If this is the evidence, the evidence must be wrong"

When deciding on treatments, the options we will consider are influenced by our prior beliefs. Suppose you firmly believe any displaced fracture in a long bone should be reduced anatomically and fixed. In that case, you can hardly imagine a study leading to a change in your belief. If a treatment does not align with common practice, more supporting evidence is requested. This raises the question of how much evidence is needed to adopt or abandon a treatment. Are ten randomized trials finding no benefit from surgery sufficient to abandon surgical treatment, or do we need another ten? Who has the burden of proof?

The surgeons who establish a surgical procedure without high-quality evidence, or those who want to de-implement the same procedure based on results from randomized trials?

Another strategy is to wait for a study to report the superiority of surgery. Such a study can be expected for purely statistical reasons. With a conventional level of statistical significance ($p = 0.05$), we will, on average, reach a false-positive result in every 20 repeated trials. Such a trial can be interpreted as decisive, providing the first proper conclusion, superseding previous findings.

Finally, if the available data in existing randomized trials do not support surgical treatment, the data can be misinterpreted in favor of the preferred treatment—*spin* occurs. This phenomenon can be found in several randomized trials on shoulder fractures [2, 3].

Statement Two: "The procedure works perfectly well in my hands, and I have very few complications in my clinic"
Orthopedic surgeons deliver timely and effective surgical interventions for musculoskeletal trauma and tend to have high confidence in their surgical capabilities. As surgeons, we are often aware of surgical failures at other institutions but may not recognize our own. We remember exceptional results and patients who complain, while those with outcomes between these extremes are forgotten if not systematically recorded. Very little is known about patients who receive non-surgical treatment outside of control groups in randomized trials. Therefore, it is crucial to systematically record outcomes for all fracture patients regardless of their treatment.

Statement Three: "If surgery is no better than no surgery, or the implant does not perform better than no implant, we need to improve the surgery or modify the implant"
Following dismal reports of outcomes after surgery, a firm belief in the benefits of surgery may lead to a search for other surgical procedures or modifications of current procedures. In orthopedic lingo, statements like *a surgical problem has a surgical solution* are standard. Besides being a truism, this claim overlooks the possibility that some issues in orthopedic surgery may have a non-surgical solution. We still need to see a procedure that performs better than non-surgical treatment for shoulder fractures. Surgical developments should be demonstrated to be superior to no surgery and not only to a competing surgical procedure or implant.

The many attempts to modify locking plates to reduce failure rates demonstrate the strength of this belief (Table 12.2). Surgeons often overlook the possibility that the patient may be better off without an implant. Similarly, the steep increase in reverse shoulder arthroplasty in fractures lacks supporting high-quality evidence. We only have two small trials, reporting no clinically relevant benefits from surgery (Chap. 13). Ongoing trials may add new knowledge on the effect of reverse arthroplasty in fracture treatment. Until high-quality supporting evidence is available, we must collect data on patient-reported outcomes and complications from all fracture patients treated with reverse shoulder arthroplasty.

Statement Four: "If two-, three-, and four-part fractures in older people should not be operated on, then at least the rest should"
This statement assumes surgery to be the *default* treatment option for displaced shoulder fractures—an assumption that has not been justified. Patients and fracture morphologies not covered by current evidence should be regarded as unsolved clinical questions and should be systematically followed up or, ideally, included in multicenter randomized trials. Injuries not covered by randomized trials include isolated tuberosity fractures, fractures in younger persons, fracture-dislocations, articular surface fractures, and high-energy trauma.

16.3 Can Orthopedic Surgeons Change Behavior?

How many orthopedic surgeons have changed their treatment preferences and, ultimately, their practice to accommodate evidence from randomized trials? This question can be answered by surveying surgeons or by retrieving data on surgical activity before and after certain events. Important events in shoulder fracture management include the publication of the ProFHER trial in 2015 [4], the publication of the updated Cochrane review later in 2015 [1], and subsequent national guidelines based on these publications [5].

A survey was conducted among members of the British Orthopaedic Association and British Elbow and Shoulder Society, resulting in 265 responses [6]. Approximately half of the responders reported changing their practice because of the ProFHER trial. Among those who did not change their practice, a third had already accommodated the evidence before the trial. The survey found that those who changed their practice tended to be slightly younger specialist shoulder surgeons rather than trauma surgeons. Overall, the respondents expressed support for evidence-based practice.

A study conducted at a single British hospital looked at the treatment of shoulder fractures before and after the ProFHER trial [7]. The study reported that after the trial, fewer patients were sent to shoulder surgeons, and the rate of surgery decreased by half. Non-shoulder specialists were more likely to manage the patients without involving a shoulder specialist or resorting to surgery.

In a registry-based study of 137,436 shoulder fracture cases in the Danish National Patient Register, my colleagues and I found that the operation rates declined from 17% in 2013 to 11% in 2018 [8]. Although causal associations cannot be derived from the registry data, there appears to be a chronological connection between the decline of surgery and the ProFHER study, the Cochrane review, and a national guideline informed by these sources [9].

16.4 What Happens If We Do Not Operate?

Reporting outcomes following nonoperative treatment for displaced fractures is rare outside randomized trials. In randomized trials, non-surgically treated patients are observed in an experimental setting. Over the past 15 years, 10 randomized trials have included only 350 non-surgically treated patients as controls [10]. Randomized trials are designed to establish baseline comparability and reduce biases. While they can provide valuable information for clinical decision-making, their application to large, unselected patient populations is less known. Prospective cohort studies collecting patient-reported outcomes can help validate evidence-based recommendations in large populations. Surgeons tend to focus on evaluating the outcome of patients who have undergone surgery. Prospective cohort studies ideally encompass the entire population of fracture patients, regardless of the treatment methods used. A predefined protocol for this study should include a list of the variables that will be recorded and the planned analyses. It is essential to remember that prospective cohort studies are non-comparative because they cannot control differences in patients, surgeons, and indications at baseline. While regression models can help address known prognostic factors, residual confounding remains challenging. Prospective cohort studies can report patient-reported outcomes and clinical failures based on shoulder function or quality of life following assessment in a nonexperimental setting. Below is a summary of cohort studies that report patient-reported outcomes after non-surgically treated shoulder fractures.

16.5 Previous Prospective Cohort Studies

Between 1992 and 1996, a cohort of 1027 consecutive patients with shoulder fractures from an urban population in Edinburgh were followed up prospectively for a year [11]. The patients were evaluated using a composite, observer-administered outcome instrument (Neer Score), translated into a four-part ranking scale (*excellent*, *good*, *fair*, or *poor*) and according to fracture categories in a series of reports. A multiple regression analysis found that age and pre-fracture ability determined the outcome [12]. In the minimally displaced group ($n = 507$), 88% of the patients had an excellent or good result after a year. From the same cohort, 81% of 125 patients with impacted valgus fractures obtained excellent or good outcome after nonoperative treatment [13]. The authors concluded that operative fixation is unnecessary in this fracture pattern regardless of the degree of displacement.

A report enlarging the above cohort (n = 1027) by adding patient data from 2000 (n = 337) and 2007 (n = 516) investigated whether socioeconomic status influenced the functional outcome measured by Constant-Murley Score (CMS). First, socioeconomically deprived patients were at increased risk of sustaining a shoulder fracture. Second, social deprivation was an independent predictor of worse CMS [14]. From the first Edinburgh cohort, 637 fractures in 629 patients aged 65 or above were retrospectively studied. The mean CMS was 64. They concluded that factors associated with social independence were more predictive of outcome than age [15].

Several prospective cohort studies on two-part fractures were performed in the late 1990s. Court-Brown and McQueen reported a cohort of 232 two-part fractures and fracture-dislocations [16]. After a 1-year follow-up, the mean nonadjusted CMS was 65. The most common two-part patterns, A2.2 (varus impacted) and A3.2 (translated), were reported separately [17, 18]. In 99 varus-impacted two-part fractures, they noted that nonoperative treatment may increase varus angulation [18]. However, they also reported that decreased shoulder function was associated with increasing age but not with increasing varus angulation. All fractures united. After 1 year, the mean Neer score was 79% after omitting the radiographic sub-score. Interestingly, they failed to demonstrate the usefulness of physiotherapy. Moreover, 126 patients with translated two-part fractures were treated nonoperatively [17]. Half the patients had more than 66% of displacement on the initial AP radiographs. Twelve patients had a more than 100% translation of the humeral shaft. The results in these patients did not differ from those with less displaced fractures. Surgery did not improve the outcome, regardless of the degree of translation. They found no correlation between translation or angulation and the ability to return to daily activities. The nonunion rate was 5%. The authors suggested that nonoperative treatment should be the *default* position for treatment of this group [16]. It should be mentioned that the study was conducted before the introduction of locking plates. In a review from 2007, Court-Brown and McQueen expressed their concern about the rapidly increasing use of locking plates and suggested that "we must balance the understandable initial enthusiasm with proven success" [16].

Between 2014 and 2015, Goudie [19] followed up 774 patients with shoulder fractures aged 18 or above in Edinburgh for a year using Oxford Shoulder Score (OSS) and quality of life with EQ-5D-3L. The authors aimed to report functional outcome after nonoperative treatment. They studied a mixed population, including minimally displaced fractures, young patients, and a relatively high prevalence of surgery. Furthermore, 22 fracture-dislocations and 11 isolated tuberosity fractures were considered unsuitable for inclusion, while another 54 patients were excluded due to primary operative treatment. An additional 33 patients were treated operatively within the cohort within the first year due to complications. Nonunion was radiographically defined as no radiographic consolidation, fracture gap widening, scalloping, or progressive varus deformity. The primary conclusion was a considerable variation in shoulder function and quality of life. In a multivariate analysis, three negative predictors were identified: high levels of dependency, social deprivation, and mood disorders. Social dependency and psychosocial factors had more influence than fracture-related factors. Younger patients were less satisfied despite higher OSS. Also, 31% had an OSS ≤ 24 (half of a total shoulder function), and 16% had a *worse-than-death* EQ-5D-3L score. A ceiling effect was reported for both outcomes.

Patient-reported outcomes can be found in other prospective cohort studies of non-surgically treated patients. Table 16.1 summarizes outcome data from cohorts reporting OSS and EQ-5D-3L. Baker [20] prospectively followed up 103 patients selected for non-surgical treatment. They were assessed at 3 and 12 months with

Table 16.1 Oxford Shoulder Score and EuroQoL 5D-3L after 6 and 12 months in prospective cohort studies of non-surgically treated patients with shoulder fractures

Author	Nonoperative (n)	Age (mean and range)	Female/male	Fx category (n and %)	OSS 6 months (mean and %)	OSS 12 months (mean and %)	EQ-5D 6 months (mean)	EQ-5D 12 months (mean)
Baker (2008)	103	61.4 (15–85)	80/23	1 part:33 2 part:39 3–4 part: 31	–	22.72[a] (76%) SD 11.68 Range 56–12	–	–
Jayakumar (2019)	177	66 (18–95)	128/49	2-part: 70 3–4 part: 69 Greater tuberosity: 38	34.8[b] (71%) SD 11.3 Range 14–48	–	0.75 SD 0.25 Range 0.14–1	–
Goudie (2021)	774	66 (18–98)	571/203	Displaced: 238 Surg. Neck: 569	–	33.2[b] (67%) (95% CI: 32.2 to 34.2)		0.58 (95% CI, 0.55 to 0.61)
Brorson (2024)[c]	627	75 (60–101) SD 8.5	493/134	1 part: 187 2-part: 279 3-part: 99 4-part: 26 Art surf: 18 Fx-disloc:14	35.7[b] (74%) SD 8.8	37.3[b] (78%) SD 10.0	0.77 SD 0.16	0.81 SD 0.15

[a]12–60 (12 best)
[b]0–48 (48 best)
[c] preliminary data

OSS. After 12 months, the mean OSS was 76% of full shoulder function. Health-related quality of life was not reported. Jayakumar [21] prospectively followed 177 patients for 6 to 9 months, with 10% being treated surgically. The mean OSS was 71% of a full shoulder function. Several demographic, psychological, and social variables were recorded, and a multivariate regression analysis was performed. Kinesiophobia after a week was the strongest predictor for limitations at 6 months.

16.6 The Danish Cohort

My colleagues and I prospectively followed up a cohort of patients referred to a Danish university hospital with displaced shoulder fractures using patient-reported outcomes for shoulder function (OSS) and quality-of-life (EQ-5D-3L). All patients aged 60 or above with displaced shoulder fractures followed a predefined protocol (Fig. 16.1) [22]. Questionnaires were completed after 6 and 12 months and collected by staff not involved in patient treatment. All patients were seen in the outpatient clinic within 3 weeks of injury. The fractures were classified by consensus according to the Neer classification (16 categories) and the AO classification (9 groups). According to Neer's definition, patients with minimally displaced fractures were excluded for two reasons. First, among surgeons, it is widely agreed that these fractures can be treated without surgery. Second, we had ethical concerns about additional follow-up visits at the hospital without potential clinical consequences. Patients with concomitant fractures (most commonly hip, wrist, or spine) and pathological fractures (except for osteoporosis), and patients unable to answer a questionnaire were excluded. The cohort was validated annually by manually retrieving all patients with a discharge diagnosis of a proximal humerus diagnosis from the institution. Patients under 60 years were excluded.

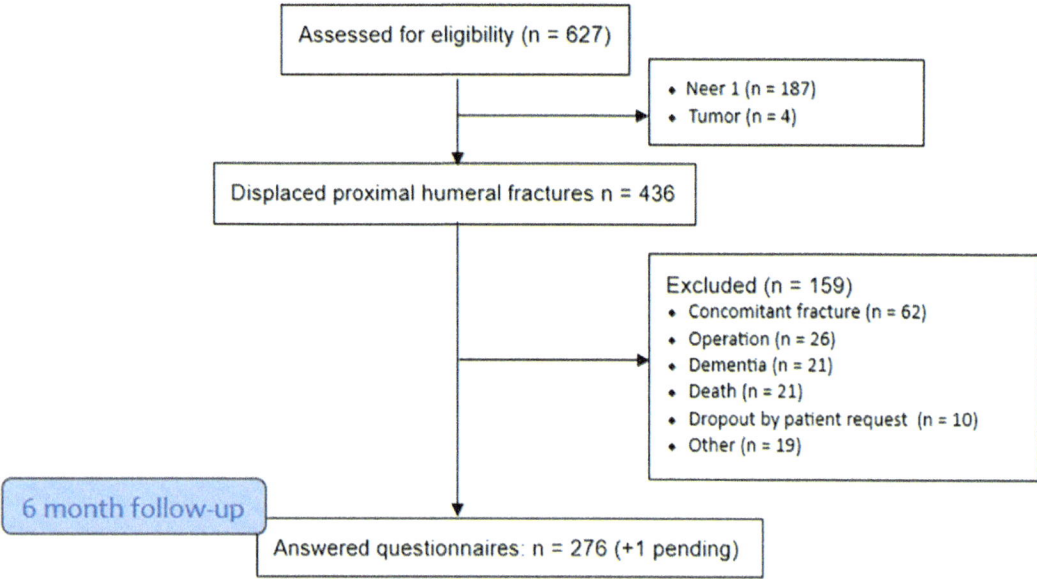

Fig. 16.1 Flowchart for the Danish cohort, including patients aged 60 or above who were seen within 3 weeks of injury between January 1, 2021, and December 31, 2023. Data for the 6-month follow-up is shown

All patients with displaced fractures were seen again in the outpatient clinic 6 weeks after injury. The chosen time points were not evidence-based, but we found them practical. If the patient suffered severe pain and wished for surgery at 6 weeks, a reverse shoulder arthroplasty was offered regardless of the fracture morphology. Operation within 6 weeks after injury was preferred due to the potential for tuberosity refixation and rotator cuff reconstruction.

16.7 Preliminary Outcome Data from the Danish Cohort

Within 36 months, 627 patients aged 60 and above received treatment at our clinic (Table 16.2). The average age was 75, with females accounting for 79% of the patients. Two-part fractures were the most commonly reported pattern, making up 45% of the cases. Minimally displaced fractures accounted for 29%, which differs from the rates reported by Charles Neer

Table 16.2 Demographics and distribution of fracture patterns in the Danish cohort

	Baseline
Number	627
Age (mean and SD)	75 (8.5)
Gender	
Male	134
Female	493
Neer category	
Minimally displaced	187
2-part	275
3-part	99
4-part	26
Fracture-dislocation	14
Articular surface	18
AO group	
A1	70
A2	265
A3	74
B1	153
B2	7
B3	2
C1	6
C2	37
C3	8

16.7 Preliminary Outcome Data from the Danish Cohort

Table 16.3 Patient-reported outcome (OSS and EQ-5D-3L) after 6 months according to fracture category and age

Six months	OSS Mean (SD) % of full score[a]	EQ-5D Mean (SD)[b]
(n = 276)	35.7 (8.8) 74%	0.77 (0.16)
Fracture category		
2-part (n = 168)	37.2 (8.1) 78%	0.79 (0.16)
3-part (n = 77)	34.4 (9.4) 72%	0.74 (0.16)
4-part (n = 15)	28.2 (8.1) 59%	0.72 (0.08)
Fract.-disloc. (n = 11)	32.6 (10.1) 68%	0.73 (0.15)
Articular fract. (n = 5)	36.6 (6.8) 76%	0.82 (0.14)
Age groups		
60–69 (n = 65)	36.6 (7.6) 76%	0.78 (0.16)
70–79 (n = 130)	36.0 (8.9) 75%	0.79 (0.14)
80–89 (n = 72)	34.5 (9.9) 72%	0.76 (0.18)
90–99 (n = 8)	36.8 (6.1) 77%	0.68 (0.10)
100+ (n = 1)	–	–

SD standard deviation
[a]Normal values for OSS in females aged 71–80: 82%, calculated from [23]
[b]Danish population norm for EQ-5D-3L in females aged 70–79: 0.82 [24]

Table 16.4 Patient-reported outcome (OSS and EQ-5D-3L) after 12 months according to fracture category and age

12 months	OSS Mean (SD) % of full score[a]	EQ-5D Mean (SD)[b]
(n = 202)	37.3 (10.0) 78%	0.81 (0.15)
Fracture category		
2-part (n = 123)	39.2 (8.9) 82%	0.82 (0.14)
3-part (n = 58)	34.7 (11.2) 72%	0.79 (0.18)
4-part (n = 9)	30.6 (10.6) 64%	0.80 (0.16)
Fract.-disloc. (n = 8)	34.6 (9.2) 72%	0.75 (0.11)
Articular fract. (n = 4)	37.5 (14.1) 78%	0.86 (0.18)
Age groups		
60–69 (n = 42)	39.6 (8.1) 83%	0.83 (0.15)
70–79 (n = 102)	37.2 (10.3) 78%	0.82 (0.15)
80–89 (n = 51)	36.1 (10.2) 75%	0.79 (0.15)
90–99 (n = 56)	33.8 (13.8) 70%	0.79 (0.13)
100+ (n = 1)	–	–

SD standard deviation.
[a]Normal values for OSS in females aged 71–80: 82%, calculated from [23]
[b]Danish population norm for EQ-5D-3L in females aged 70–79: 0.82 [24]

[23] but is not far from later epidemiological studies (Table 2.1). In the AO classification, A2 fractures accounted for 42%, followed by B1 fractures at 24%.

A ceiling effect was observed for both outcome measures. At 6 months, the mean OSS was 74% (Table 16.3), increasing to 78% of the total score after 12 months (Table 16.4). The normal value for females aged 71–80 has been calculated to be 82% [23]. Patients with two-part fractures had the best shoulder function, achieving an OSS of 78% after 6 months, which increased to 82% after 12 months. The mean value for health-related quality of life (EQ-5D-3L) in all patients was 0.77 at 6 months (Table 16.3), increasing to 0.81 at 12 months (Table 16.4). The population norm for EQ-5D-3L in females aged 70–79 was 0.82 [24]. Patients with two-part fractures had the highest score of 0.79, increasing to 0.82 at 12 months [25].

Treatment failure of nonoperative treatment was defined as the need for surgery, an OSS at 24 or below, or an EQ-5D-3L below 0. Twenty-eight patients out of 627 (4%) needed surgery, while 26 out of 202 (13%) of the patients with displaced fractures had an OSS ≤ 24 at 12 months. No patients had an EQ-5D-3L below 0.

Prospective cohort studies have strengths and limitations. While they can help evaluate the implementation of evidence and provide estimates for patient outcome, they cannot provide data to compare treatment effects between subgroups, treatments, or other cohorts. Another weakness is the lack of translatability between the Neer and the AO classifications in outcome reporting. For example, using the complete AO form for two-part fractures, six subgroups (A2.1, A2.2, A2.3, A3.1, A3.2, A3.3) cover most morphologies, including varus and valgus impaction, angulation, translation, and comminution. However, without a definition of displacement, we cannot translate these patterns into Neer two-part surgical neck fractures [26]. We have chosen the Neer classification for our reporting because we find the definition of displacement clinically useful. This choice is, however, at the cost of a detailed reporting of the morphology.

16.8 Perspectives

Older people with displaced shoulder fractures seem to recover well after evidence-based treatment. Mean values for patient-reported shoulder function and health-related quality of life are close to those of the background population after a year, with an overall operation rate of 4%. Nonsurgical treatment should serve as the default position in older people, with a few exceptions of fracture-dislocations and head-splitting fractures. Although follow-up schedules have not been tested in randomized trials, I have suggested follow-up after 2 and 6 weeks. The Danish cohort reported that most patients undergoing delayed surgery had two-part surgical neck fractures without bony contact. We hypothesize that providing a joint replacement with a reverse arthroplasty in these patients after 6 weeks will reduce the number of symptomatic nonunions.

The optimal timing of reverse arthroplasty is unknown, and outcome reports from observational studies can be challenging to interpret. Patients are rarely comparable at baseline. The patients offered a primary reverse arthroplasty often differ from those offered a late reverse arthroplasty and are operated on different indications. Determining the ideal time for surgery in a randomized trial is challenging as a relatively small population can be randomized to early or late surgery. At baseline, we do not know if there will be an indication of late surgery. Moreover, it should first be demonstrated that reverse is better than no reverse. We are awaiting data from ongoing studies [27, 28], adding to previous reports [3, 29].

The widespread use of early reverse prostheses may result in a good outcome if patients with high activity and independence are operated on. The drawback is the likely performance of unnecessary surgery and the revision burden in the long run. Differences in favor of early reverse arthroplasty reported from observational studies do not justify increased surgery rates. On the other hand, surgery performed months after the injury is demanding. It may still offer pain relief, but the rotator cuff has retracted, and the functional result is often disappointing,

I recommend restraint regarding early surgery in the elderly, except in a few cases of fracture-dislocations and head-splitting fractures. As only a minor part of the fracture population needs surgery after 6 weeks, the operation can be postponed to that time. The window for successful insertion of a fracture prosthesis has widened from about 2 weeks post-injury for hemiarthroplasty to about 6 weeks for reverse arthroplasty. This window can be utilized to decrease the number of redundant surgeries.

Systematic outcome collection from large cohorts of patients with shoulder fractures suggests that an evidence-based and non-surgical approach in older people is safe and leads to a level of shoulder function and quality of life close to the background population, with an operation rate of about 4%. Data from large cohort studies covering all treatment modalities may contribute to bridging the evidence-practice gap among orthopedic surgeons hesitant to de-implement surgical interventions and help avoid unnecessary surgery.

References

1. Handoll HH, Brorson S. Interventions for treating proximal humeral fractures in adults. Cochrane Database Syst Rev. 2015;11:CD000434. Available from: http://doi.wiley.com/10.1002/14651858.CD000434.pub4
2. Olerud P, Ahrengart L, Ponzer S, Saving J, Tidermark J. Hemiarthroplasty versus nonoperative treatment of displaced 4-part proximal humeral fractures in elderly patients: a randomized controlled trial. J Shoulder Elb Surg. 2011;20(7):1025–33.
3. Miquel J, Cassart E, Santana F, Martínez R, Valls L, Salomó-Domènech M, et al. Reverse shoulder arthroplasty or nothing for patients with displaced proximal humeral fractures. A randomized controlled trial. J Shoulder Elb Surg. 2024;S1058-2746(24):00224-6.
4. Rangan A, Handoll H, Brealey S, Jefferson L, Keding A, Martin BC, et al. Surgical vs nonsurgical treatment of adults with displaced fractures of the proximal humerus: the PROFHER randomized clinical trial. JAMA. 2015;313(10):1037–47. Available from: https://jamanetwork.com/journals/jama/fullarticle/2190987
5. National Institute for Health and Care Excellence. Fractures (non-complex): assessment and management. 2016; Available from: https://www.nice.org.uk/guidance/ng38

References

6. Jefferson L, Brealey S, Handoll H, Keding A, Kottam L, Sbizzera I, et al. Impact of the PROFHER trial findings on surgeons' clinical practice: an online questionnaire survey. Bone Joint Res. 2017;6(10):590–9. Available from: https://boneandjoint.org.uk/article/10.1302/2046-3758.610.BJR-2017-0170
7. Dwijen Roy K, Poyser E, Raj S, Boktor J, Mehta H. Has the ProFHER trial changed the Orthopaedic surgeons? Decision making and treatment of proximal humeral fractures? Ortop Traumatol Rehabil. 2022;24(6):393–7.
8. Brorson S, Viberg B, Gundtoft P, Jalal B, Ohrt-Nissen S. Epidemiology and trends in management of acute proximal humeral fractures in adults: an observational study of 137,436 cases from the Danish National Patient Register, 1996–2018. Acta Orthop. 2022;93:750–5. Available from: https://actaorthop.org/actao/article/view/4578
9. Danish Orthopaedic Association: [Surgical versus non-surgical management of displaced proximal humeral fractures in elderly]. 2015. Available from: https://www.ortopaedi.dk/wp-content/uploads/2019/10/Prox-humerusfraktur_Final.pdf
10. Handoll HH, Elliott J, Thillemann TM, Aluko P, Brorson S. Interventions for treating proximal humeral fractures in adults. Cochrane Database Syst Rev. 2022;(6, 6):CD000434. Available from: https://www.cochranelibrary.com/cdsr/doi/10.1002/14651858.CD000434.pub5/abstract
11. Court-Brown CM, Garg A, McQueen MM. The epidemiology of proximal humeral fractures. Acta Orthop Scand. 2001;72(4):365–71. Available from: https://actaorthop.org/actao/article/view/20079
12. Gaebler C, McQueen MM, Court-Brown CM. Minimally displaced proximal humeral fractures: epidemiology and outcome in 507 cases. Acta Orthop Scand. 2003;74(5):580–5. Available from: https://actaorthop.org/actao/article/view/19797
13. Court-Brown CM, Cattermole H, McQueen MM. Impacted valgus fractures (B1.1) of the proximal humerus. The results of non-operative treatment. J Bone Joint Surg Br. 2002;84(4):504–8.
14. Clement ND, McQueen MM, Court-Brown CM. Social deprivation influences the epidemiology and outcome of proximal humeral fractures in adults for a defined urban population of Scotland. Eur J Orthop Surg Traumatol. 2014;24(7):1039–46.
15. Clement ND, Duckworth AD, McQueen MM, Court-Brown CM. The outcome of proximal humeral fractures in the elderly: predictors of mortality and function. Bone Joint J. 2014;96-B(7):970–7. Available from: https://boneandjoint.org.uk/article/10.1302/0301-620X.96B7.32894
16. Court-Brown CM, McQueen MM. Two-part fractures and fracture dislocations. Hand Clin. 2007;23(4):397–414. v. Available from: https://www.sciencedirect.com/science/article/abs/pii/S0749071207000856?via%3Dihub
17. Court-Brown CM, Garg A, McQueen MM. The translated two-part fracture of the proximal humerus. Epidemiology and outcome in the older patient. J Bone Joint Surg Br. 2001;83(6):799–804.
18. Court-Brown CM, McQueen MM. The impacted varus (A2.2) proximal humeral fracture: prediction of outcome and results of nonoperative treatment in 99 patients. Acta Orthop Scand. 2004;75(6):736–40. Available from: https://actaorthop.org/actao/article/view/19601
19. Goudie EB, MacDonald DJ, Robinson CM. Functional outcome after nonoperative treatment of a proximal humeral fracture in adults. J Bone Joint Surg Am. 2022;104(2):123–38.
20. Baker P, Nanda R, Goodchild L, Finn P, Rangan A. A comparison of the constant and Oxford shoulder scores in patients with conservatively treated proximal humeral fractures. J Shoulder Elb Surg. 2008;17(1):37–41.
21. Jayakumar P, Teunis T, Williams M, Lamb SE, Ring D, Gwilym S. Factors associated with the magnitude of limitations during recovery from a fracture of the proximal humerus: predictors of limitations after proximal humerus fracture. Bone Joint J. 2019;101-B(6):715–23.
22. Brorson S, Borg SA IZ. Research Registry®: a global repository for all study types involving human participants (6502). researchregistry6502. Available from: https://www.researchregistry.com/browse-the-registry#home/registrationdetails/6013f116dd32e900213ab89c/
23. Clement ND, Court-Brown CM. Oxford shoulder score in a normal population. Int J Shoulder Surg. 2014;8(1):10–4. Available from: https://www.ncbi.nlm.nih.gov/pmc/articles/PMC4049034/
24. Sørensen J, Davidsen M, Gudex C, Pedersen KM, Brønnum-Hansen H. Danish EQ-5D population norms. Scand J Public Health. 2009;37(5):467–74.
25. Brorson S, Borg SA, Houkjær LL, Holtz KB, Issa Z. Patient-reported outcome was close to the Danish background population 6 months after non-surgical treatment of Neer 2-part surgical neck fractures: a prospective cohort study in patients aged 60 or above. Acta Orthop. 2024;95:619–24. Available from: https://actaorthop.org/actao/article/view/42301
26. Brorson S, Eckardt H, Audigé L, Rolauffs B, Bahrs C. Translation between the Neer- and the AO/OTA-classification for proximal humeral fractures: do we need to be bilingual to interpret the scientific literature? BMC Res Notes. 2013;6(1):69. Available from: https://www.ncbi.nlm.nih.gov/pmc/articles/PMC3610277/
27. Smith GCS, Bateman E, Cass B, Damiani M, Harper W, Jones H, et al. Reverse Shoulder Arthroplasty for the treatment of Proximal humeral fractures in the Elderly (ReShAPE trial) : study protocol for a multicentre combined randomised controlled and observational trial. Trials. 2017;18(1):91. Available from: http://trialsjournal.biomedcentral.com/articles/10.1186/s13063-017-1826-6
28. Launonen AP, Fjalestad T, Laitinen MK, Lähdeoja T, Ekholm C, Wagle T, et al. Nordic innovative tri-

als to evaluate osteoPorotic fractures (NITEP) collaboration: the Nordic DeltaCon trial protocol—non-operative treatment versus reversed total shoulder arthroplasty in patients 65 years of age and older with a displaced proximal humerus fracture: a prospective, randomised controlled trial. BMJ Open. 2019;9(1):e024916. Available from: http://bmjopen.bmj.com/lookup/doi/10.1136/bmjopen-2018-024916

29. Lopiz Y, Alcobía-Díaz B, Galán-Olleros M, García-Fernández C, Picado AL, Marco F. Reverse shoulder arthroplasty versus nonoperative treatment for 3- or 4-part proximal humeral fractures in elderly patients: a prospective randomized controlled trial. J Shoulder Elb Surg. 2019;28(12):2259–71.

Open Access This chapter is licensed under the terms of the Creative Commons Attribution 4.0 International License (http://creativecommons.org/licenses/by/4.0/), which permits use, sharing, adaptation, distribution and reproduction in any medium or format, as long as you give appropriate credit to the original author(s) and the source, provide a link to the Creative Commons license and indicate if changes were made.

The images or other third party material in this chapter are included in the chapter's Creative Commons license, unless indicated otherwise in a credit line to the material. If material is not included in the chapter's Creative Commons license and your intended use is not permitted by statutory regulation or exceeds the permitted use, you will need to obtain permission directly from the copyright holder.

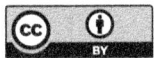

Part VI

Conclusions

Shoulder Fractures in Context: The Academic Bonesetter

17.1 Introduction

The practice of bringing broken bones together is a human trait found throughout history. The principle of restoring the anatomy has been passed down through generations. In recent decades, a growing number of randomized trials have been unable to demonstrate the superiority of surgical interventions for shoulder fractures in older people. Surprisingly, this has not led to an adjustment of the treatment recommendations but, rather, to an increase in surgeries and implants.

All surgeons wish the best for their patients—but, unfortunately, evidence is not always part of clinical decision-making. Surgeons cannot assume surgery to be beneficial without systematic testing. Before routine use, new procedures and implants must undergo clinical testing in randomized trials with non-surgically treated control groups to evaluate their benefits and harms. Without rigorous testing, there is a risk of multiple biases taking over thinking and practice, potentially leaving patients with unnecessary or harmful treatments. The widespread use of locking plate osteosynthesis in osteoporotic shoulder fractures is a conspicuous example (Chap. 12). Randomized trials have unambiguously reported no clinical benefits from locking plates compared to non-surgical treatment. However, the implant is widely used despite failure rates of around 30%, leading to pain, loss of function, and revision surgery with inferior outcomes [1, 2].

This chapter first introduces *the historic bonesetter*, an important but poorly described practitioner in historical populations and developing countries. Next, I will present some examples of historical writers' accusations against uneducated practitioners regarding the treatment of shoulder fractures. As an alternative to the historic bonesetter, I will sketch some of the preferred qualities of the modern orthopedic surgeon, termed the *academic bonesetter*. Finally, I will propose potential avenues for future research and evidence-based treatment for patients with shoulder fractures.

17.2 The Historic Bonesetter

> A Bonesetter is an empirical practitioner who claims the power of diagnosing and setting fractures, reducing dislocations, and relieving painful and stiff joints. The bone-setter differs from the cultist in that his craft is entirely empirical; bone-setters have made no effort to elaborate on theory to support or justify their practice [3]

Bonesetters have played an important role in providing medical services in historical communities as part of folk medicine. In Europe, the Church prohibited clerics from performing surgery from the eleventh and twelfth centuries, leading to several procedures being performed by illiterate folk practitioners [3]. Among these, bonesetting survived the changes in medicine, including the emergence of French hospital medicine in the late eighteenth century (Chap. 5). Bonesetters have continued to practice even after educated medical writers abandoned the Hippocratic principles of forceful reduction of shoulder fractures. In countries without access to educated practitioners, bonesetting remains a common practice. The actual practice of bonesetting throughout history is not well-documented, however, and it may have differed substantially from the dogmatic tradition passed down in written sources.

A few prominent bonesetter families from the eighteenth and nineteenth centuries have been recorded, like the Welsh family of Thomas and the Sweet family in the United States. Bonesetting was considered a natural and innate gift. The craft of bonesetting runs in families but has not been restricted to a profession, and the practitioners have often been considered quacks. In low-income countries or rural areas, they have represented an available and less costly alternative to fracture care by healthcare professionals. Traditionally, bonesetters have been poorly esteemed by academic writers, although their practice and contributions to public health may have been substantial.

The success of bonesetting has not been recorded, but it must have required some basic anatomical knowledge. A few practical handbooks on anatomy have survived, including Waterman Sweets' book, published in 1844, *Views on Anatomy and Practice of Bone-Setting by a Mechanical Process Different from All Book Knowledge* [4].

A fundamental principle in bonesetting is that aligning a fractured bone benefits the patient. This principle has been incorporated into modern orthopedics as the principle of anatomical reduction. A substantial aspect of modern orthopedics and traumatology concerns aligning fractured long bones, followed by bracing or internal or external operative fixation. In the first lecture on orthopedic surgery, aspiring orthopedic surgeons learn that anatomical reduction is the initial step in treating displaced long bone fractures and, conversely, that surgical intervention is necessary for nonanatomical conditions.

17.3 Poor Practice and Iatrogenic Injury

Strong opinions regarding the proper treatment of shoulder fractures are not new. While there is almost no evidence of bonesetters and their treatment results, there are written sources from learned medical writers who criticized their learned colleagues, surgeons, and uneducated practitioners for their poor practices. The key areas of disagreement included the technique for realigning the fracture, the amount of force applied, the proper tightness of bandages and splints, and ethical issues. In this section, I will sketch the historical controversy. A general introduction to the historical sources can be found in Part II. It is important to note that the discussion between learned medicine and medical practitioners is biased because only one side's opinion has been preserved for posterity.

The forceful Hippocratic maneuver for reducing shoulder fractures and dislocations (c. 415 BCE) (Figs. 5.5 and 17.1) remained remarkably unchanged for over two millennia with only minor modifications. Galen (c. 129–215 CE) added that reduction should be performed with the patient sitting in a high position. A patient sitting high would be subjected to less damage than a patient sitting low because a change in position would only slightly impact the reduction [5] (pp. 422–6).

During the early eighteenth century, Jean-Louis Petit (1674–1750) further developed the Hippocratic traction method, suggesting that an assistant should perform powerful counter-extraction on the opposite arm. Samuel Cooper (1781–1848) condemned this method for causing harm by applying much more power than required for reduction:

> This method is liable to three kinds of inconveniences. It fatigues and even pains the patient, it lessens the extensive power by bringing them near to the moveable point, it irritates such muscles as proceed from above to the lower end of the fracture, and thus increases their disposition to contract [7]. (pp. 298–9)

Not until the late eighteenth century was the Hippocratic method of reduction and bandaging

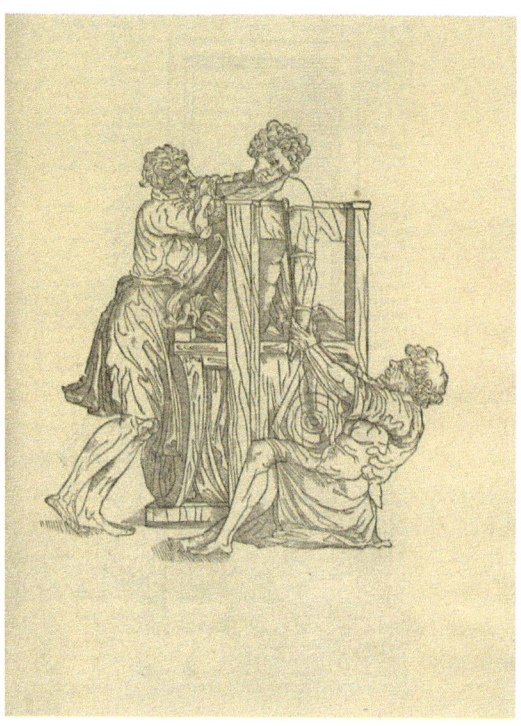

Fig. 17.1 Renaissance interpretation of the Hippocratic method for extension and reduction of the shoulder and upper arm [6]. (With permission from Bibliothèque nationale de France)

substantially criticized. Pierre-Joseph Desault (1744–1795) argued that if reduction was done according to Hippocrates, it could cause ecchymoses and secondary displacement. His justification was biomechanical:

> These means, in general, besides being insufficient, are liable to a further objection, in consequence of their acting on the edges of the pectoralis major, latissimus dorsi, and teres major, which being thus forced upwards, draw the fragments on which they adhere in the same direction, and thereby constitute an obstacle to the reduction [8]. (p. 75)

The Hippocratic application of bandages and splints is illustrated in Fig. 5.6. The Hippocratic writer described the adverse effects of bandages applied too tightly at the upper arm, causing pressure wounds [9] (*On Joints*, XXVI). The Roman medical writer Celsus (25 BCE–50 CE) suggested that multiple turns of a bandage were more effective than tightening it, as it could lead to gangrene [10] (VIII, 10). Paul of Aegina (c. 625–690 CE) expressed concerns about applying splints over the shoulder. He also cautioned against excessive splinting on the inner side of the upper arm as it may lead to ulcers and inflammation [11] (VI, 99). Early modern sources include the criticism of uneducated bonesetters and barber-surgeons applying bandages. William Salmon (1644–1713) recommended stretching the elbow every time dressings of the humerus were changed. By gentle loading of the injured arm, contraction could be prevented:

> The shrinking of Tendons (which Barbers, and ignorant Chirurgeons call the Shrinking of the Nerves or Sinews,) may yet easily be cured in ten or twelve Weeks time, if you cause the Patient to carry every day, some fit or proportional Weight [12]. (p. 1266)

17.4 Professional Ethics

Since the time of the Hippocratic writings, allegations of malpractice can be found. The Hippocratic request on non-maleficence was bound to professional ethics. If there was a risk of doing more harm than good, the advice was to refrain from the intervention: "As to diseases, make a habit of two things – to help, or at least to do no harm" [13] (Epidemics I).

Less noble motives were expressed by the Arab surgeon Albucasis (936–1013), who advised fellow surgeons to refrain from treating difficult cases: "Use your utmost diligence; keep clear of entering upon a course with a dangerous outcome. … For this will best ensure the continuance of your prestige and safeguard your good name. God willing" [14] (p. 836).

Limiting the practice to the handling of easy cases alone was one method of preserving reputation and income. In cases of humerus malunion, Albucasis cautioned against refracturing the humerus, a practice discussed in Middle Ages sources. Referencing the practices of the Ancients, Albucasis criticized the methods employed by bonesetters:

> What some ignorant bone-setters do is to break the bone again if at first the repair is not as it should and has mended crookedly. This operation of theirs is mistaken and dangerous; if it were right the Ancients would undoubtedly have spoken of it in their books and would have used it [14]. (p. 696)

Fig. 17.2 Failed staple osteosynthesis of a surgical neck fracture [17]. (With permission from the Wellcome Collection)

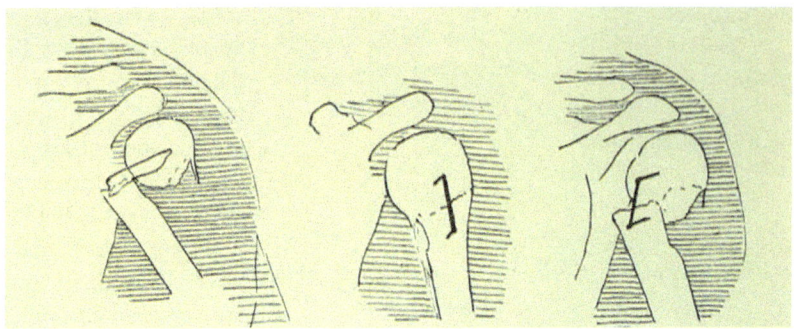

Several nineteenth-century sources expressed concerns about professional ethics in treating shoulder fractures. In 1847, Robert William Smith (1807–1873) urged his colleagues to avoid misleading prognostic statements regarding shoulder fractures, writing that "the prudent surgeon will never omit to announce to the patient that a certain degree of impairment of the motions of the joint will be a permanent result of the injury" [15] (p. 190).

In 1839, Sir Astley Cooper (1768–1841) described fracture-dislocations of the shoulder as "a formidable accident" (Fig. 6.1). He acknowledged the poor prognosis following fracture-dislocations and reprimanded his colleagues collegially. Instead of blaming colleagues for failing to reduce the fracture-dislocation due to incompetence:

> These cases should teach the members of our profession to be kind, generous, and liberal towards each other; and not to impute to ignorance or inattention that which is the result of a generally incurable accident. It too often happens, that, when every trial has been made to restore the parts, and without success, the patient goes to some other surgeon, to whom he shews his arm, and points out its uselessness and want of motions. A jealous and illiberal medical man might say, "Yes, this is a dislocation which has not been reduced. I wish I had seen it at first; but now it is too late for a successful attempt to replace it." However, any intelligent well-informed surgeon will now confess, that no knowledge, or exertion of skill, could have prevented the deformity and loss of the natural motion which results from this formidable accident [16]. (p. 277)

The introduction of internal fixation of shoulder fractures in the early twentieth century (Chap. 7) opened the door to various new complications and treatment failures. The pioneer of osteosynthesis, Albin Lambotte (1866–1955), reported very few failures after osteosyntheses. However, in 1907, he presented a failed osteosynthesis of the proximal humerus (Fig. 17.2) [17]. The failure was attributed to the patient leaving the clinic too early: "Only stupid indocility made the patient leave the bed and leave the clinic on the fifth day" [17] (p. 84).

This is probably not the only time a patient has been blamed for a failed osteosynthesis.

17.5 The Academic Bonesetter

The conflict between learned medicine and clinical practitioners can be found in the Greek philosopher Philo of Alexandria (c. 10 BCE–c. 40 CE), who unflatteringly described the competencies of the medical practitioners of Alexandria: "those who are clever with words, excellent expositors of the signs, causes, and therapies that make up the art of medicine, but who are hopeless at assisting the sick" [18].

The modern bonesetter is no longer illiterate. Academia is an integral part of the orthopedic curriculum. However, there is a widespread belief that surgeons with strong academic backgrounds may not be skilled practitioners. At the same time, those with excellent surgical skills may not feel the need to follow the evidence. Modern orthopedic surgeons must excel in both disciplines and build bridges between them. Evidence-based practice is an integrative process that includes clinical experience (including surgical skills), the best evidence available, and patient values and preferences [19].

When advancing modern orthopedics, the main obstacle is not the development of surgical skills, procedures, or implants. The real challenge lies in the tendency of surgeons to focus on minor differences between almost identical implants and procedures, often ignoring clinical evidence. The companies funding clinical orthopedic research have a legitimate interest in maximizing their profits—but surgeons have an unlimited responsibility to create value for patients now and in the future. Craftsmanship and evidence-based practice are perfectly compatible. Poorly performed surgery on the right indications does not add value to patients, nor does well-performed surgery on the wrong indications. If we continue performing surgical procedures without considering the evidence, we cannot differentiate ourselves from uneducated bonesetters and quacks. We can improve by re-evaluating our current surgical practice by including the best evidence and the patient's preferences in clinical decision-making.

17.6 Future Directions

In this section, I will suggest a few directions to improve the treatment of future patients with shoulder fractures.

As an essential initial step, we must revisit the principles governing the management of long bone fractures in osteoporotic proximal humerus fractures. We need to recognize that the shoulder differs from the hip, and the humerus differs from the femur. The differences in weight-bearing and the ability to tolerate nonanatomical healing require unique approaches. We should not perform surgery on older people with shoulder fractures based solely on findings of nonanatomical conditions on radiographs; this is contrary to the best available evidence, and, often, it is not to the patient's preferences. In the future, we need to involve patients more actively in clinical decision-making and the assessment of treatment outcomes.

Patient-reported outcomes should be collected for all patients regardless of the treatment provided. Using appropriate qualitative methods, we must develop and validate patient-derived, condition-specific outcome-measuring tools (Chap. 14). A future core outcome set should be determined and validated to improve clinical relevance and comparability of research and quality assessment.

To ensure completeness and coverage of collected outcomes, national arthroplasty registries could be broadened to include data on patients treated with head-preserving surgical techniques or without surgery. Alternatively, and in accordance with Codman's *end result idea*, large consecutive prospective cohort studies should gather outcome data, including complication data, for quality assessment (Chap. 7). The outcome collection should include the suggested core event set for treatment complications (Chap. 15).

To minimize research waste, future clinical research should concentrate on populations and treatments not addressed in previous randomized trials. Key areas for consideration include the treatment of isolated tuberosity fractures, high-energy trauma, and fractures in younger individuals. Although such trials are currently underway, there is an urgent need for trials examining the benefits and harms of reverse shoulder arthroplasty in fractures.

Future trials evaluating surgical treatments should include a non-surgically treated control group. While industry-sponsored studies investigating minor modifications in implants already on the market may offer research funding, they may provide limited patient benefits until surgical procedures are proven superior to non-surgical treatment. The surgeon's armamentarium may be composed of advanced surgical procedures and implants—but they do not necessarily benefit patients. We need to focus more on patient value than surgeon or company value. From a global perspective, performing redundant surgery is not an option.

17.7 Perspectives

A century ago, surgical treatment of shoulder fractures was not a common practice and was only offered to a select few patients. A century later, in the first two decades of the twenty-first century, there was an increase in the popularity of osteosynthesis, leading to a substantial increase in surgery rates. Using reverse arthroplasties in fracture cases further allowed surgeons to broaden the indications for surgery. In some countries, surgery has been offered to almost every patient with a displaced fracture, with only a few unfit for surgery being excluded. But the growing disparity between the best available evidence and the actual practice has led to a questioning of the benefits of surgery. Surgery has been found to be no more beneficial than non-surgical treatment and has high failure rates. In that case, the default position should be non-surgical, and surgery should only be considered in exceptional cases.

It is essential to collect outcomes systematically in medical practices. It is questionable whether Codman's end result idea of systematically following up on outcomes for all patients treated at a hospital has ever been implemented for shoulder fractures. More than a century later, most patients with shoulder fractures do not have their outcomes collected, except those involved in a few clinical trials or recorded in national arthroplasty registries. The surgeon's responsibility does not end with the postoperative radiograph. A systematic follow-up of all patients, regardless of their treatment, could have reduced the suffering of older people with shoulder fractures.

Surgery is often the easy choice in patients with displaced shoulder fractures. The surgeon demonstrates the power of action, adheres to basic surgical principles, acts as a peer, and often provides improved radiographs. But in most cases of shoulder fractures, surgeons and patients have time to think twice and to reconsider the treatment options. After 2 weeks, the fracture is still accessible for surgery, pain is under control, muscle spasms have decreased, and swelling has subsided. Patients and care providers are ready for reflection and shared decision-making. Few older people strongly wish to undergo surgery, especially if confronted with the evidence. The easy part of surgical decision-making is assigning an implant to a radiograph. The challenging part is assigning the appropriate treatment to the patient.

In this book, I have argued for reintegrating non-surgically treated fracture patients into orthopedic care. In line with the Hippocratic writer, we should refrain from intervention if there is a risk of doing more harm than good. Leaving the majority of shoulder fracture patients without orthopedic care because they do not benefit from surgery, however, is not proper practice.

Evidence-based practice does not neglect surgery; too often, surgeons neglect the evidence.

References

1. Barlow JD, Logli AL, Steinmann SP, Sems SA, Cross WW, Yuan BJ, et al. Locking plate fixation of proximal humerus fractures in patients older than 60 years continues to be associated with a high complication rate. J Shoulder Elb Surg. 2020;29(8):1689–94.
2. Kristensen MR, Rasmussen JV, Elmengaard B, Jensen SL, Olsen BS, Brorson S. High risk for revision after shoulder arthroplasty for failed osteosynthesis of proximal humeral fractures. Acta Orthop. 2018;89(3):345–50. Available from: https://actaorthop.org/actao/article/view/7206
3. Peltier LF. Fractures: a history and iconography of their treatment. San Francisco: Norman Publishing; 1990.
4. Sweet W. Views on anatomy and practice of bonesetting by a mechanical process different from all book knowledge. I Riggs; 1844. Available from: https://wellcomecollection.org/works/kpswh9uj
5. Claudius Galenus C. In: Kühn CG, editor. Galeni opera omnia (II). Lipsiae; 1821.
6. Vidio V. Chirurgia e Greco in Latinum conversa Vido Vidio Florentino interprete cum nonnullis ejus dem Vidii commentariis. Lutetiæ Parisiorum. 1544; Available from: https://archive.org/details/BIUSante_00248
7. Cooper S. A dictionary of practical surgery: containing a complete exhibition of the present state of the principles and practice of surgery, collected from the best and most original sources of information, and illustrated by critical remarks. London; 1809.
8. Desault P-J. A treatise on fractures, Luxations, and other affections of the bones. Project Gutenberg; 1805. Available from: https://wellcomecollection.org/works/pa6vyz7y
9. Hippocrates, Withington ET (Edward T. Hippocrates. Volume III: On wounds in the head. In the surgery. On fractures. On joints. Mochlicon. Cambridge, MA: Harvard University Press; 1928. (Loeb Classical Library;149).

References

10. Celsus AC. De medicina. In: Spencer WG, editor. De medicina. London: Heinemann; 1935. Available from: https://archive.org/details/sevenbooksofpaul02pauluoft/page/n15/mode/1up.
11. Paulus A. The seven books of Paulus Ægineta (translated by Francis Adams). Project Gutenberg; 1844. Available from: https://archive.org/details/sevenbooksofpaul02pauluoft/mode/2up
12. Salmon W. Ars chirurgica a compendium of the theory and practice of chirurgery. In seven books. London: J. Dawks; 1699.
13. Hippocrates, Jones WHS. Hippocrates. Volume I: Ancient Medicine. Airs, Waters, Places. Epidemics 1 and 3. The Oath. Precepts. Nutriment. Cambridge: Harvard University Press; 1923. (Loeb Classical Library;147).
14. Spink MS, Lewis GL. Albucasis. On surgery and instruments. Berkeley: University of California Press; 1973.
15. Smith RW. A treatise on fractures in the vicinity of joints and on certain forms of accidental and congenital dislocations. Dublin: Hodges and Smith; 1847. Available from: https://wellcomecollection.org/works/msz6zwcq
16. Cooper A. Of the dislocation of the os humeri upon the dorsum scapulæ, and upon fractures near the shoulder joint. Guys Hosp Rep. 1839;IV:265–84.
17. Lambotte A. L'intervention opératoire dans les fractures récentes et anciennes envisagée particulièrement au point de vue de l'ostéo-synthèse avec la description de plusieurs techniques nouvelles. Paris: A. Maloine; 1907. Available from: https://wellcomecollection.org/works/ufsrbypb/items
18. Nutton V. Galen and Egypt. In: Galen und das hellenistische Erbe. Sudhoffs Arch Beihefte. 1993;11–31.
19. Sackett DL. Evidence-based medicine and treatment choices. Lancet. 1997;349:570.

Open Access This chapter is licensed under the terms of the Creative Commons Attribution 4.0 International License (http://creativecommons.org/licenses/by/4.0/), which permits use, sharing, adaptation, distribution and reproduction in any medium or format, as long as you give appropriate credit to the original author(s) and the source, provide a link to the Creative Commons license and indicate if changes were made.

The images or other third party material in this chapter are included in the chapter's Creative Commons license, unless indicated otherwise in a credit line to the material. If material is not included in the chapter's Creative Commons license and your intended use is not permitted by statutory regulation or exceeds the permitted use, you will need to obtain permission directly from the copyright holder.

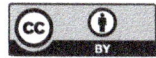

The manufacturer's authorised representative in the EU is Springer Nature Customer Service Centre GmbH, Europaplatz 3, 69115 Heidelberg, Germany. If you have any concerns regarding our products, please contact ProductSafety@springernature.com

Printed and bound by CPI Group (UK) Ltd, Croydon, CR0 4YY

26/03/2026

02078996-0001